T0238582

EMPOWERING DECISION-MAKING IN MIDWIFERY

Decision-making pervades all aspects of midwifery practice across the world. Midwifery is informed by a number of decision-making theories, but it is sometimes difficult to marry these theories with practice.

This book provides a comprehensive exploration of decision-making for midwives irrespective of where in the world they practice or in which model of care. The first part critically reviews decision-making theories, including the Enhancing Decision-making Assessment in Midwifery (EDAM) tool, and their relevance to midwifery. It explores the links between midwifery governance, including professional regulation and the law, risk and safety and decision-making as well as how critical thinking and reflection are essential elements of decision-making. It then goes on to present a number of diverse case studies, demonstrating how they interrelate to and impact upon optimal midwifery decision-making. Each chapter presents examples that show how the theory translates into practice and includes activities to reinforce learning points.

Bringing together a diverse range of contributors, this volume will be essential reading for midwifery students, practising midwives and midwifery academics.

Elaine Jefford is a midwifery academic and researcher at Southern Cross University, Australia. Elaine is a UK-trained nurse and midwife who immigrated to Australia in 2005. Her primary research focus is within the field of midwifery decision-making and abdicating one's professional accountability, the impacts of this in relation to risk, safety and quality of care provision on maternal and neonatal health, midwives and the midwifery profession. She has also been involved in national and international curriculum development in midwifery.

Julie Jomeen is a Professor of Midwifery and Dean of the Faculty of Health Sciences at the University of Hull, UK. Julie currently co-leads a Research Group for Maternal, Reproductive Health within the Faculty. A key focus of her work is exploring issues of perinatal mental health and psychological health in childbearing women. Other research interests include women's choice and decision-making and practitioner decision-making.

EMPOWERING DECISION-MAKING IN MIDWIFERY

A Global Perspective

Edited by Elaine Jefford and Julie Jomeen

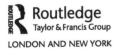

Routledge
Taylor & Francis Group

LONDON AND NEW YORK

First published 2020
by Routledge
2 Park Square, Milton Park, Abingdon, Oxon OX14 4RN

and by Routledge
52 Vanderbilt Avenue, New York, NY 10017

Routledge is an imprint of the Taylor & Francis Group, an informa business

British Library Cataloguing-in-Publication Data
A catalogue record for this book is available from the British Library

Library of Congress Cataloging-in-Publication Data
A catalog record for this book has been requested

ISBN: 978-0-367-02726-1 (hbk)
ISBN: 978-0-367-02728-5 (pbk)
ISBN: 978-0-429-39817-9 (ebk)

Typeset in Bembo
by Apex CoVantage, LLC

This book is dedicated to the global family of midwives to which we belong, and to the student midwives we walk beside. Together we strive to provide quality and safe care in sometimes complex and challenging situations and environments, yet our focus remains on working in partnership so we can support women's choices and decision-making to enhance their childbirthing experience.

CONTENTS

PART III
Decision-making within the context of the socially and culturally constructed maternity care environment

ILLUSTRATIONS

Figures

Tables

Boxes

CONTRIBUTORS

Renee Adair, Cert IV Doula Support Services, Cert IV TAE, Qualified Childbirth and Parenting Educator, Dip Aroma, Founder and Director Australian Doula College, Australia. Renee first began working with women and babies in 1994 and since then has been a regular contributor in pregnancy and parenting publications and websites. She has worked for the Red Cross and currently sits on the Consumer Advisory Board of the Australian College of Midwives. Renee worked in collaboration to create the first doula research. Renee has trained thousands of doulas and continues to doula families through birth, the post-natal period and end of life.

Amanda Burleigh, RGN, RN, BSc Hons, Midwifery Consultant UK. Amanda's main area of interest is optimal cord clamping. She has been a midwife for over 30 years. Midwife of the Year UK 2012 (Yorkshire Evening Post) + 2015 (British Journal of Midwifery) for work in optimal cord clamping. Co-inventor of the Basics/Lifestart trolley. Founder of the #Waitforwhite campaign.

Amanda Carter, Midwife, PhD, MMid, IBCLC, BaHlthSc, Bachelor of Midwifery Program Director, Griffith University Australia. Amanda has been a midwife for over 30 years and worked in a variety of midwifery clinical, management, leadership, education and academic roles. Her philosophy of teaching stems from her philosophy of midwifery with a strong synergy between the two. As a midwife, Amanda's clinical practice is always centred on the woman and she has now transferred that philosophy of being woman-centred to being student-centred.

Hannah Dahlen, RN, BN (Hons 1st), MCommN, Grad cert Mid (pharm), PhD, FACM. Professor of Midwifery, Higher Degree Director, Western Sydney University, Australia. Hannah has been a midwife for nearly 30 years and still practices. She is one of the first midwives in Australia to gain eligibility and access to a Medicare provider number following government reforms in 2010. In 2017 Hannah gained one of the first clinical privileging positions to provide care in a hospital as a Visiting Midwife. Hannah works in a group practice with five other private midwives called Midwives at Sydney and beyond.

Lorna Davies, PhD, RM, RN, MA, BSc (Hons), PGCEA Ara, Associate Head of Midwifery and Principal Lecturer, Institute of Canterbury, Christchurch, New Zealand. Research areas: sustainability and healthcare, physiological birth and midwifery workforce issues. Lorna is a UK-educated midwife who is now based in New Zealand. She has edited and co-edited a number of midwifery textbooks, has contributed chapters to several others and has written many articles relating to midwifery practice and research. She is married, has three adult children and a home-birthed granddaughter.

Daniela Drandić, BA Hons., Master's Student, University of Dundee (Maternal and Infant Health), Reproductive Rights Program Lead, Roda – Parents in Action (Croatia). Daniela is a pro-choice researcher and advocate working in the field of maternity care in Croatia and the Central and Eastern European Region and is passionate about antenatal education, maternal choice and autonomy. She is a board member of Human Rights in Childbirth and has headed social media campaigns on improving maternity care in Croatia. She is the principal author of the Expecting mobile app for pregnant women and is mum of three children.

Lyn Ebert, RN, RM, Graduate Certificate in Neonatal Nursing, Grad Dip in Adult Education, Master of Nursing, MPhil in Midwifery, PhD in Midwifery. Lyn is the Deputy Head of School-Teaching and Learning and Head of Discipline-Midwifery in the School of Nursing and Midwifery, Faculty of Health and Medicine at the University of Newcastle, Australia. Her research areas include woman-centred care, maternal health and midwifery education.

Claire Foord is a mother, artist, educator and advocate. Claire learned of the leading cause of death in children in Australia, in what some would consider the hardest possible way, through the term stillbirth of her healthy baby girl. She became a passionate advocate for change and founded Still Aware, Australia's first charity dedicated to awareness and education of stillbirth in pregnancy. Claire's efforts have been recognised when she was awarded South Australia's Local Hero in the 2016 Australian of the Year Awards. A qualified educator she has taught students in schools, tertiary institutions and career-based learning.

Mari Greenfield, MA Social Sciences, MA Social Policy Research Associate at the University of Hull, UK. Mari's research focus is investigating traumatic birth and perinatal choices. Mari has worked as a doula and breastfeeding counsellor for over 10 years, and is passionate about using research to improve the experiences of those giving birth.

Joyce Hendricks, Associate Professor in the School of Nursing, Midwifery and Social, Sciences at Central Queensland University. She is the Head of Courses – Post Graduate Studies and supervisor several PhD students. Joyce research interests include care of the adolescent mother through pregnancy and motherhood.

Elaine Jefford, PhD, MSC (healthcare policies and practice), Post Graduate Diploma Teaching and Learning, BSC (Hons) Midwifery, BSC (Hons) nursing, Midwifery academic and researcher at Southern Cross University, Australia. Elaine is a UK-trained nurse and midwife immigrating to Australia in 2005. Her primary research focus is within the field of midwifery decision-making and abdicating one's professional accountability, the impacts of this in relation to risk, safety and quality of care provision on maternal and neonate health, midwives, and the midwifery profession. She has also been involved in national and international curriculum development in midwifery.

Julie Jomeen, PhD, MA, RGN, RM, PGCHE. Julie is a Professor of Midwifery and Dean of the Faculty of Health Sciences at the University of Hull, UK. A key focus of her research is exploring issues of perinatal mental health and psychological health in childbearing women – a programme of research which has led to strong collaborations in national and international research, service development and practitioner training initiatives. Other research interests include women's choice and decision-making and practitioner decision-making. She has also been involved in national and international curriculum development in midwifery, has held several editorial positions and was Chair of the Society for Reproductive and Infant Psychology from 2014 to 2017.

Catriona Jones, RM, MSc, BSc (Hons), PGCE, Senior Research Fellow in maternal and reproductive health within the Faculty of Health Sciences, University of Hull, UK. She is a midwifery lecturer, a registered midwife, and holds an honorary contract with the local NHS Trust. Her various roles have included Programme Leader (Midwifery), and Deputy and Acting Lead Midwife for Education. She has a growing research and publications portfolio in the area of maternal and reproductive health. Since 2008, she has seen a number of funded research projects through to successful completion.

Sigfríður Inga Karlsdóttir, PhD, Associate Professor at the School of Health Sciences, University of Akureyri, Iceland. Her main research areas have been women's experiences of childbirth, women's attitude and experience of pain and pain management in childbirth, childbearing women's perspective on caring and uncaring encounters with midwives and other health professionals, and the primacy of the good midwife in midwifery services. She is a Registered Midwife and Nurse with broad clinical experience and she has worked in labour wards, antenatal clinics, assisted women in home births and organised and held antenatal classes for expectant parents for many years.

Janet Kelly, PhD, LLB (Hons) (Bachelor of Laws Degree), MA, Postgraduate Certificate in Higher Education, Diploma in Health Service Management, Senior Lecturer in Healthcare Law and Ethics, Head of Department for Midwifery and Child Health, University of Hull, UK. Janet is a peer reviewer of several international journals including the *Lancet, Nursing Ethics, Nurse Education, Women and Birth* and the *Journal of the Australian College of Midwives.* Janet is also a Registrant Chair for the UK's Nursing Midwifery Council's, Fitness to Practise Conduct and Competence Committees sitting for both nursing and midwifery registrants.

Mary Kirk, Director of Nursing and Midwifery and Chief Executive Officer of the Queen Elizabeth II Family Centre. Mary is a life member of the Australian College of Midwives and Vice-President of the International Confederation of Midwives. Mary holds invaluable experience and expertise in health service governance, leadership and professional regulation. She has exemplary professional contributions as Board Member and Deputy Chair of the Nursing and Midwifery Board of Australia, Board Member of ACM, Executive Board Member of ICM, Health Adviser on the National Council of Women Australia, President and Board Member of the Australasian Association of Parenting and Child Health, and Founding President of Safe Motherhood for all Australia.

Hildur Kristjánsdóttir, RM, RN, MEd, Diploma in Public Health, Associate professor, Department of Midwifery, University of Iceland. Midwife for 40 years, worked in many fields of childbirth care, mostly in antenatal care. Worked for several years as Chief midwifery officer at the Directorate of Health in Iceland. Has been active in the Icelandic Midwives Association and president of the Nordic Midwives Association (NJF) since 2007. Was made an honorary member of Iceland's Midwives Association in 2014. Manager and investigator of the Childbirth and Health study in Iceland and was Iceland co-ordinator in the BIDENS six country study.

Magdalena Kurbanović, Bachelor's Degree in Midwifery and Master's in Nursing, International Board Certified Breastfeeding Consultant (IBCLC). She works as a midwife on the labour and delivery ward at Pula General Hospital (Croatia). She teaches antenatal and breastfeeding classes at the hospital but also as part of an independent midwifery organisation called Midwife and Family. Magdalena's master's research focused on midwifery education and midwives' professional autonomy in Croatia.

Shahna Mailey, Bachelor of Psychological Science (Hons), School of Health and Human Sciences, Southern Cross University Student Psychology.

Claire Marshall, Specialist Perinatal Mental Health Nurse, Clinical Lead with the Hull and East Yorkshire Perinatal Mental Health Liaison Team, Humber Teaching NHS Foundation Trust, NIHR Clinical Academic Fellowship with the University of Hull. She has worked collaboratively with researchers at the University of Hull across 12 years to improve service delivery by resolving the challenges which exist in everyday practice. In addition, she has a key role in designing and delivering the degree and masters level perinatal mental health module provided by the University of Hull.

Robyn Maude, PhD, MA (Midwifery), BN, RM, RN, PGCHELT, Senior Lecturer and Midwifery Programme Lead at the Graduate School of Nursing, Midwifery and Health (GSNMH) at Victoria University of Wellington (VUW), New Zealand. Robyn's research interests are focused on activities that promote and protect normal physiological birth. These include monitoring fetal well-being, water immersion for labour and birth, the use of probiotics in pregnancy, medico-legal aspects of the provision of care, knowledge translation, Knowledge-to-Action process, quality improvement and clinical effectiveness, continuity of midwifery care, standards of midwifery practice, models of midwifery and midwifery leadership.

Eveline Mestdagh, PhD, Masters in Medical and Social Sciences, Bachelor of Midwifery, Head of the Midwifery Department (AP), post-doctoral researcher at Artesis Plantijn University College Antwerp, Belgium and the Centre for Research and Innovation in Care at the University Antwerp, Belgium. Eveline is also a juridical expert in nursing and midwifery.

Tina Morrison, Masters of Midwifery, Graduate Diploma of Midwifery, Bachelor of Nursing is Midwifery Unit Manager Women's Care Unit, Grafton Base Hospital Northern NSW Local Health District, NSW, Australia. Tina has a passion for teaching and mentoring the next generation of midwives in an increasingly complex maternity space. She has an interest in the role of clinical reasoning and decision-making in the clinical environment and an evolving fascination for the impact of culture in the workspace on the delivery of safe care to women and babies.

Marianne Nieuwenhuijze, RM PhD MPH, Professor of Midwifery, Head of the Research Centre for Midwifery Science, Academy for Midwifery Studies, Zuyd University, the Netherlands. Her research areas include shared decision-making, physiological childbirth and ethics in midwifery care. As a researcher and educator, my main interest is in women's participation in their care around childbirth to contribute to a fair and positive experience for all women.

Elizabeth Newnham, PhD. Elizabeth is a midwife academic whose research interests centre on cultural and political analysis of birthing practice, and the role of midwives in promoting physiological and humanised birth. She is a passionate midwifery advocate and has held roles in the Australian College of Midwives, including state Committee Chair, and was also active within the Midwives Association of Ireland while working at Trinity College Dublin. She is currently Lecturer in Midwifery at Griffith University, Brisbane.

Samantha Nolan, RM, PhD. Sam is an academic/researcher with affiliations to Central Queensland University and Southern Cross University, Australia. Sam is a UK-trained midwife with 22 years' experience, predominantly in outreach roles providing continuity of care, advocacy and liaison for adolescent mothers and their families. Sam now teaches Bachelor of Midwifery students and is involved in research projects that include exploring ways to enhance midwifery students' learning experiences.

Steve Provost, PhD School of Health and Human Sciences, Southern Cross University Academic – Psychology.

Thejal Rupnarain, Bachelor of Psychological Science (Hons), School of Health and Human Sciences, Southern Cross University, Student Psychology.

Ruth Sanders, RM, BSc (Hons), MA, BA (Hons) University of East Anglia UK, Midwifery Lecturer Kings College London, Midwifery Teaching Fellow. Her research areas are pain management, decision-making and health communication. She is on the RCM Magazine Editorial Board Member. Her contribution to this book was supported by Wellbeing of Women (grant number ELS503).

Mandie Scamell, BA in Anthropology, MRes in Medical Anthropology, MA in Social Research Methods, PhD in Health Policy and RM, Senior lecturer, post graduate programme director at the Maternal and Child Health Research Centre at City, University of London. Her interest in the work midwives do around risk and physiological birth originated out of a mixture of her medical anthropological academic background, her embodied experience of becoming a mother, as well as her identity as practicing midwife in the UK. She is passionate about strengthening compassion and kindness in midwifery practice through both my research and teaching.

Kendra Short, Bachelor of Midwifery. Kendra is a mother of four. She works in a small practice of self-employed community midwives who support women to birth at home or in the local base hospital in South Canterbury, New Zealand. The majority of women in her caseload live in rural locations, which brings many interesting and varied challenges.

Anna Smyth, Bachelor of Psychological Science (Hons), School of Health and Human Sciences, Southern Cross University, Student Psychology.

Jennifer Stevens, DrPHc, MS, CN, UNFPA, Bangladesh. International Midwifery Specialist in midwifery centres in low resource areas. Her focus is on standards for quality, midwifery led care, human rights implementation, participatory action research and midwifery education. Keeping the voice of those we serve at our heart and centre, makes the path forward clear.

Jeroen van Dillen, MD, PhD, DTM&H Amalia Childrens Hospital, Radboudumc, Nijmegen Netherlands Consultant obstetrician. His research area is quality and organisation of (inter) national maternity care, with special interest in patient centred care and interprofessional collaboration.

Amanda Wain, RM, MSc, BSc (Hons), PGCHE, FHEA is an Assistant Professor of Midwifery at the University of Nottingham UK. Her interests in teaching and learning centre upon clinical practice, reflection and also pregnancy loss and bereavement care. She was awarded a Lord Dearing Award for Teaching and Learning Excellence in 2017. She has conducted research into midwives experiences during preceptorship, and has a strong interest in preceptorship and mentoring. She has a growing portfolio of educational scholarship and is currently leading a postgraduate mandatory programme for Senior Midwives to endorse quality improvement for maternity services in the UK.

Harvey Ward, BScMed MBChB DMCOG FCOG(SA) MMed O&G (Stell) LMCC FRANZCOG, Departmental Head OBGYN, Coffs Harbour Health Campus, New South Wales, Australia Associate Professor University NSW Rural Clinical School. His research areas are surgical audit, obesity in pregnancy and autoimmune disease related to vaccines. Harvey is a passionate teacher and student mentor. He has been a fetal welfare assessment, obstetric emergencies and neonatal resuscitation training instructor and is the ITP training supervisor for 13 yrs. He has a large private practise in Coffs Harbour, Australia.

Jane Warland, RM, PhD. Jane is a registered midwife and associate professor in Nursing and Midwifery at the University of South Australia. Since suffering the unexplained full term stillbirth of daughter Emma, she has been a passionate researcher into preventative and modifiable risk factors for stillbirth as well as promoting public and maternity care provider awareness of stillbirth. Her program of research is STELLAR (stillbirth, teaching, epidemiology, loss, learning, awareness and risks). She is regularly called upon to present her research at national (Australian) and international conferences. She has more than 90 publications many in the area of stillbirth.

Jinguo Helen Zhai, PHD, RN, RM. Head of the Midwifery Department of School of Nursing, Southern Medical University China. She was a visiting fellow at Baylor College of Medicine and Texas Children's Hospital. Currently, she is deputy chair of Chinese Women's and Children's Association of Midwifery branch and the Chinese Continuing Education Committee of OBGYN. She is the expert member of the Chinese Nursing Association. Dr Zhai won first prize of national higher education micro lecture competition (Medicine group) and Guangdong micro-lecture competition of using computer software for education (higher education group) and the best midwife honour in Guangdong province.

FOREWORD

My interest in and passion for all things maternity spans more than two decades, from the days when I was a Health Minister in the House of Lords, through the National Maternity Review, which published its report *Better Births* in 2016, to the present day. I have witnessed huge changes in healthcare, and I have sought to encourage and enable change in maternity care. Despite the increasing numbers and complexity of births, the quality and outcomes of maternity services have improved significantly over the last decade – the stillbirth and neonatal mortality rate in England has fallen by over 20%. Yet, of course, there is more to do to achieve a personal and safe experience for all women, babies and families.

Beyond the statistics, the starkest change is in the fact that choice and control are now being firmly embedded in maternity care and rightly regarded as key factors in the quality and safety of care and in each woman's satisfaction with her birth experience. I first made the argument for women's choice and control in my 1993 report *Changing Childbirth*. My hope was that one day we would be in a position where maternity services would be defined by personalised care, centred on the woman, her baby and her family, centred around their needs and their decisions, where they have genuine choice, based on unbiased information. It has taken a while, but I am thrilled that this is now becoming a reality.

Choice is undeniably about good information, but it is more than that. It is about how women are supported by and form a partnership with their midwives to understand information, consider their options and preferences and assess risks.

Understanding midwives' decision-making, the regulatory frameworks in which they operate and their high degree of professional accountability is central to appreciating the change we have seen in recent years.

Drawing on over a decade's worth of experience, the authors of this book have done exactly that. They have drawn together work from a diverse range of authors and settings to explore theoretical, regulatory and empirical findings and considerations with specific reference to midwifery.

The authors take us on a journey, tracing a woman's path through maternity services and encounters in particular clinical contexts, while exploring midwives' role in relation to others involved in the woman's maternity journey.

Collecting all these perspectives together for a midwifery audience in one publication provides an immensely valuable resource for practising and academic midwives, midwifery students, and others who work in maternity settings.

Baroness Julia Cumberlege CBE
Chair, UK National Maternity Review

INTRODUCTION

Elaine Jefford and Julie Jomeen

As academics teaching undergraduate and postgraduate midwifery programmes we have found there are very limited texts related to decision-making for midwives. What is offered has predominately been 'borrowed' from other disciplines so not grounded within midwifery philosophy. Following completion of our PhDs, exploring women's choices in maternity care and midwifery decision-making, we have continued to work in the national and international decision-making space and come together to explore this issue.

The idea for this book was conceived at the International Confederation of Midwives (ICM) 31st triennial congress in Toronto in 2017. It was born out of the need to share how decision-making can empower midwives around the globe to work in partnership supporting women's choice and enhancing their maternity experience. The gestation period for the book has been longer than 40 weeks and has had a few bumps along the way. Yet with international contributors from nine countries and multiple disciplines, such as midwifery, medicine, clinicians, doula, psychology, nursing and academia, the book has arrived.

The book has two parts. Part I critically reviews decision-making theories, frameworks and tools, including midwifery specific ones. The next few chapters explore the links between international midwifery governance including professional regulation, the law, risk and safety and decision-making. The concept of 'Midwifery Abdication', which is provocative and may be regarded as somewhat unpalatable, is introduced. 'Midwifery Abdication' occurs when a midwife, consciously or unconsciously, acts outside the parameter of our recognised midwifery governance frameworks. This is followed by chapters exploring how critical thinking and reflection are essential elements of decision-making.

Part II of the book is in two subsections. Fundamental to these two subsections and interwoven in each chapter is the partnership relationship with the woman, and the need for collaboration with the wider multidisciplinary team to ensure the woman feels and retains choice and is consequently the final decision-maker. The chapters are applied to all income countries and the diversity of midwifery models of care provisions within all three income levels (high, middle and low), and draws on midwifery governance including professional regulation and the law, risk and safety.

The first subsection describes how authors have explored decision-making empirically in different areas of practice and demonstrate how that relates to and impacts upon midwifery decision-making. This journey begins, as you might expect, with the antenatal context and a chapter focusing on the importance of the relationship between the midwife and other professionals in the circumstance of perinatal mental health and associated decision-making. Other areas explored are stress urinary incontinence in pregnancy, care for pregnant and parenting adolescents and the complexity of midwifery decision-making when transferring a woman from a birth centre to a hospital. Labour and birth is next, with chapters exploring pain-management, fetal monitoring, third stage of labour and optimal cord clamping, traumatic birth and stillbirth.

The second subsection critically explores midwifery decision-making within the context of the socially and culturally constructed maternity care environment. It critically reviews how a midwife behaves and how these factors influence relationships with women, with each other and with the wider multidisciplinary team including doulas. Some of the similarities, differences, strengths and limitations between a midwife and other practitioners are highlighted and how at times this leads to tension, yet the need for collaboration is critical. Threading through this subsection are decision-making frameworks, and the need for the midwife to feel valued and safe in order to facilitate successful interaction with women across her childbearing experience. The final two chapters discuss how proactive behaviour can be applied in midwifery education and practice and how it should be a prerequisite of shared decision-making between the woman and the midwife. This begins with how student midwives learn to understand and use practice-based reasoning by being introduced to a broad spectrum of approaches and strategies within their undergraduate education.

Decision-making in midwifery is a complex process that shapes and underpins our practice and to a large extent, the quality of care that we provide. We hope this book enables you to reflect on decision-making in relation to your own practice, wherever that may be around the world, but also on how as midwives we can truly work in partnership with women in decision-making to enhance their birth experience.

PART I

Influencing factors underpinning midwives' decision-making

1

MIDWIFERY AND DECISION-MAKING THEORIES

Elaine Jefford

Chapter overview

The focus of this chapter will be on the following decision-making theories/models and frameworks/tools: medical clinical reasoning, a non-midwifery specific shared decision-making model (USA and UK), a midwifery-specific decision-making model (UK), decision-making tool (Australia and UK), decision-making flowchart (Ireland) and Page's (UK) five steps of evidence-based midwifery. These will be critically appraised for their ability to provide a teachable framework for midwifery clinical reasoning that is consistent with the philosophy of midwifery and their utility to midwifery practice.

Introduction

The International Confederation of Midwives (ICM) represent approximately 500,000 midwives across 113 countries via its 132 midwives associations. The ICM mandates the required level of education, professional responsibilities and clinical skills a midwife is to demonstrate, irrespective of geographical location or model of care. The ICM's explicit aim is to promote and safeguard the safety of women and babies, thus holding midwives to account for their clinical reasoning, decisions, resultant actions and any related outcomes (International Confederation of Midwives, 2017, 2018). This accountability has been accepted and incorporated in many countries' regulatory documents, such as Australia (Nursing and Midwifery Board of Australia, 2018b), the UK (Nursing and Midwifery Council, 2014), New Zealand (Midwifery Council New Zealand, 2007, 2010), Iceland (Ministry of Welfare, 2012), and the Netherlands (Gezondheidszorg, 1993; Verloskundige, 2008), but yet not in others, for example Mexico, Bangladesh and India. Although outside the scope of this chapter, it is worth acknowledging midwifery decision-making accountability has not transferred into practice within some countries, such as in Central and Eastern Europe (Mivsek et al., 2016).

There are numerous decision-making theories, models, frameworks, tools and aids within the disciplines of medicine and nursing. In the past, midwifery has drawn upon these as well as from other disciplines. Yet how well suited they are to midwifery is debatable. In 2011,

Jefford, Fahy and Sundin explored the strengths and limitations of several decision-making theories/framework and their usefulness to midwifery (Jefford et al., 2011). This paper drew on Jefford's (2012) PhD thesis. The authors of the paper and Jefford concluded no decision-making theories embraced the midwifery philosophy so could not meet the needs of midwifery (Jefford et al., 2011; Jefford, 2012). The information presented in those publications remains relevant to midwifery today, despite the passage of time.

As new context-specific knowledge has emerged and the landscape of contemporary midwifery has changed, it is timely to explore more recent decision-making theories/models and frameworks as well as to revisit two older ones. The first part of this chapter will briefly refer to medical clinical reasoning and present a synopsis of a non-midwifery-specific shared decision-making model (USA and UK). This will be followed by a midwifery-specific decision-making model (UK), a decision-making tool (Australia and UK), a decision-making flowchart (Ireland) and Page's (2000, 2006) five steps of evidence-based midwifery (UK). The second part of the chapter will be a critical appraisal of these for their ability to provide a teachable framework for midwifery clinical reasoning that is consistent with the philosophy of midwifery and their utility to midwifery practice. The final part of the chapter will offer the reader an opportunity to engage in a clinical reasoning learning activity.

Medical clinical reasoning

Medical clinical reasoning derives from the analytical or rational approach to decision-making – hypothetico-deductive theory. As such, this theory and medical clinical reasoning favours the technical rational approach, relying on empirical data such as randomised controlled research and quantifiable clinical data obtained from the five senses. Over time it's clearly defined steps, albeit with slight variations, have been well documented (Elstein et al., 1978; Elstein and Schwartz, 2000; Elstein et al., 1978; Jefford et al., 2011, 2016; Chodzaza et al., 2018). The clinical reasoning steps are documented in a linear way and consist of:

- Cue acquisition
- Cue clustering
- Cue interpretation or hypothesis generation
- Focused cue acquisition
- Diagnosis
- Evaluate treatment options
- Implement or prescribe treatment
- Evaluate treatment outcomes.

Three-talk model for shared decision-making

This model was first published in 2012 (Elwyn et al., 2012) and revised in 2017 following feedback. The original model was linear and lacked elements around risk, patient preferences and the relational psychosocial dimensions of care (Elwyn et al., 2017). Medical practitioners are the intended audience of this model. Yet as you will see as you read different chapters within this book, midwives are using it.

The three-talk model for shared decision-making has three key steps embedded within an active listening and deliberation ethos: *Team Talk, Option Talk* and *Decision Talk*. The aim of the *Team Talk* step is to establish what outcomes the patient wants around their health. The medical practitioner then offers 'reasonable options' of care provision using a variety of media such as email. Discussion led through risk communication principles guide the next step: *Option Talk*, which is a collaborative, reciprocal, face-to-face meeting between the medical practitioner and the patient. Care options are reviewed, patient understanding is clarified and a patient decision support tool is utilised. The final step in this shared decision-making model is *Decision Talk*. Medical practitioners elicit what matters and what is valued by the patient and how this fits within the decided upon care provision option.

This midwifery-specific decision-making model sits within the physical, legal, political, cultural and societal environmental boundaries within which women and midwives live and work. This includes midwifery professional standards and national and local policies. These elements influence the four areas of evidence: *from the woman, from resources, from the midwife* and *from research*, which in turn impact upon the partnership evidence-informed decision-making at the centre of the model (Menage, 2016a, 2016b).

Evidence from the woman has three components: (1) a midwife employing a technical rational approach gathering quantifiable clinical data using her/his five senses; (2) a midwife exploring and understanding what the woman's psychological and social health is and her needs; (3) establishing a reciprocal woman/midwife partnership based on equality. *Evidence from resources* focuses on the midwife's knowledge about the boundaries or scope of practice each member of a multidisciplinary team has and the ability to access such professionals. It also requires the midwife to have the capability and capacity to draw on her knowledge in order to offer the woman a multidisciplinary care approach as and when necessary. Encapsulated within

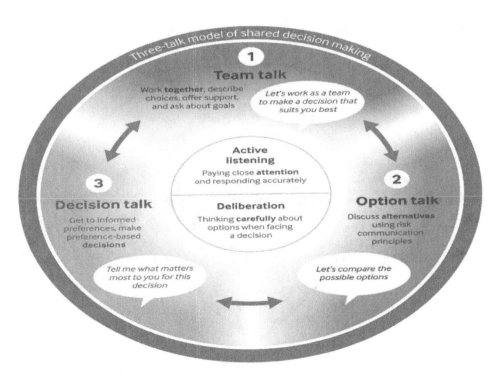

FIGURE 1.1   Three-talk model for shared decision-making

the *evidence from midwife* area is time to enable a dialogue so informed decisions can be made. A midwife's need to reflect on her/himself as a professional and person, including any limitations and how these impact upon her/his role within the woman/midwife partnership, is also noted to be an important part of this area of evidence. *Evidence from research* relies on qualitative and quantitative research as well as evidence from the other three areas of this model.

Enhancing Decision-making and Assessment in Midwifery (EDAM)

This midwifery specific decision-making tool arose from etic and emic data. Midwives from all states and territories in Australia representing all models of maternity care provision were part of an original decision-making framework (Jefford, 2012). Etic data was drawn from theoretical literature around decision-making, for example Hamm (1988a, 1988b) and Hammond (1980) and specifically medical clinical reasoning (Elstein et al., 1978; Elstein and Schwartz, 2000; Elstein et al., 1978, Jefford et al., 2011, 2016; Chodzaza et al., 2018), birth territory theory (Fahy et al., 2008) and midwifery professional, regulatory and legal documents (International Confederation of Midwives, 2011, 2017, 2018; Nursing and Midwifery Board of Australia, 2018a, 2018b).

In 2016, following international testing, the original Jefford (2012) decision-making framework was changed and EDAM (Jefford et al., 2016) was born. EDAM (Jefford et al., 2016) has been verified as a robust, valid and reliable psychometric instrument for measuring midwifery decision-making.

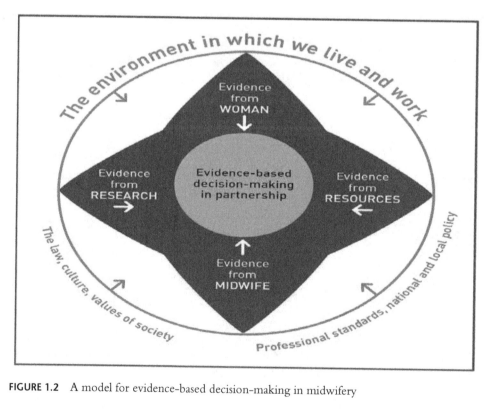

FIGURE 1.2 A model for evidence-based decision-making in midwifery

EDAM has two domains: *Clinical Reasoning* and *Midwifery Practice*. The Clinical Reasoning domain reflects the steps of medical clinical reasoning as noted earlier. Yet unlike medical clinical reasoning it has two distinct subscales: the *clinical reasoning process* emphasises the theoretical aspect of hypothetico-deductive theory and arriving at a hypothesis, whilst the *integration and intervention* subscale focuses more on nursing models of clinical reasoning and the inclusion of intuition and reflection.

The Midwifery Practice domain embraces the midwifery philosophy within the boundaries of midwifery professional frameworks (International Confederation of Midwives, 2011, 2017, 2018). The subscale *women's relationship with the midwife* centres on knowing what matters and what is important to the woman, trusting the physiological process of birth and being present with the woman – in other words, the philosophy of midwifery (International Confederation of Midwives, 2014a). *General midwifery practice* links with how the midwife enacts the professional frameworks to support decision-making.

TABLE 1.1 Clinical reasoning

Clinical Reasoning	
Clinical Reasoning Process	*Integration and Intervention.*
1. Cue acquisition[†] – appears to be comprehensive	6. Evaluates treatment options relevant to the diagnosis – if relevant
2. Cue clustering[††] –appears to be comprehensive	7. Prescribes and/or implements planned care
3. Cue Interpretation[†††] – Generating multiple hypotheses – if relevant	8. Evaluates outcomes
4. Focused cue acquisition – if needed and relevant to hypothesis	9. Uses intuition to aid decision-making
5. Ruling in and ruling out hypotheses – if relevant	

Midwifery Practice	
Woman's relationship with midwife	*General midwifery practice*
1. Stays in the room with the woman in labour	4. Honest and complete information sharing with woman/partner
2. Shares a common, known goal with the woman	5. Accountability for own professional behaviour in accordance with professional frameworks
3. Trusts the woman and her body	6. Skills in negotiating with medical staff or senior midwifery staff
	7. Assumes appropriate responsibility for woman/baby's well-being in labour
	8. Shows reflexive practice
	9. When the woman and midwife disagree about care, takes appropriate action (documentation and consultation)
	10. The woman is the final decision-maker

[†] Cue Acquisition: Sensory data that is collected; signs and symptoms
[††] Cue Clustering: Cues that are possibly related are considered together; pulse and respiration with blood pressure
[†††] Cue Interpretation: Using knowledge to understand the meaning of cues, to explain the cue cluster/s (provisional & differential diagnosis)

Scope of practice decision-making flowchart

This type of flowchart is not unique to Ireland, with countries such as Australia (Nursing and Midwifery Board of Australia, 2010) and the Netherlands (Expertgroep Zorgstandaard Integrale Geboortezorg Expertteam Care standard Integral Maternity Care, 2016) offering versions which focus on decision points. For this section, however, the Nursing and Midwifery Board of Ireland has a decision-making flowchart within their Scope of Nursing and Midwifery Practice Framework (Nursing and Midwifery Board of Ireland, 2015), which was why it was chosen by the author. This framework is encased within midwifery professional documents such as the Code of Professional Conduct and Ethics for Registered Nurses and Registered Midwives and the Scope of Practice framework (Nursing and Midwifery Board of Ireland, 2014, 2015). The flowchart aims to ensure patient safety by posing key questions which ask nurses and midwives to accept responsibility and accountability for their role and/or activity including collaboration or referral to other healthcare providers. It does this through four key questions:

1 Does the role/activity sit within the values and definitions of the (above) professional documents?
2 Are you competent to perform the role/activity?
3 Is this role/activity support by the clinical environment (legislation, policy, evidence)?
4 Are you willing to accept responsibility and accountability for your role and/or activity?

The nurse/midwife may proceed if these questions are answered positively. If the answer is negative at any step, then collaboration or referral to other healthcare providers is required.

Five steps of evidence-based midwifery

In 2000, Page (2000) put forward these five steps with the aim of interlinking the sensitivity (art) and scientific evidence (science) within midwifery. In 2006, Page (2006) again published her five steps using a scenario to illustrate how to apply it (pp. 360–371). Although Page (2000, 2006) does not explicitly refer to the five steps of evidence-based midwifery as a decision aid, it is considered as one by many midwives. The rationale is that in order to provide evidence-informed care, a midwife must enter into a relationship whereby a sharing of information occurs, thus enabling the woman to be the decision-maker about her care. During such sharing, the midwife must engage in these five steps:

1 Finding out what is important to the woman and her family
2 Using information from the clinical examination
3 Seeking and assessing evidence to inform decisions
4 Talking it through
5 Reflecting on the outcomes, feeling and consequences (Page, 2006, p. 360).

Having read the brief synopsis of the other theories/models and frameworks descriptions, it becomes evident that they and the five steps offered by Page (2000, 2006) are intrinsically linked.

Strengths and limitations of the presented decision-making theories/models and frameworks

Decision-making is complex, multi-dimensional and influenced by multiple factors. Within midwifery, unlike other professions, an added complexity is the mother-baby dyad. Any decision made ultimately has the potential to impact upon not only the childbearing women (hereinafter referred to as the woman), but also her (unborn) baby. Midwifery acknowledges and embraces a woman's autonomy and the need for her to be central in all decision-making (International Confederation of Midwives, 2014a; Department of Health, Public Health England, 2014).

Global healthcare reforms focus on a people-centred healthcare approach (World Health Organization, 2007). This has led to changing societal expectations of healthcare service delivery and patients' expectation that they will be part of the decision-making process about their care. The principle of a woman (patient) and doctor equally sharing power, collaboratively discussing care options which focus on the woman's needs and preferences, then planning and implementing that care is far removed from the patriarchal risk-dominated lens of healthcare and childbirth. Consequently, within medicine a flurry of shared decision-making models have been produced, one of which is the model by Elywn et al. (2012).

The strength of the three-talk model for shared decision-making as presented by the circle is that it provides an opportunity to go back to any stage for further discussion (Elwyn et al., 2017). Good relationships where women feel they are supported and can express their views and preferences and get the information they need are of the utmost importance in this process (Elwyn et al., 2012). The strength therefore lies in the fact this is an empowering model whereby women are encouraged to make informed decisions about their care as an ongoing conversation with healthcare providers. A limitation, however, of this model (2012) is that there was no consumer participation in its design or development; instead it was designed solely by medical practitioners and researchers in the UK and USA. There are five recorded consumer participants within the 2017 revised version; the other participants were medical practitioners in six clinical specialist areas, one of which was obstetrics (Elwyn et al., 2017). The authors do acknowledge that although patients are the recipients of the role and/ or actions the medical practitioner chooses to enact within the collaborative model, they are not the intended audience. This then raises the question, if community-based participatory engagement or research was not part of this shared decision-making model, how do we know the model is cognisant of what is relevant to women in relation to maternity care options and decisions that impact upon them? This limitation is highlighted further by the first step in the model, *Team Talk*, where face-to-face interaction is not deemed necessary when establishing what matters and what is important to each individual woman and what care options are available. During this step, authors note the core elements of shared decision-making is one where the medical practitioner puts forward what they perceived as risk averse options as 'shared decision-making is easier when options are reasonable' (Elwyn et al., 2017, p. 1).

This model, therefore, would sit well within a fragmented model of care where the lens is predominately medical, where a woman's agency, autonomy and ability to adequately articulate and co-lead decision-making is severely limited. Women's agency is further limited within the medical risk and harm communication principles with no face-to-face interaction. The challenge for midwives using this model therefore lies within the fundamental ethos of midwifery, which firmly asserts birth is a normal physiological, social, cultural and spiritual event of which they are the experts (or guardians) (Fahy et al., 2008). This ethos is evident in the midwifery philosophy where trust within the mother-midwife relationship acts as a catalyst for facilitating and supporting women as decision-makers irrespective of perceived risk. If childbearing becomes complex and the need to draw on medical expertise is required, then together midwives and other health professionals must facilitate the woman to make an informed decision based upon information, within a framework of what matters and what is important to her as an individual so she is the final decision-maker. Consequently a model of shared decision-making that does not include the community it is to serve, in this case child-bearing women, in its design, does not displace the patriarchal 'doctor knows best' assumption and does not embrace the philosophy within which midwives practice, arguably therefore it is not transferrable to midwifery. Nevertheless, some midwives would argue the three talk elements of the model intend to promote equal collaboration and exchange between the people involved in the decision-making process. All three talks may take place within one consultation if there is a time pressure. However, people often need more time to process information, therefore preferably more time is allowed and the conversation can spread over two or more consultations/visits. Ultimately, the model focuses on a medical practitioner rather than a midwife.

A strength of the model for evidence-based decision-making in midwifery (Menage, 2016b) is that it draws upon shared decision-making between the midwife and woman at its centre, thus removing the 'expert knowledge' imbalance noted in the Elwyn model (2017). Building a trusting, reciprocal partnership where empirical and psychosocial evidence can be gained is the focus of the evidence from the women area part of the model. Continuity of care from a known midwife is noted by Menage (2016a) as the ideal approach to facilitate such a relationship. The benefits of such a continuous midwifery-led model of care are well documented (Sandall et al., 2016), yet unfortunately the majority of women are unable to access such a model at the present time. Rather most women enter a fragmented model of care where it is possible she will meet more than one midwife during her labour. This is not a unique challenge to this decision-making model, instead it is the reality all midwives attempt to circumnavigate when working in a fragmented system. Nevertheless, it is unclear within the 'most radically different aspect of this model' proposed by Menage (2016b, p. 139) how a midwife navigates the fragmented model of care in order to provide evidence from herself through a reciprocal relationship with the woman. This is further complicated when a midwife is caring for more than one woman in labour at one time. Under the evidence from resources area, a midwife is to discuss with the woman how insufficient resources such as staffing impact upon the woman's needs and what care options can be realistically provided. This approach therefore has the ability to limit women's care options, much the same as obstetricians who view childbirth through a risk lens limit women's care options (Dove, 2013; Dannaway and Dietz, 2014; Scamell, 2014) as noted in Elwyn et al.'s model (2017). It could therefore be suggested that such an approach is not cognisant with the ethos of continuity of care or being woman-centred expounded in the evidence from the woman area of this model.

The evidence from research area, within the Ménage (2016b) model, relies upon midwives having the capability to seek and critically analyse both quantitative and qualitative research. Whilst all midwives should be competent to undertake such tasks, it is unrealistic to assume anyone can be across all literature for all clinical scenarios or even has time within the clinical environment when scenarios arise to undertake a literature search. Ménage (2016b) does suggest reliance on high-quality clinical guidelines as one way to support and improve care provision. Many high-income countries have national guidance they can rely upon to be current for many conditions, for example the National Institute of Clinical Excellence (UK) Diabetes in Pregnancy: Management from Preconception to the Postnatal Period (National Institute of Clinical Excellence, 2015). Unfortunately, however, this is not universal or global and evidence is ever evolving, thus creating a challenge for up-to-date guidance.

The lack of information on what community-based participatory engagement or research was undertaken when designing, developing and validating this model for evidence-informed decision-making in midwifery is, however, this model's most fundamental limitation. How were the needs and preferences of women, including those marginalised from lower social and economic backgrounds, taken into consideration by the author? Does this midwifery specific model (Menage, 2016b) mirror the Three-Talk Model for Shared Decision-Making (Elwyn et al., 2012), replacing the patriarchal 'doctor knows best' assumption with a matriarchal 'midwife knows best' one? If so, despite it, in principle, embracing the midwifery philosophy, this may not be the reality and therefore one needs to question if this model is suitable for midwifery until these issues have been addressed.

A limitation of the EDAM framework was its ability to be used as a validity and reliability assessment tool, hence limiting its utility within the clinical setting. A further limitation was that, like the Three-Talk Shared Decision-Making model (Elwyn et al., 2017) and the model for Evidence-Based Decision-Making in Midwifery (Menage, 2016b), it failed to engage women during any stages of development. In 2016, the first of these limitations was addressed through a study which enabled psychometric testing of the framework facilitating its development as an assessment tool for decision-making. The Enhancing Decision-making Assessment in Midwifery (EDAM) was verified as a robust, valid and reliable psychometric instrument for measuring midwifery decision-making (Jefford et al., 2016).

A strength of EDAM is that it draws on medical clinical reasoning, thus offering midwives clearly defined and agreed steps of clinical reasoning. These steps appears linear, however movement can be back and forth. EDAM's clinical reasoning domain permits midwives to demonstrate the transparency of their decision-making thus supporting their accountability and justification of their decisions, resultant actions and any related outcomes (International Confederation of Midwives, 2018). In other words it permits consensual checking of the midwife's knowledge and reasoning against clinical reasoning steps that can be tested (Chodzaza et al., 2018; Crow et al., 1995; Elstein et al., 1978; Elstein and Schwartz, 2000; Lawson, 2000; Thompson and Dowding, 2009). These clearly articulated steps of clinical reasoning are missing in the other decision-making models/flowcharts reviewed here, rather a midwife or doctor is instructed to make a decision without guiding them through the analytical steps involved (Elwyn et al., 2017; Menage, 2016b; Nursing and Midwifery Board of Ireland, 2015). A limitation of medical clinical reasoning, however, is the lack of the subjective 'self' or other decision-making theories such as the intuitive-humanistic. Instead empirical data that can be rationalised within scientific (quantitative) research is valued. In 1977 and 1984 the intuitive-humanistic theory (Benner, 1984; Dreyfus and Dreyfus, 1977) was recognised as an important part of nursing and later midwifery practice. This theory acknowledges health professionals can, with experience, undertake an automated assessment: identifying cues, rejecting those not perceived as important and drawing hypotheses (Benner, 1984). As a profession, midwifery cannot rely solely on such an approach to decision-making, because one can't necessarily articulate or justify the reasoning and resultant decision. To address this limitation of clinical reasoning, EDAM incorporates intuition within the integration and intervention subscale of clinical reasoning as the authors believe intuition is acceptable only if midwife then engages in medical reasoning to support her intuitive hypothesis/decision. Yet if medical clinical reasoning, even incorporating intuition is limited if it is not supported or situated within a midwifery philosophy.

This limitation is another strength of EDAM in that although the clinical reasoning domain can be taught separately as can the midwifery practice domain, both domains are part of an indivisible whole. Embedded within the two sub-scales of midwifery practice are fundamental elements, which are derived from the midwifery philosophy, as well as the definition of a midwife and midwifery's regulatory and professional documents (International Confederation of Midwives, 2011, 2014a, 2014b, 2017, 2018), thus firmly placing midwifery's regulatory and professional documents and the consequentialism of enacting them at the forefront of decision-making. This is also present within the Ménage (2016b) model for evidence-based decision-making, where midwives are asked if they accept both responsibility and accountability for their role/activity. Menage (2016b) incorporates or alludes to the midwifery philosophy, the definition of a midwife and midwifery's regulatory and professional documents in her explanation of the evidence from the midwife and evidence from the woman areas. The importance of midwifery regulation is discussed further in Chapter 2.

EDAM fails to recognise or refer to the potential influence of culture, as well as the physical impact the working environment/organisation may or may not have upon midwifery clinical reasoning or midwifery practice. This is not the case for the Menage (2016b) model for evidence-based decision-making in midwifery, which clearly acknowledges the physical, legal, political, cultural and societal environmental boundaries within which women and midwives live and work. The Scope of Practice Decision-Making Flowchart (Nursing and Midwifery Board of Ireland, 2015), asks midwives to consider national and local legislative documents as well as environmental policies and guideline boundaries. Although the Three-Talk Model for Shared Decision-Making (Elwyn et al., 2017) is not midwifery focused, the only tentative reference to environmental/organisational boundaries is doctors being able to offer reasonable care options.

Facilitative or hindrance for midwifery decision-making

Irrespective of where a midwife is located around the world, or the model of care she works within, the predominate feature of shared decision-making within the midwifery clinical environment as noted in some of the models, frameworks and/or tools presented here is key. The other key tenet is alignment with the philosophy of midwifery and taking into account the boundaries of midwifery professional frameworks (International Confederation of Midwives, 2011, 2017, 2018). Some of these models presented do this. Such inclusions can only therefore be facilitative in supporting midwives' decision-making around the world.

The hindrance for midwifery decision-making is their utility, in that no one model, framework or tool encompasses all the positive strengths (benefits) women and midwives require to support and facilitate best practice. It therefore becomes very important for midwifery pre- and post-graduate education or in the clinical environment to teach clinical reasoning and decision-making. One possible option is an additional learning package. Such a learning package would need to facilitate, through reflection, the acquisition of highly salient and context relevant clinical practice knowledge in contrast to 'rote' approaches. The reflective component is of particular relevance, since this psychologically anchors learning within contemporary clinical context, thus facilitating learning relevance and retention of knowledge dynamically. The online learning package would need to inspire students and midwives in innovative learning activities that have the potential to increase their engagement.

Conclusion

The explicit aim of maternity care is to promote the safety of women and babies, irrespective of whether that care provider is a midwife or medical health professional. We are accountable for the decisions we make, their resultant actions and any related outcomes. Yet midwives and doctors view childbirth through different lenses, which impact upon decision-making and care options (Dove, 2013; Dannaway and Dietz, 2014; Scamell, 2014). Earlier in this chapter the inference was that only doctors have a risk lens and was generically applied to all doctors. It is, however, not necessarily true. Neither is the assumption that all midwives use the 'normality' lens necessarily true. Some midwives and doctors are risk-takers and some are risk-averse. Multiple factors influence decision-making including psychological characteristics such as impulsivity and risk tolerance, observed or learnt behaviours, own childbirthing experiences or vicarious experiences. Some of these are discussed towards the end of this book, as is the contested space a midwife must engage in when trying to meet the needs of the woman and her birthing experience and those of the regulatory and legal systems (Chapters 2 and 3). No decision-making theory, model, tool or framework at the moment takes into consideration all these elements, variables and influencing factors, and one wonders if it is actually possible.

References

Benner, P. 1984. *From novice to expert, excellence and power in clinical nursing.* Menlo Park, CA: Addison-Wesley Publishing Company.

Chodzaza, E., Haycock-Stuart, E., Holloway, A. & Rosemary, M. 2018. Cue acquisition: A feature of Malawian midwives decision making process to support normality during the first stage of labour. *Midwifery,* 58, 56–63.

Crow, R., Chase, J. & Lamond, D. 1995. The cognitive component of nursing assessment: An analysis. *Journal of Advanced Nursing,* 22, 206–212.

Dannaway, J. & Dietz, H. 2014. Unassisted childbirth: Why mothers are leaving the system. *Journal of Medical Ethics,* 40, 817–820.

Department of Health, Public Health England. 2014. *A framework for personalised care and population health for nurses, midwives, health visitors and allied health professionals: Caring for populations across the lifecourse* [Online]. Department of Health, Public Health England. London. Available: www.health-ni.gov.uk/publications/framework-for-nurses-midwives-health-visitors-and-allied-healthwww.health-ni.gov.uk/publications/framework-personalised [Accessed 1 September 2018].

Dove, S. 2013. Enhancing choice and improving outcomes through the mediation of childbirth risk discourses within a midwifery model of care: Findings from a critical ethnography. *Women & Birth,* 26, s5.

Dreyfus, H. L. & Dreyfus, S. E. 1977. Uses and abuses of multi-attribute and multi-aspect model of decision-making. *In:* Benner, P. (ed.) *From novice to expert: Excellence and power in clinical nursing practice.* Commemorative ed. Upper Saddle River, NJ: Prentice-Hall.

Elstein, A. S. & Schwartz, A. 2000. Clinical reasoning in medicine. *In:* Higgs, J. & Jones, M. (eds.) *Clinical reasoning in the health professions.* 2nd ed. Oxford: Butterworth-Heinemann Ltd.

Elstein, A. S., Shulman, L. S. & Sprafka, S. A. 1978. *Medical problem solving: An analysis of clinical reasoning.* Cambridge, MA: Harvard University Press.

Elwyn, G., Durand, M., Song, J.J., Aarts, J.P., Barr, P., Berger, Z., Cochran, N., Frosch, D., Galasiński, D.P., Gulbrandsen, P., Han, P., Härter, M., Kinnersley, P., Lloyd, A., Mishra, M., Perestelo-Perez, L., Scholl, I., Tomori, K., Trevena, L., O Witteman, H. & van der Weijden, T. 2017. A three-talk model for shared decision making: Multistage consultation process. *British Medical Journal*, 359, 1–7.

Elwyn, G., Frosch, D., Thomson, R., Joseph-Williams, N., Lloyd, A., Kinnersley, P., Cording, E., Tomson, D., Dodd, C., Rollnick, S., Edwards, A. & Barry, M. 2012. Shared decision making: A model for clinical practice. *Journal of General Internal Medicine*, 27, 1361–1367.

Expertgroep Zorgstandaard Integrale Geboortezorg Expertteam Care Standard Integral Maternity Care. 2016. *Zorgstandaard integrale zorg [Care standard integral maternity care]* [Online]. Utrecht: College Perinatal Care [Accessed 13 September 2018].

Fahy, K., Foureur, M. & Hastie, C. 2008. *Birth territory and midwifery guardianship: Theory for practice, education and research*. Sydney: Butterworth Heinemann Elsevier.

Gezondheidszorg, W.O.D.B.I.D.I. 1993. *Act for professionals in individual healthcare* [Online]. Wet op de beroepen in de individuele gezondheidszorg. Available: http://wetten.overheid.nl/BWBR 0006251/2018-09-01# [Accessed 13 September 2018].

Hamm, R. 1988a. Clinical intuition and clinical analysis: Expertise and the cognitive continuum. *In:* Dowie, J. & Elstein, A.S. (eds.) *Professional judgment: A reader in clinical decision making*. Cambridge, MA: Cambridge University Press.

Hamm, R. 1988b. Moment by moment variation in experts' analytical and intuitive cognitive activity. *IEEE Transactions on Systems, Man and Cybernetics*, 18, 757–776.

Hammond, K. 1980. *The integration of research in judgement and decision theory*. Boulder, CO: University of Colorado, Centre for Research on Judgment and Policy.

International Confederation of Midwives. 2011. *Global standards for midwifery regulation*. The Hague: International Confederation of Midwives.

International Confederation of Midwives. 2014a. *Philosophy and model of midwifery care*. The Netherlands: International Confederation of Midwives.

International Confederation of Midwives. 2014b. *Professional accountability of the midwife*. Geneva: International Confederation of Midwives.

International Confederation of Midwives. 2017. *Definition of the midwife* [Online]. Brisbane: International Confederation of Midwives. Available: www.internationalmidwives.org [Accessed 4 September 2015].

International Confederation of Midwives. 2018. *International code of ethics for midwives: International confederation of midwives*. The Netherlands: International Confederation of Midwives.

Jefford, E. 2012. *Optimal midwifery decision-making during 2nd stage labour: The integration of clinical reasoning into practice*. PhD Research, Southern Cross University. NSW.

Jefford, E., Fahy, K. & Sundin, D. 2011. Decision-making theories and their usefulness to the midwifery profession both in terms of midwifery practice and the education of midwives. *International Journal of Nursing Practice*, 17, 246–253.

Jefford, E., Jomeen, J. & Martin, C. 2016. Determining the psychometric properties of the Enhancing Decision-making Assessment in Midwifery (EDAM) measure in a cross cultural context. *BMC Pregnancy and Childbirth*, 19, 95–106.

Lawson, A. 2000. The generality of hypothetico-deductive reasoning: Making scientific thinking explicit. *The American Biology Teacher*, 62, 482–495.

Menage, D. 2016a. Part 1: A model for evidence-based decision-making in midwifery care. *British Journal of Midwifery*, 24, 44–49.

Menage, D. 2016b. Part 2: A model for evidence-based decision-making in midwifery care. *British Journal of Midwifery*, 24, 137–143.

Midwifery Council New Zealand. 2007. *The competencies for entry to the register of midwives1*. Wellington: Midwifery Council.

Midwifery Council New Zealand. 2010. *Midwifery (Scope of practice and qualifications)*. Wellington: Midwifery Council.

Ministry of Welfare. 2012. *Regulation on the education, rights and obligations of midwives and criteria for granting of licences and specialist licences.* Akureyri's: Ministry of Welfare.

Mivsek, P., Baskova, M. & Wilhelmova, R. 2016. Midwifery education in Central-Eastern Europe. *Midwifery*, 33, 43–45.

National Institute of Clinical Excellence. 2015. *Diabetes in pregnancy: Management of diabetes and its complications from preconception to the postnatal period.* 2.1 ed. London: National Institute of Clinical Excellence.

Nursing and Midwifery Board of Australia. 2010. *Midwifery practice decision flowchart.* 2010 ed. Canberra: Nursing and Midwifery Board of Australia.

Nursing and Midwifery Board of Australia. 2018a. *Code of conduct for midwives.* Canberra: Nursing and Midwifery Board of Australia.

Nursing and Midwifery Board of Australia. 2018b. *Midwife standards for practice.* Canberra: Nursing and Midwifery Board of Australia.

Nursing and Midwifery Board of Ireland. 2014. *Code of professional conduct and ethics for registered nurses and registered midwives.* Dublin: Nursing and Midwifery Board of Ireland.

Nursing and Midwifery Board of Ireland. 2015. *Scope of nursing and midwifery practice framework.* Ireland: Nursing and Midwifery Board of Ireland.

Nursing and Midwifery Council. 2014. *Standards for competence for registered midwives.* London: Nursing and Midwifery Council.

Page, L. 2000. Putting science and sensitivity into practice. *In:* Page, L. & Percival, P. (eds.) *The new midwifery: Science and sensitivity in practice.* Edinburgh: Churchill Livingstone.

Page, L. 2006. Being with Jane in childbirth: putting science and sensitivity into practice. *In:* Page, L. & Mccandish, R. (eds.) *The new midwifery: Science and sensitivity in practice.* 2nd ed. Oxford: Elsevier Ltd.

Sandall, J., Soltani, H., Gates, S., Shennan, A. & Devane, D. 2016. Midwife-led continuity models versus other models of care for childbearing women. *Cochrane Database of Systematic Reviews* 4. CD004667. https://doi.org//10.1002/14651858.

Scamell, M. 2014. She can't come here! Ethics and the case of birth centre admission policy in the UK. *Journal of Medical Ethics*, 40, 813–816.

Thompson, C. & Dowding, D. 2009. Theoretical approaches. *In:* Thompson, C. & Dowding, D. (eds.) *Essential decision making and clinical judgement for nurses.* Edinburgh: Churchill Livingstone Elsevier.

Verloskundige, B.O.E.D. 2008. *Order on education requirements and area of expertise midwife* [Online]. The Hague: Besluit opleidingseisen en deskundigheidsgebied verloskundige. Available: https://protect-au.mimecast.com/s/-c02CoV1jZiBLPOfzHI_R?domain=wetten.overheid.nl.

World Health Organization. 2007. *People-centred health care: A policy framework.* Geneva: World Health Organization.

2

MIDWIFERY REGULATION

Global perspective

Mary Kirk

Chapter overview

The key concepts related to regulating the profession of midwifery are examined in this chapter, recognising that regulation is a social contract between the profession and society to protect the public. Safe and effective midwifery care for the woman and her newborn is central to midwifery regulation governance. To demonstrate the broader context in which the regulator operates, key regulatory relationships are highlighted demonstrating that the views of key stakeholders must be carefully analysed in the formulation of an effective governance framework. Health professional regulatory approaches that are commonly used and the reasons for the shift from self-regulation to co-regulation are also discussed. The principles of right-touch regulation are investigated to illustrate the benefit for the midwifery context. A model articulating the principal elements of a regulatory framework is provided to illustrate the complexities of regulation and guide midwives in their delivery of safe quality care.

Introduction

In September 2000 world leaders came together to adopt the United Nations Millennium Declaration. The Declaration committed nations to a new global partnership to reduce extreme poverty through a series of eight time-bound targets as the Millennium Development Goals (MDGs) with a deadline of 2015. Embedded in those targets were three particular goals that had significant impact on women and midwifery: *Promote Gender Equality, Reduce Child Mortality and Improve Maternal Health* (UNGA 2000).

The MDG's were enhanced in 2015 by the universal 2030 Agenda for Sustainable Development which 'provides a shared blueprint for peace and prosperity for people and the planet' through a common commitment to the achievement of 17 sustainable development goals (SDGs) (UNGA 2015). The continuing commitment created a global shift in policy direction and reforms in sexual and reproductive health. Of particular importance to midwifery was the focus on the 'delivery of the full continuum of care spanning sexual and reproductive health needs and rights of women and adolescents, pregnancy care, safe delivery, the first weeks of life and the early years of life' (PMNCH 2005; UN 2010).

The requirement for and benefits of a global increase in the availability of an enabled midwifery workforce are reinforced through the reports *A Universal Truth: No Health Without a Workforce* (WHO 2014) and the *State of the Worlds Midwifery* (SoWMy) reports (UNFPA 2011; UNFPA, ICM & WHO 2014). These reports are further strengthened by the needs of women and their newborns embedded in all of the SDGs (Every Woman Every Child 2015). The International Confederation of Midwives (ICM) asserts that for quality midwifery care to occur in any setting, midwives must be:

> recognised, valued, educated and regulated to global standards, working in supportive health services in which they have equal access to safe and respectful working environments with sufficient resources for them to do their work effectively and to practise to their full scope.
>
> (ICM 2017a, p. 14)

ICM holds that there are three interdependent pillars to an enabling environment for midwives: education, regulation and association (ERA). Since 2011 there have been some improvements in ERA in low- and middle-income countries, though not all elements have been implemented equally (Lopes et al. 2015). Safe, quality midwifery care across all settings requires ongoing commitment to establishing and maintaining an enabling environment through implementation of an effective regulatory regime for the profession, which is interdependent with education and association.

Protecting the public

Social contract

The regulation of health professions, including midwifery, is a social contract between a society and health professionals. The social contract is one of accountability and responsibility, and in return for the privilege to exercise the authority and autonomy to regulate itself, society expects the midwifery profession to maintain its trust and act with integrity by ensuring safe, high-quality midwifery care (Pairman & Tumilty 2016, p. 2; Calnan & Kane 2018, pp. 245–262).

Professional self-regulation may be misunderstood as a mechanism to maintain the elite nature of a profession. Exclusive requirements may serve to maintain the separate nature of a profession (WHO EMRO 2002). There is a global movement away from self-regulation dominated by members of the profession to co-regulatory models of shared decision-making, with multiple agencies charged with oversight and other responsibilities (Bennett et al. 2018; Baron 2015). Globally, models of midwifery regulation are variable. In low-, medium- and high-resourced countries there may be no regulation at all, regulation by other professions including medicine and nursing, self-regulation, and as highlighted by Staunton and Chiarella, most often co-regulation (2017, p. 238).

Regulatory mechanisms

Health professionals, including midwives, are regulated by boards, councils or professional colleges through many mechanisms such as employment conditions, remuneration and legislation relating to medicines as well as through inspection, scrutiny and audit of different aspects of their management and care (Staunton & Chiarella 2017, p. 238). Like other regulated health professions, the purpose of regulating midwifery is first and foremost to protect the public by ensuring that only midwives who are properly educated and qualified to practise in a competent and ethical manner are certified and re-registered to practise (ICM 2011; Pairman & Tumilty 2016; Roche 2018, p. 77).

Midwifery regulation that enables midwives:

- Works in partnership with women and industry to support access to services provided by midwives in all healthcare environments including the home, community, hospitals, clinics or health units (ICM 2017a);
- Facilitates the provision of high-quality education of midwives;
- Carries out the assessment of fitness to practise for internationally qualified midwives;
- Minimises harm by enabling the continuous development of a flexible, responsive and sustainable midwifery workforce;
- Helps midwives to practise safely through the promotion of innovation in the education of and service delivery by midwives.

Protection of the title

Foundational to the regulation of any profession are definition and protection of the title; definition of the scope of practice; and clarification of the work of the profession. For the effective regulation of midwifery and to promote access to care, it is critical that midwifery is recognised as a distinct profession with a unique philosophy and its own scope of practice. Country-based legislated acknowledgement of the title is essential, including a definition of the midwife and scope of practice based upon the ICM definition of the midwife (Box 2.1).

BOX 2.1 ICM DEFINITION OF THE MIDWIFE

A midwife is a person who has successfully completed a midwifery education programme that is based on the ICM Essential Competencies for Basic Midwifery Practice and the framework of the ICM Global Standards for Midwifery Education and is recognised in the country where it is located; who has acquired the requisite qualifications to be registered and/or legally licensed to practice midwifery and use the title 'midwife'; and who demonstrates competency in the practice of midwifery.

Scope of Practice

The midwife is recognised as a responsible and accountable professional who works in partnership with women to give the necessary support, care and advice during pregnancy, labour and the postpartum period, to conduct births on the midwife's own responsibility and to provide care for the newborn and the infant. This care includes preventative measures, the promotion of normal birth, the detection of complications in mother and child, the accessing of medical care or other appropriate assistance and the carrying out of emergency measures. The midwife has an important task in health counselling and education not only for the woman but also within the family and the community. This work should involve antenatal education and preparation for parenthood and may extend to women's health, sexual or reproductive health and child care. A midwife may practise in any setting including the home, community, hospitals, clinics or health units.

Revised and adopted at the ICM Council Meeting, ICM 2017b

Global attention was drawn to the needs of women and their newborns through the MDGs and subsequently through the SDGs, where the term 'midwifery' was used in research reports to describe the work of all health professionals who provide maternal and newborn healthcare (UNFPA 2011). In 2017, the ICM approved the ICM definition of midwifery in response to concerns raised by communities and midwives relating to potential confusion about identification of maternity service providers. The ICM definition provided the requisite clarification for users of midwifery services, midwives, health service providers, policy makers and health service planners as well as midwifery regulators (Box 2.2).

BOX 2.2 ICM DEFINITION OF MIDWIFERY

Midwifery is the profession for midwives; only midwives practice midwifery. It has a unique body of knowledge, skills and professional attitudes drawn from disciplines shared by other health professions such as science and sociology, but practised by midwives within a professional framework of autonomy, partnership, ethics and accountability.

Midwifery is an approach to care of women and their newborn infants whereby midwives:

- Optimise the normal biological, psychological, social and cultural processes of childbirth and early life of the newborn;
- Work in partnership with women, respecting the individual circumstances and views of each women;
- Promote women's personal capabilities to care for themselves and their families;
- Collaborate with midwives and other health professionals as necessary to provide holistic care that meets each woman's individual needs.

Midwifery care is provided by an autonomous midwife. Midwifery competencies (knowledge, skills and attitudes) are held and practised by midwives, educated through a preservice/preregistration midwifery education programme that meets the ICM global standards for midwifery education.

In some countries where the title 'midwife' is not yet protected, other health professionals (nurse and doctors) may be involved in providing sexual, reproductive, maternal and newborn healthcare to women and newborns. As these health professionals are not midwives, they do not possess the competencies of a midwife and do not provide midwifery skills, but rather aspects of maternal and newborn care.

Adopted at ICM Council Meeting, ICM 2017a

The ICM definitions and core regulation documents aim to 'allow for clear, transparent and diligent oversight by a regulatory body with robust procedures and processes, helping build trust with women, other health professionals, and the wider community by providing high quality, safe care' (Pairman & Tumilty 2016, p. 6).

Regulatory theories

There has been a global trend towards responsive models of regulation that help practitioners to practise safely. In these models, regulation moves away from the 'command and control approach' to unlawful or inappropriate conduct to using the 'every case on its own merit' approach. This change has resulted in individual and situation circumstances being taken into consideration to secure compliance rather than punishment (Bennett et al. 2018; Ayers & Braithwaite 1992).

A number of contemporary regulatory theories inform models applied by regulators that include:

- Responsive regulation
- Risk regulation
- Right-touch regulation (Parker 2013).

Right-touch regulation builds upon responsive and risk models of regulation and was first introduced as a concept by the United Kingdom Better Regulation Executive and built upon by the Professional Standards Authority (PSA) in 2010 (Box 2.3). The right-touch approach has attracted international appeal across many regulated sectors from that time (PSA 2015a, 2015b). The right-touch approach is 'based on a proper evaluation of risk, is proportionate and outcome-focused; creates a framework in which professionalism can flourish and organisations can be excellent' (Bennet et al. 2018). Irrespective of the model of health professional regulation adopted in a country, the PSA principles of right-touch regulation are worthy of consideration when contemplating a new midwifery regulatory system or reform of an existing framework and system undergoing renewal (Box 2.3).

BOX 2.3 PRINCIPLES OF RIGHT-TOUCH REGULATION

Proportionate: regulators should only intervene when necessary. Remedies should be appropriate to the risk posed, and costs identified and minimised.

Consistent: rules and standards must be joined up and implemented fairly.

Targeted: regulation should be focused on the problem, and minimise side effects.

Transparent: regulators should be open, and keep regulations simple and user friendly.

Accountable: regulators must be able to justify decisions, and be subject to public scrutiny.

Agile: regulation must look forward and be able to adapt to anticipate change.

Professional Standards Authority 2015

Partnerships for effective regulation

The global growth of co-regulatory models in health professional regulation has emerged following significant governance failures by health services and regulators resulting in loss of confidence in health organisations and regulatory bodies (CHRE 2012; Francis 2013). Whilst co-regulatory models may challenge professional autonomy to self-govern, they may also provide opportunity to enhance partnerships to manage inevitable risks and clarify the regulatory responsibilities for safe, high-quality healthcare services, including midwifery (Cayton & Webb 2014). Co-regulation can result in professional regulation that works in the public interest and helps midwives flourish as they work in partnership with women to assess risks for themselves to inform good choices (Hills 2015).

In striving to achieve a midwifery regulatory framework, ICM encourages midwives to 'seek opportunity to strengthen midwifery regulation and to work collaboratively with governments, regulators and policy makers' (Global Standards for Midwifery Regulation 2011, p. 7). Whilst ICM advocates for autonomous practise by midwives, it recognises by its very nature that midwifery works in partnership with women. In line with contemporary regulation practises, ICM promotes consumer representation on midwifery regulatory authorities (Partnership Between Women and Midwives 2017d; Midwifery Regulation and Collaboration with Women 2017c).

Women

Effective midwifery regulation is predicated on working in partnership with women. As service users take advantage of unprecedented access to information, they are also more thorough and informed about their health and choices for healthcare. As they become informed they demand transparency, accountability and integrity from their health systems, services and providers (PWC 2017). ICM advocates for the active participation of women as users of midwifery services in the regulation of the profession in its Position Statement on Midwifery Regulation and Collaboration with Women (ICM 2017d).

Professional midwifery associations

The principal role of professional association is to benefit members by advocating for, leading and developing the profession by engaging in activities such as promoting the interest of midwifery, providing education, and leading the strategic policy and research agendas within the country. The role of the regulator is to protect the public and maintain public confidence in the profession by exercising authority delegated by law. The regulatory authority establishes, maintains and develops standards of qualification, practice and conduct (Balthazar 2017a). Whilst there may appear to be a tension between the two roles, they are not mutually exclusive. Both share the common goal of wanting midwives to thrive and work in partnership with women to achieve best health outcomes for them and their newborns. As the regulator is responsible for establishing, implementing and evaluating standards, codes and guidelines, its key informant on the best contemporary midwifery care, education, research, management and policy is the profession itself and the women who experience the services of midwives. This is best achieved through a genuine commitment to collaboration and a robust and formal program of consultation and feedback.

ICM asserts the requirement for appropriate legislation relating to the practice of midwives in all countries (Legislation to Regulate Midwifery Practice 2014). However, in contexts where there is no regulatory framework, the professional association may fulfil a dual role in an effort to protect the public by mandating the knowledge, skills and practise of the profession and, in some circumstances, maintaining registers. It takes great mindfulness to effectively separate the role of advocate and regulator, and whilst they do not have a statutory mandate to regulate the profession, those professional associations should be applauded for their efforts until the opportunity arises to transition the regulatory functions to a mandated midwifery regulatory authority.

Governments

Governments often struggle with competing demands, with society and the media calling for fewer controls or regulations while at the same time demanding governments to do more. In the case of health professional regulation, there has been a global shift from self-regulation to shared regulation through co-regulatory models. Contemporary models of health professional regulation often have government agencies as key partners forming a secretariat or an oversight body. This evolution to partnership or co-regulatory models of professional regulation has meant that the regulatory authority or board comprises profession members and a significant number of consumers or lay members. The intention is for boards to focus on strategic objectives rather than operational matters which are handled by a government agency (Cayton & Webb 2014). In most jurisdictions co-regulation already occurs through regulations relating to drugs, privacy, remuneration and other matters which impact on the work of health professionals, including midwives.

Industry

The midwifery regulator has a responsibility to support access to services provided by midwives in all healthcare environments including the home, community, hospitals, clinics or health units. This cannot be done unless it works in partnership with the health service industry, both public and private, to ascertain their unique perspectives on regulatory opportunities and barriers that restrict midwives ability to work to their full scope of practice in enabling environments. A deep understanding of the health service environment and cooperation of service providers is also necessary for the formulation of sound decisions in disciplinary matters.

Education providers

The facilitation of high-quality education of midwives through the development of nationally consistent pre-service education standards and accreditation standards is a core responsibility of the midwifery regulator. An effective collaborative relationship based upon mutual respect is key to the achievement of innovation in education and the governance responsibilities of both the regulator and education providers. In some jurisdictions, midwifery students may also be registered and the cooperation of the providers is an essential element of their successful registration and regulation. Education providers may also provide declarations of fitness to practise at the completion of pre-service programs, and their understanding of their own obligations and the responsibilities of the board is critical for this arrangement to provide for protection of the public.

Health policymakers and planners

Given an enabling environment, midwives can deliver the majority of the essential interventions for safe and effective maternal and newborn healthcare, including the elements for basic emergency obstetrics and neonatal care required for safe, effective and respectful maternity care (Homer et al. 2014, p. 1146). In partnership with health policymakers and planners, regulators can assist, through an enabling regulatory framework, in the continuous development of a flexible, responsive and sustainable midwifery workforce, educationally prepared and skilled to work in innovative models of care within a functional health system.

Regulatory framework

Balthazard defines professional regulation as 'anything and everything that is done with the genuine intent of promoting and protecting the public interest by reducing, suppressing, mitigating or eliminating harms or potential harms stemming from the practice of a profession' (2017). Governance of health professional regulation refers to the framework used to conduct the legitimate affairs of the regulatory authority and describes the processes by which the regulatory authority carries out its functions. Foundational to effective midwifery regulation is enabling legislation which provides the regulator with legitimate authority to regulate the profession. Enabling legislation also calls upon the regulator to use a model of regulation which is liberal enough to facilitate the autonomy of the midwife to practice within their full scope of practice in evolving healthcare environments. The regulator's role is also to promote excellence in practice.

The conceptual model (Figure 2.1) depicts the principal elements of comprehensive regulatory governance for midwifery. It comprises three core components:

- Protecting the public
- Partnerships for effective regulation
- Regulatory framework.

Midwifery decision-making

Midwives, as autonomous practitioners, are accountable for their clinical reasoning, their decisions and the care they provide (Jefford & Jomeen 2015). Quality midwifery care is reliant upon midwives making a multiplicity of decisions with every woman, every day. The nature of the collaborative environment between midwives and other maternity care providers and locally developed protocols dominates midwives' clinical decision-making (Daemers et al. 2017).

Jefford et al. (2011) identified that best practice midwifery clinical decision-making theory needs to give guidance about:

1 Effective use of cognitive reasoning processes
2 How to include contextual and emotional factors
3 How to include the interests of the baby as an integral part of the woman
4 Decision-making in partnership with woman
5 How to recognize/respond to clinical situations outside the midwife's legal/personal scope of practice.

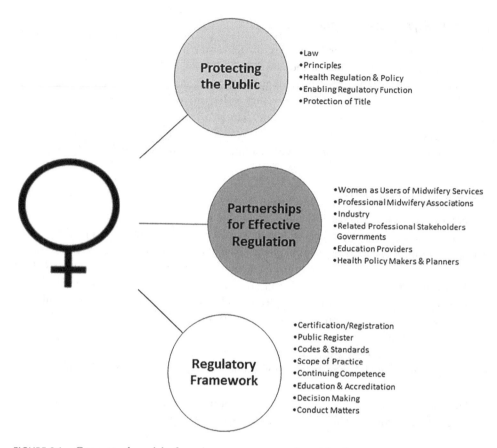

FIGURE 2.1 Conceptual model of regulatory governance for midwifery

Midwives may find themselves conflicted about meeting the needs of the woman and the demands of the operating environment and its protocols and complying with their professional obligations under the law. As autonomous professionals they are accountable for their decisions, and the midwifery regulator has a responsibility to provide clear guidance to midwives that will assist them in their clinical decision-making for woman-centred, respectful midwifery care.

Conclusion

The SDG era is a dynamic and exciting time for the profession of midwifery. More importantly, it has brought to global attention the human rights of woman and their newborns to respectful, quality maternity care. It has also made transparent the positive effect universal midwifery care could have if appropriately qualified and skilled midwives worked in enabling environments within functional health systems. ICM and other global agencies such as WHO and UNFPA recognise that an enabling midwifery regulatory framework is critical for the midwife to practice to her full scope of practice in dynamic environments. Midwives and midwifery regulators cannot do this alone. Success is predicated on the implementation of enabling regulatory legislation and a framework that recognises the distinct nature of the profession and all stakeholders working in partnership with midwives and women for the achievement of best health outcomes for the woman and her newborn.

When midwifery regulation is established in a jurisdiction, it is usually within a broader regulatory context. Alteration in the social contract from self-regulation to co-regulation has occurred in response to changing community and government expectations (Staunton & Chiarella 2017; Cruess, Johnston & Cruess 2002). In many jurisdictions, despite the attempts to achieve a right-touch regulation approach, these reforms have resulted in an increase of pluralism within the health professional regulation arena with a number of agencies sharing the former role of health professions boards (Bennett et al. 2018).

References

Ayres, I. & Braithwaite, J. (1992). *Responsive regulation: transcending the deregulation debate.* Oxford University Press. Oxford.

Balthazard, C. (2017a). *Defining professional regulation.* Human Resources Professional Association. https://www.hrpa.ca/.

Balthazard, C. (2017b). *The four types of professional organisations.* Human Resources Professional Association. https://www.hrpa.ca/.

Baron, R.J. (2015). Professional self-regulation in a changing world: old problems need new approaches. *Journal of the American Medical Association* 313(18):1807.

Bennett, B., Carney, T., Chiarella, M., Walton, M., Kelly, P., Satchell, C. & Beaupart, F. (2018). Australia's national registration and accreditation scheme for health practitioners: a national approach to polycentric regulation. *Sydney Law Review* 7–40(2).

Calnan, M. & Kane, S. (2018). Trust and the regulation of health systems: insights from India. In *Professional health regulation in the public interest*, eds. Chamberlain, J.M., Dent, M. & Saks, M. Policy Press University of Bristol. Bristol.

Cayton, H. & Webb, K. (2014). The benefits of a 'right touch' approach to health care regulation. *Journal of Health Services Research & Policy* 19(4):198–199.

Council for Healthcare Regulatory Excellence. (2012). *Strategic review of the nursing and midwifery council.* CHRE. London.

Cruess, S.R., Johnston, S. & Cruess, R.W. (2002). Professionalism for medicine: opportunities and obligations. *Medical Journal of Australia* August 19, 177(4):208–211.

Daemers, D., van Limbeek, E., Wijnen, H., Nieuwenhuijze, M. & de Vrie, S.R. (2017). Factors influencing the clinical decision-making of midwives: a qualitative study. *BMC Pregnancy and Childbirth* 17:345.

Every Woman Every Child. (2015). *Every woman every child strategy for women's, children's and adolescents' health 2016–2019.* UN. Geneva.

Francis, R. (2013). *Report of the Mid Staffordshire NHS foundation trust public inquiry: executive summary.* The Stationary Office Ltd.

Hills, C. (2015). *Right-touch regulation revised.* Lexology.

Homer, C., Friberg, I., Bastos Dias, M., ten Hoope-Bender, P., Sandall, J., Speciale, A.M., & Bartlett, A. (2014). The projected effect of scaling up midwifery. *Midwifery*, 384(0048):1146–1157.

International Confederation of Midwives. (2011). *Global standards for midwifery regulation.* ICM. The Hague.

International Confederation of Midwives. (2014). *Position statement: legislation to regulate midwifery practice.* ICM. The Hague.

International Confederation of Midwives. (2017a). *Definition of midwifery.* ICM. The Hague.

International Confederation of Midwives. (2017b). *International definition of the midwife.* ICM. The Hague.

International Confederation of Midwives. (2017c). *Position statement: midwifery regulation and collaboration with women.* ICM. The Hague.

International Confederation of Midwives. (2017d). *Position statement: partnership between women and midwives*. ICM. The Hague.

International Confederation of Midwives. (2017e). *Strategy 2017–2020*. ICM. The Hague.

Jefford, E., Fahy, K. & Sundin, D. (2011). Decision-making theories and their usefulness to the midwifery profession both in terms of midwifery practice and the education of midwives. *International Journal of Nursing Practice* 17(3):246–253.

Jefford, E. & Jomeen, J. (2015). Midwifery abdication: a finding from an interpretive study. *International Journal of Childbirth* 5(3):116–125.

Lopes, S. C., Nove, A., ten Hoope-Bender, P., de Bernis, L., Bokosi, M., Moyo, N. T. & Homer, C.S.E. (2016). A descriptive analysis of midwifery education, regulation and association in 73 countries: the baseline for a post-2015 pathway. *Human Resources for Health* June 8, 14:37.

Pairman, S. & Tumilty, E. (2016). *ICM regulation toolkit*. ICM. The Hague.

Parker, C. (2013). Twenty years of responsive regulation: an appreciation and appraisal. *Regulation & Governance* 7(1):2–13.

The Partnership for Maternal, Newborn & Child Health is the title of the document and was presented at the The 6th Global Conference on Health Promotion, organized by the World Health Organization and the Ministry of Public Health, Thailand, was held at the United Nations Conference Centre in Bangkok, on 7–11 August 2005.

Price Waterhouse Cooper. (2017). *The empowered consumer: more demanding and discerning consumers are opening doors for new entrants in healthcare provision*. PwC. London.

Professional Standards Authority. (2010). *Right touch regulation*. PSA. London.

Professional Standards Authority. (2015a). *Right-touch regulation revised*. PSA. London.

Professional Standards Authority. (2015b). *Right-touch regulation – international perspectives*. PSA. London.

Roche, W. (2018). Medical regulation for the public interest in the United Kingdom in *Professional health regulation in the public interest: international perspectives*, eds. Chamberlain, J.M., Dent, M. & Saks, M. Policy Press University of Bristol. Bristol.

Staunton, P. & Chiarella, M. (2017). *Law for nurses and midwives*. Elsevier Australia. Chatswood.

United Nations. (2010). *Global strategy for women and children's health*. United Nations. Geneva.

United Nations General Assembly. (2000). *Resolution A/RES/55/2 United Nations millennium declaration*. UNGA. New York.

United Nations General Assembly. (2015). *Resolution A/RES/70/1 transforming our world: the 2030 agenda for sustainable development*. UNGA. New York.

United Nations Population Fund. (2011). *State of the world's midwifery: delivering health, saving lives*. UNFPA. Geneva.

United Nations Population Fund, International Confederation of Midwives & World Health Organization. (2014). *The state of the world midwifery: a universal pathway. A woman's right to health*. UNFPA, ICM, WHO. Geneva.

World Health Organization. (2002). *Midwifery: a guide to professional regulation*. Nursing Technical Series. EMRO. No 27:11. Geneva.

3

LEGAL ISSUES IN MIDWIFERY CARE

Janet Kelly

Chapter overview

Using worked examples, this chapter focuses on legal issues and women's options for childbirth globally as well as the implications for midwives irrespective of the midwifery model of care. If the midwife accepts the responsibility and undertakes the care of a woman in childbirth, that midwife is then accountable to that woman. The chapter will also focus on the midwife's legal implications of meeting a woman's wishes and the midwife's legal duty of care and accountability. A distinction is also made between a woman who is competent to make decisions herself in being able to refuse care as opposed to demanding certain types of care, which is not a legal requirement although where possible, midwives will try and accommodate a woman's choices in childbirth. Using international documents and policies and UK case law, emphasis will be made on the concept of a duty of care owed by midwives to women and the standard of care that ought to be applied globally without distinction. A woman's choices in childbirth can be dependent on availability of resources, expertise and environmental factors, and therefore choices often become options. This inevitably puts pressure on midwives when women do not receive the care they believe they ought to receive. The chapter also covers meeting a woman's expectations in a legal context. If a woman has a poor birth outcome or if they suffer any adverse consequence as a result of childbirth, the midwife is very often the first person to be blamed for any harm suffered. This chapter will therefore focus on the concept of vicarious liability and clinical negligence. Emphasis will also be placed on how a midwife can best protect herself legally through the importance of accurate record keeping.

Introduction

The three vignettes presented in this chapter are similar to cases that a midwife may be presented with in a home, community or hospital environment. Using the vignettes this chapter will explore the relevant legal issues using UK case law and also recognition of international policies and documents.

The Office of the United Nations High Commissioner for Human Rights (OHCHR, 2010) places fundamental commitments on states to ensure that women survive pregnancy and are able to live a life of dignity. Further, the World Health Organization (WHO) places responsibility on states to ensure that there is 'health for all' (2008). The Universal Declaration of Human Rights (1948) recognises that all patients are equal and should receive care without prejudice and discrimination. Specifically, Article 25(2) states that 'Motherhood and childhood are entitled to special care and assistance'. Further, despite different social and cultural norms within different jurisdictions, it is universally accepted that all healthcare professionals owe their patients a duty of care, regardless of the location or the circumstances in which they give this care (WHO, n.d.). The term 'patient' is used as opposed to client to distinguish the legal terminology of a legal client.

Activity 1

Please read these three vignettes: one involves late pregnancy, one is intrapartum focused and one involves postnatal care. The location of each vignette represents the predominate models of care a midwife may work in irrespective of whether practising in a high-, middle- or low-income country. These vignettes will be discussed later in the chapter.

BOX 3.1   VIGNETTE 1 – LINKED ACTIVITY 1

Patient A is pregnant for the first time. She wishes to birth at home and wants it to be a natural birth. However, when she attends her antenatal appointment at 38 weeks and is seen by her usual community midwife, Midwife A, she presents with hypertension and proteinuria. Patient A also has some swelling of her ankles. Patient A is diagnosed with pre-eclampsia but refuses all medical treatment and goes home instead. She fully understands the risks. A few days later she starts to go into labour and contacts Midwife A from her home to request that she come and care for her. Midwife A, is very unhappy with the situation and is uncertain to know what is the best cause of action. Midwife A is worried that if she refuses to attend and asks Patient A to go to the local hospital instead, she will not be respecting Patient A's wishes. Conversely, Midwife A is concerned that if she does attend it will be in the knowledge that Patient A and her unborn baby's health and well-being could be compromised.

BOX 3.2   VIGNETTE 2 – LINKED ACTIVITY 1

Patient B is being cared for by Midwife B. Midwife B is an inexperienced midwife. Patient B is a multiparous woman in advanced labour at 40 weeks' gestation with her second baby at her local midwife-led unit. Her previous birth was two years ago, when she gave birth to a healthy baby boy at 39 weeks. This pregnancy has been normal. However, yesterday Patient B came into the unit for a check-up due to reduced fetal movements and was then later discharged having been reassured that everything was normal. Her birth plan states: *she wishes to use relaxation and breathing techniques for as long as possible; then gas and air, Pethidine and an epidural in that order, if needed. She does not wish to have continuous monitoring if at all possible, only intermittent monitoring*. Midwife B agrees to this without checking Patient B's notes or being aware of the earlier check-up for reduced fetal movements. Midwife B is also caring for another women on the labour ward who has just given birth and is due to be discharged home. She also gets asked to do other tasks by the labour ward co-ordinator due to midwifery staff shortages caused by sickness. Midwife B is feeling pressured. This results in Midwife B not being physically present with Patient B over long periods of time and she does not monitor the fetal heart as frequently as she ought to do. Further, as she is rushing, the notes that she does make are difficult to decipher. As labour progresses Patient B requests Pethidine, which is given intramuscularly. Midwife B forgets to monitor the fetal heart afterwards as she is busy doing these other tasks. Approximately 30 minutes after the Pethidine was given, Patient B suddenly presses the patient buzzer requesting help as she notices that her waters have broken. When Midwife B enters the room, she observes that Patient B is very distressed and there is thick meconium. She listens to the fetal heart via a sonicaid and it is approximately 60 bpm. Midwife B immediately seeks medical intervention from the medical practitioner who is on call for the midwifery-led unit. The decision is to expedite delivery. Patient B is immediately transferred to a nearby hospital and undergoes an emergency lower segment caesarean section. Sadly, the birth outcome is poor and despite vigorous resuscitation at birth, the baby girl dies.

BOX 3.3   VIGNETTE 3 – LINKED ACTIVITY 1

Patient C is a woman who has given birth for the third time at home in a rural environment to a baby boy at 40 weeks' gestation. Patient C is being cared for by Midwife C, her community midwife. The pregnancy and birth were normal as were her pervious pregnancies and birth. However, shortly after birth, Patient C starts to have a postpartum haemorrhage. Midwife C gives appropriate and immediate care to Patient C but due to limited resources is unable to get Patient C to the local medical facility. Despite summoning transportation, it does not arrive in time and unfortunately, Patient C dies. Midwife C is distraught and blames herself for Patient C's death.

Duty of care

Despite different social and cultural norms with different jurisdictions, it is universally accepted that all healthcare professionals, which includes midwives, owe their patients a duty of care, regardless of the location or the circumstances in which they give this care (WHO, n.d.). In the United Kingdom, Mr Justice Hewart affirmed the duty of care relationship between healthcare practitioner and patient in the case of *R v Bateman* (1925 at paragraph 49), where he stated 'if he [the doctor] accepts the responsibility and undertakes the treatment and the patient submits to his direction and treatment accordingly, he owes a duty to the patient'. The concept of owing a duty of care to a patient, therefore, provides a framework that ensures all healthcare professionals are accountable to their patients (Witting, 2005; Tye and Dent, 2018). Moreover, it arises when a person who is trained to undertake tasks are deemed competent to perform those tasks (Yamin, 2010). In a midwifery context, therefore, it means doing what a midwife is trained and expected to do.

A duty of care arises between two people when one person is directly affected by the other person's acts or omissions. This is known as the neighbour principle, where a duty is imposed if it is reasonably foreseeable that the claimant may be injured as a result of the defendant's negligence. As indicated by Allen (2009) and Golden (2018), at common law, an omission to perform an act is not unlawful in itself, as a person is not obliged to act as the Good Samaritan in the absence of a duty of care. However, where a midwife or any healthcare professional is acting in the course of their employment, they may face professional disciplinary proceedings if they fail to act accordingly, as they could be breaching the fundamental tenets of their profession (Nursing Midwifery Council (NMC), 2015).

The law and professional guidelines are clear. This is, if a midwife gives care, treatment, or advice to a woman, they then owe that woman a duty of care (NMC Advice Sheet: Duty of Care, 2008; Royal College of Nursing, RCNa, n.d.). The duty of care and the legal responsibility begins, as earlier emphasised by Lord Justice Denning in *Cassidy v Ministry of Health* (1951), 'whenever they accept a patient for treatment'. Clearly, therefore, the duty of care concept is comprehensive and goes to the very essence of ensuring that it sets clinical boundaries for all midwives globally (Water, 2017). This is important so that the midwife remains accountable for their acts or omissions and are liable for the consequences of careless and or reckless behaviour (RCNa, n.d.).

Legal implications and the vignettes

It is clear that all three midwives in the vignettes owe a duty of care to their patient, irrespective of the environment and/or global location where this care is given. In addition, irrespective of Patient A's determination to give birth to her baby at home against medical and midwifery advice, this does not mean a midwife can relinquish her duty of care to her patient. In determining if Midwives A, B, and C owe a duty of care to each woman in their care respectfully, it first needs to be determined if a legal relationship exists between each of them (Witting, 2005; Tye and Dent, 2018). The incremental approach to determine this arose from the House of Lords case, *Caparo Industries v Dickman* (1990). This conceptual framework established three factors that need to be taken into consideration as discussed below.

First, the harm must be reasonably foreseeable. The test of foreseeability is that of the 'reasonable man'. Accordingly, in relation to midwifery care, a midwife must act as the 'reasonable midwife' whatever their environment and wherever they are practising midwifery. In addition, the 'reasonable midwife' must realise that if they fail to give immediate midwifery attention to a woman in need of maternity care or appropriate care in any environment, the woman, her foetus and/or her newborn baby's health condition may deteriorate. Clearly, from the vignettes it is reasonably foreseeable that all three midwives meet this criterion.

Second, there must be a relationship of sufficient 'proximity'. In a maternity context, this is proximity between the midwife and her patient. Although this test can appear to be ambiguous, 'proximity' refers to legal as opposed to geographical proximity (*Muirhead v Industries*

Tank Specialities, 1985). Proximity means 'close and direct relations that the act complained of directly affects a person whom the person alleged to be bound to take care would know would be directly affected by his careless act'. Accordingly, in a midwifery context, if there is proximity between the midwife and the patient, a duty of care may be assumed. Again, as the three midwives in the three different vignettes are providing direct care to the women, it can be seen that there is sufficient 'legal' proximity. Further, it can be argued that the midwifery co-ordinator in vignette 2 also owes a duty of care to Patient B because they have indirect legal proximity. Moreover, Patient B is affected by the co-ordinator's acts and omissions in co-ordinating the overall care. The co-ordinator could be responsible for the acts and or omissions of Midwife B as in certain circumstances another person in the workplace can be vicariously liable for the acts and omissions of its workers (Anselmi, 2012). This would mean that the employer would be liable to pay any compensation for any wrongdoing proved against the patient (Griffith, 2012).

Third, even when the first two factors are satisfied, it must be fair, just and reasonable to impose a duty of care on the midwife. This part is directed to public policy considerations relevant to whether there should be liability in a given situation (Fedele, 2018).

As mentioned earlier, a midwife is not obliged to be a Good Samaritan (RCNa, n.d.). A duty to act will not usually impose a duty of care on that person (Green, 2006). However, if a midwife fails to respond to a woman in need of maternity care, then that person may be in breach of their professional code of practice (NMC, 2015). However, it will rarely be difficult, except perhaps in an emergency, to establish a duty to treat in such circumstances (Brazier and Cave, 2016). Nonetheless, the scope of the duty of care is very broad. As mentioned by Lord Diplock in *Sidaway v Bethlem Royal Hospital* (1985), which confirmed the leading case of *Bolam v Friern Hospital Management Committee* (1957) (*Bolam*), his Lordship stated, 'A single comprehensive duty covering all the ways in which you are called on to exercise skill and judgement in the improvement of the physical and mental condition of the [mothers and babies]'.

Standard of care

General standard of care

The general standard of care expected by the reasonable man is an objective one. Thus, Lord Alderson in *Blyth v Birmingham Water Works* (1843–60 at paragraph 480), stated 'negligence is the omission to do something which a reasonable man, guided upon those considerations which ordinarily regulate the conduct of human affairs, would do, or doing something which a prudent and reasonable man would not do'. His Lordship further added, 'A reasonable man would act with reference to the average circumstances of the temperatures in ordinary years' (*Blyth v Birmingham Water Works*, 1843–60 at paragraph 480). The standard therefore expected is not to reach perfection, but only a reasonable standard. However, a breach of a standard of care will occur when the defendant has not taken the steps that a reasonable man would be expected to take in the circumstances at that time.

Professional standard of care

Experts and professionals such as midwives with particular skills are judged by the standards of the 'reasonable man' with those specialist skills. The leading case of *Bolam* (1957, at paragraph 112) affirms the point, where Mr Justice McNair stated it is 'not the test of the man on the top of a Clapham omnibus'. It is 'the ordinary skilled man exercising and profess- ing to have that special skill. A man need not possess the highest expert skill' (Bolam, 1957 at paragraph 112). Therefore, in relation to the vignettes; the standard of care that Midwife A should give to Patient A is the ordinary skilled midwife in the community giving antenatal care and advice; Midwife B to Patient B is the ordinary skilled midwife on the labour ward; and Midwife C to Patient C is the ordinary skilled midwife in the community assisting in a home birth. All three midwives (including the labour ward co-ordinator) are professionally responsible for their own acts and omissions (NMC, 2015; RCNa, n.d.). All must be judged by the standard of the reasonable and competent midwife. Therefore, the question in each vignette is not did Midwife A, B and C give reasonable care to each of their patients. Instead, it is what would a reasonable midwife in those environments and situations have done, and did each midwife meet the required standard when giving care to their respected patients?

Regarding Midwife A, she is worried that if she refuses to attend Patient A at her home and prefers that she goes to the local hospital instead, she will not be respecting Patient A's wishes. Although a competent adult can refuse treatment and may make decisions that healthcare professionals think unwise or eccentric in English law, 'even when his or her own life depends on receiving medical treatment, an adult of sound mind is entitled to refuse it' (*St George's Healthcare NHS Trust v S, R v Collins and others, Ex Parte S*, 1998). In this sense, Patient A is legally entitled to give birth to her baby at home. Conversely, there is no legal obligation for any healthcare professional to give treatment to a patient demanding the type of treatment they wish. Irrespective of the legal position, it places the midwife in an ethical dilemma as to what course of action to take. Midwives are frequently faced with moral dilem- mas, and experts have differing views (Barker, 2014). A fundamental role of a midwife, how- ever, is to empower women to make their own birth choices; yet, there is no universal way to deal with any ethical dilemma (Kelly and Welch, 2016). Patient A is acting autonomously as she fully understands the risks but nonetheless still desires to have her baby at home. Golden (2018) remarks that the question is how to keep midwives safe professionally in such chal- lenging circumstances and whether employers can do more to protect them using legislation.

Regarding Midwife B, the reasonable midwife would have ensured that she did check her patient's notes prior to agreeing not to perform continuous monitoring especially with a his- tory of reduced fetal movements. The reasonable midwife would also always check a patient's notes before giving any care or treatment. The importance of accurate keeping was addressed in the Court of Appeal hearing of *Prendergast v Sam and Dee Ltd and others* (1989), where the court said that poor writing was a breach of a duty of care because it began a chain of events that led to patient harm. The court stated that handwriting must be 'to a standard of legibility which reduces the possibility of it being misread by a careless or busy person'. Clearly, a poor or a lack of handwriting can cause significant risk towards safe patient care and accurate and legible handwriting is part of a midwife's standard of care (Griffith, 2015). Midwife B has failed to keep accurate records. Failures in record keeping and failing to adequately monitor a fetal heart not only places patients at risk but also damages the reputation of the midwifery profession. Consequently, it is imperative, irrespective of location and model of care, that all midwives keep clear and accurate records relevant to their practice (NMC, 2015).

Further, the 'reasonable midwife', despite how busy they are, would not forget to monitor a fetal heart after giving Pethidine. The 'reasonable midwife' who felt they were too busy to deliver safe and competent care would raise a concern and not wait for something untoward to happen (RCNb, n.d.). It could therefore be argued that Midwife B breached her duty of care to Patient B by giving sub-standard care to Patient B in this respect. It would however, be for a court to determine if the midwife caused the death of the baby. In the case of *Whitehouse v Jordan* (1981 at paragraph 277), Lord Edmund-Davies confirmed Mr Justice McNair's point from Bolam succinctly when he said, 'If a surgeon fails to measure up to the standard in any respect ("clinical judgment") he has been negligent'. This means that if Midwife B's standard of care when caring for Patient B in the vignette fell below that of the ordinary skilled midwife in the same environment and situation in 'any respect', they would have breached their duty of care and could be negligent. At the House of Lords, Lord Scarman in *Maynard v West Midlands Regional Health Authority* (Maynard, 1985, at paragraph 639) further endorsed Mr Justice McNair's views by stating, 'a doctor who professes to exercise a special skill must exercise the ordinary skill of his speciality'. Therefore, this would suggest that Midwife B and all the midwives in the vignettes must also exercise the ordinary skill of their specialty expected in the context of their environment.

Inexperience

In *Nettleship v Weston* (1971), the court found that inexperience was not a defence as a practitioner is expected to be competent at the point of registration. The standard of care remains objective, even for an inexperienced midwife such as Midwife B. Lord Winn in *The Lady Gwendolene* (1965 at paragraph 300) demonstrated the objective reasonable man test where he stated 'the law must apply a standard which is not to cater for [the defendants'] factual ignorance of all activities'. Thus, carelessness is not measured by ascertaining if a professional fell below their standard of conduct, but by that of the reasonable person's conduct. In affirming this, Lord Mustill in *Wilsher v Essex Area Health Authority* (1986 at paragraph 814) (*Wilsher*) stated 'this notion of a duty tailored to the actor, rather than to the act which he elects to perform, has no place in the law of tort'. Moreover, Lord Denning in *Nettleship v Weston* (1971, at paragraph 700), when referring to inexperience, stated 'the learner driver may be doing his best, but his incompetent best is not good enough'. For student midwives this means that whilst they are not accountable to their regulator for their acts and omissions whilst in training as a student, they do nonetheless remain responsible for any harm and could be to sued for any breach of a standard of care. In other words, they are accountable legally but not professionally. This is because as students they are not registered by a regulatory body such as the NMC (Guy, 2010). The NMC only holds a register for qualified nurses and midwives and not students. This, however, is not the case is all countries; for example, in Australia a student midwife is registered by a regulatory body, the Australian Health Practitioner Regulation Agency (AHPRA), and therefore is accountable legally and professionally.

However, this objective approach can create tensions, as clearly recognised by Lord Mustill in *Wilsher*. When considering the performance of the healthcare professional, His Lordship stated that the 'proper response cannot be to temper the wind to the professional man. If he assumes to perform a task, he must bring to it the appropriate care and skill' (*Wilsher* at paragraph 811). He further stated 'the standard is not just that of the averagely competent and well-informed junior houseman (or whatever the position of the doctor) but of such a person who fills a post in a unit offering highly specialised service' (*Wilsher* at paragraph 814). For student midwives and those who have just qualified it means a sophisticated understanding is required that ordinarily could only ever be achieved through clinical practice thereby gaining appropriate experience (Blake, 2012). Further, it suggests that no leniency or account can be taken of how experienced or inexperienced (as in the case of Midwife B) a midwife is in his or her role, as he or she must still perform at the standard the role dictates, and not of a lower standard. Nonetheless, in *Wilsher* Lord Mustill was also careful to protect inexperienced defendants in negligence cases and muddied the waters by judging on activities of the post and the person who would normally undertake them. He stated that as long as the professional man 'had provided an adequate service on average, he should not be held liable for occasions when his performance fell below the norm' (*Wilsher* at paragraph 811). Moreover, His Lordship implied that where treatment is technically difficult and the chances of success are uncertain, 'the courts can . . . constantly bear in mind . . . in those situations which call for the exercise of judgment, the fact that in retrospect the choice actually made can be shown to have turned out badly is not in itself a proof of negligence, and to remember that the duty of care is not a warranty of a perfect result' (*Wilsher* at paragraph 811). Furthermore, 'the court should . . . be particularly careful not to impute negligence simply because something has gone wrong' (*Wilsher* at paragraph 813). Concerning Midwife C, despite giving appropriate and immediate care, Patient C dies. Despite this tragic outcome, this does not mean that Midwife C has breached her duty of care and given sub-standard of care as the care given was appropriate and immediate.

The law on experience is therefore clear. For Midwife B, it means that she must conform to the general practice of the midwifery profession. Irrespective of the midwife's inexperience in dealing with Patient B, who went on to have an emergency procedure, she must not perform at a lower standard. Consequently, in spite of Midwife B being under pressure due to her workload, no allowance or mitigation can be given for their inexperience, which caused them to forget to monitor the fetal heart after giving Pethidine.

Emergencies

In contrast to inexperience not being considered as mitigation for sub-standard care, in emergencies, it can be difficult for any healthcare professional to give the same standard of care that might be normally expected. The law caters for such circumstances. Midwives wherever an emergency may arise must offer anyone at risk the assistance they could reasonably be expected to provide. In *Wilsher* (at paragraph 813), Lord Justice Mustill stated,

> I accept that full allowance must be made for the fact that certain aspects of treatment may have to be carried out in what one witness . . . called 'battle conditions'. An emergency may overburden resources and, if an individual is forced by circumstances to do too many things at once, the fact that he does one of them incorrectly should not lightly be taken as negligence.

This re-affirms Lord Macmillan's dictum in *Glasgow Corporation v Muir* (1943 at paragraph 49), thus further emphasising that although the standard remains objective and is not variable, it can be flexible in an emergency.

Consequently, this may mean that although Midwife B may argue successfully that she forgot to monitor the fetal heart after giving Pethidine. Further, maintain accurate records because they were very busy and had other equally important pressing tasks to complete, they cannot nonetheless, argue that in those circumstances, when under pressure, they do not have to monitor the fetal heart in the first instance and maintain accurate records. The NMC code is clear in that a nurse and midwife must 'Keep clear and accurate records relevant to your practice' (2015, paragraph 10). This is a notion that is to be applied to all locations around the world where midwives practise and is irrespective of the model of care adopted.

Midwife B must still act 'reasonably' and exercise the ordinary skill of a midwife in emergency circumstances. The law, even in an emergency, will not allow different and variable standards of care. Nevertheless, it does, as stated by Lord Justice Asquith in *Daborn v Bath Tramways Motor Co Ltd and Trevor Smithey* (1946, at paragraph at 337) (*Daborn*), establish that 'the standard of reasonable care' that should be given is that 'which is reasonably to be demanded of him in the circumstances'. For Midwife B, the circumstances that need to be taken into account are those of a busy labour ward and a midwife undertaking multiple tasks. As Lord Justice Asquith further stated, 'the importance of the end to be served by behaving in this way or in that' (*Daborn* at paragraph at 337). It should, therefore, not always be deemed as the ideal care or care that was actually achieved, but the most reasonable care that could be achieved given the circumstances. The courts may, therefore, consider that Midwife B did not give sub-standard care in her interventions with Patient B. Nonetheless, regarding record keeping, Midwife B has failed to keep accurate records. Failures in record keeping and failing to adequately monitor a fetal heart in labour not only places patients at risk but also damages the reputation of the midwifery profession. Consequently, it is imperative, irrespective of location and model of care, that all midwives must keep clear and accurate records relevant to their practise (NMC, 2015).

In conclusion, the primary function of the midwifery professional is to protect patients and the wider public interest, which includes maintaining confidence in the midwifery profession and upholding proper standards of conduct and performance (NMC, 2015). The overarching objectives of midwives is to protect, promote and maintain the health and safety and well-being of their patients (Griffith et al., 2010). The public would be shocked if a midwife who had caused harm and suffering to their patient was not found to have their clinical practice deemed unprofessional and impaired.

References

Allen, N. (2009) Saving Life and Respecting Death: A Savage Dilemma, *Medical Law Review*, 17(2), 262–273.

Anselmi, K.K. (2012) Nurses' Personal Liability vs. Employer's Vicarious Liability, *Medical-Surgical Nursing*, 21(1), 45–48.

Barker, K. (2014) The Changing Climate of Legal and Ethical Issues in Maternity Services, *British Journal of Midwifery*, 22(12), 842.

Blake, D. (2012) Newborn Examination: The Student's Role? *British Journal of Midwifery*, 20(12), 892–896.

Blyth v Birmingham Water Works [1843–60] All ER Rep 478 at 480.

Bolam v Friern Hospital Management Committee [1957] 2 All ER 118 at 122.

Brazier, M. and Cave, E. (2016) *Medicine, Patients and the Law (Contemporary Issues in Bioethics)*, Manchester: Manchester University Press.

Caparo Industries v Dickman [1990] 2 WLR 358.

Cassidy v Ministry of Health [1951] 1 All ER 574 at 586.

Daborn v Bath Tramways Motor Co Ltd and Trevor Smithey [1946] 2 All ER 333 at 337.

Fedele, R (2018) The Broad Value of Professional Indemnity Insurance, *Australian Nursing and Midwifery Journal*, 25(9), 18.

Glasgow Corporation v Muir [1943] 2 All ER 44 at 49.

Golden, P. (2018) Who Has a Duty of Care to Keep Midwives Safe? *British Journal of Midwifery*, 26(1), 62–63.

Green, S. (2006) Coherence of Medical Negligence Case, *Medical Law Review*, 14(1), 1–14.

Griffith, R. (2012) Accountability in Midwifery Practice: Answerable to the Employer, *British Journal of Midwifery*, 20(10), 753–754.

Griffith, R. (2015) Standard of Handwriting Is Part of a Midwife's Duty of Care, *British Journal of Midwifery*, 23(7), 522–523.

Griffith, R., Tengnah, C. and Patel, C. (2010) *Law and Professional Issues in Midwifery*, Exeter: Learning Matters.

Guy, H. (2010) Accountability and Legal Issues in Tissue Viability Nursing, *Nursing Standard*, 25(7), 62–67.

Kelly, J. and Welch, E. (2016) Ethical Decision-Making Regarding Infant Viability: A Discussion, *Nursing Ethics*. Available Online: https://journals.sagepub.com/doi/10.1177/0969733016677869.

The Lady Gwendolene [1965] 2 All ER 283 at 300.

Maynard v West Midlands Regional Health Authority [1985] 1 All ER 635 at 639.

Muirhead v Industries Tank Specialities [1985] 3 All ER 705.

Nettleship v Weston [1971] 2 Q.B. 691.

Nursing Midwifery Council. (2008) *Advice Sheet: Duty of Care*, London: Nursing Midwifery Council.

Nursing Midwifery Council. (2015) *The Code*, Prioritise People, para 1, London: Nursing Midwifery Council.

The Office of the United Nations High Commissioner for Human Rights. (2010) *On Discrimination Kills, Maternal Mortality and Human Rights* (OHCHR LOGO Dur: 6:44" 17 June 2010). Geneva. Available online: https://lib.ohchr.org/_layouts/15/WopiFrame.aspx?sourcedoc=/SPdocs/Press/VideoMaternalMortality.doc&action=default&DefaultItemOpen=1 [Accessed 17/12/2018].

The Office of the United Nations High Commissioner for Human Rights and The Universal Declaration of Human Rights. (1948) *Article 25 (2)*. Available online: www.ohchr.org/EN/UDHR/Documents/UDHR_Translations/eng.pdf [accessed 17/12/2018].

Prendergast v Sam and Dee Ltd [1989] 1 Med LR 36.

Royal College of Nursing. (n.d.a) *On Duty of Care*. London. Available Online: www.rcn.org.uk/get-help/rcn-advice/duty-of-care#Legal%20duty%20of%20care [Accessed 17/12/2018].

Royal College of Nursing. (n.d.b) *On Raising a Concern*. Available Online: www.rcn.org.uk/employment-and-pay/raising-concerns/guidance-for-rcn-members [Accessed 17/12/2018].

R v Bateman [1925] All ER Rep 45 at 49.

Sidaway v Bethlem Royal Hospital [1985] 1 All ER 643.

St George's Healthcare NHS Trust v S, R v Collins and Others, Ex Parte S, [1998] 3 All ER 673.

Tye, J. and Dent, B. (2018) From Accountability to Ownership, *Reflections on Nursing Leadership*, 44(1), 152–164.

Water, T. (2017) Nursing's Duty of Care: From Legal Obligation to Moral Commitment, *Nursing Praxis in New Zealand*, 33(3), 7–20.

Whitehouse v Jordan [1981] 1 All ER 267 at 277.

Wilsher v Essex Area Health Authority [1986] 3 All ER 801 at 814.

Witting, C. (2005) Duty of Care: An Analytical Approach, *Oxford Journal of Legal Studies*, 25(1), 33–63.

World Health Organization. (2008) *On the Right to Health, Fact Sheet 31, Monitoring the Right to Health and Holding States Accountable*, page 31. Geneva. Available online: www.refworld.org/docid/48625a742.html [Accessed 17/12/2018].

World Health Organization. (n.d.) *Genomic Resource Centre: Patients' Rights*. Geneva. Available online: www.who.int/genomics/public/patientrights/en/ [Accessed 17/12/2018].

Yamin, A.E. (2010) Toward Transformative Accountability: Applying a Rights-Based Approach to Fulfil Maternal Health Obligations, *International Journal on Human Rights*, 7(12), 95–122.

4

DOING GOOD

Ethics of decision-making in midwifery care

Marianne Nieuwenhuijze

Chapter overview

In this chapter, we explore decision-making in midwifery care from an ethical perspective, reflecting on what 'doing good' means for midwives around the globe when engaging with a woman in the decision-making process during the perinatal period. The ethical virtue of 'doing good' is universal, even though the enabling environment of midwives to support women in the decision-making process may differ per circumstance, setting and country.

First, I will discuss the various dilemmas midwives may encounter when supporting a woman in decision-making. Subsequently, I will introduce ethical perspectives on decision-making with specific attention to 'care ethics', building from the grounding work of Gilligan (1982/2016) and Tronto (1993/2009). Finally, I will reflect on what considerations this ethical perspective on care can add to dealing with the dilemmas in everyday midwifery care, both for the individual midwife and the political agenda of midwifery.

Introduction

In the last two decades, there has been a growing understanding that decisions in midwifery care are shared between a midwife and a woman, similar to all other areas of healthcare (Elwyn et al., 2010). The woman's right to informed decision-making and self-determination are regarded an essential component of the worldwide philosophy of midwifery care, concentrating on the individual woman's circumstances and needs and giving each woman an active say in what happens to her and her child (ICM, 2014). Midwives can contribute to woman-centred care by proactively exploring women's preferences throughout pregnancy and birth, supporting women in developing well-informed choices and facilitating these choices to happen.

Studies in countries around the world show that women want to be involved in decisions during the life-changing transition period of childbirth (Hendrix et al., 2009; Downe et al., 2016, 2018). Women want to make their own choices and take responsibility for their health and that of their baby (Seefat-van Teeffelen et al., 2011). However, the degree of involvement may vary depending on women's individual preferences and circumstances as well as the support she gets from her midwife or significant others (Noseworthy et al., 2013).

Shared decision-making was defined as:

> an approach where a clinician and patient share the best available evidence when faced with the task of making decisions, and where the patient is supported to consider options to achieve informed preferences.
>
> *(Elwyn et al., 2010)*

Over time, it has become clear that not just evidence is part of coming to a decision; values, preferences, earlier experiences, the immediate environment, society and other issues important to quality of life influence decisions of both women and care providers in the perinatal period (Nieuwenhuijze & Kane Low, 2013). This is particularly significant for midwifery care because having a baby is more than a medical procedure; it affects the whole lives of those intimately involved and carries significant meaning for the woman, her family, and the community (de Vries, 2005; ICM, 2014). Becoming a mother is a major life event that affects a woman, her baby and her family in physical, emotional and social ways.

In this context, decision-making is a complex process that brings different perspectives to the table. It may confront care providers and women with ethical dilemmas that need to be considered in order to provide 'good' midwifery care, including 'good' decision-making, tailored to a woman's needs.

Ethical considerations around decision-making in midwifery care

Ethical dilemmas are defined as 'decision-making problems involving two or more courses of action, neither of which are unambiguously acceptable or preferable' (Oxford English Dictionary, 2019). This suggests complicated situations with vital issues, but also apparently small disagreements in care between a woman and her midwife have an impact on a woman's experience of 'good' midwifery care.

One of the most attention-grabbing dilemmas of decision-making in midwifery care is balancing the welfare of the mother and her child when confronted with a decision in pregnancy or birth that implies different benefits for each of them. Although rare, these situations can emerge because a medical reason presses the need of an intervention for either the woman or the baby that is potentially harmful for the other. Another reason might be a mother's preference, which she seeks for personal reasons, and that is interpreted by the midwife or doctor as enhancing the chances of harm to her baby. What is the best way to move forward in these situations: pressure the mother to undergo an intervention she does not want (e.g. a forced caesarean section) or accept that a choice might increase the chances of fetal harm by a certain margin?

Beside this demanding dilemma, other issues can complicate shared decision-making, such as establishing the right balance between empowering a woman's autonomy and concerns about abandoning her with the burden of a decision. A woman can be vulnerable in pregnancy and childbirth for various psychological, social or medical reasons (Noseworthy et al., 2013). Having to make the final decision by herself can be a huge responsibility for a woman in certain situations and around certain decisions. Making important decisions about health and safety often involves contemplating the regret that may arise if a decision turns out badly

(Koch, 2014). If outcomes are uncertain or the woman is left alone, 'anticipated regret' may be the woman's leading motive to make a certain choice (Dugas et al., 2012).

Another concern is the power imbalance between a woman and her midwife in access to certain choices or knowledge. When a midwife offers a woman a choice but subsequently does not support the woman in fulfilling that choice (e.g. a birth without epidural), there is no genuine shared decision-making. Demands from the institution can also inflict a midwife with dilemmas around supporting women to make their own decisions, if she is forced to adhere to strict institutional policies and not free to offer certain options (Newnham & Kirkham, 2019).

Shared decision-making also implies an open dialogue with honest and unbiased information. However, this open dialogue can be jeopardised by framing information in a particular way to obtain a preferred choice (Declercq et al., 2013) or by ideas about a woman's capability to be involved in decision-making. These ideas may be translated in the assumption that a less educated woman or a woman with a certain cultural background finds it less important to be involved in decision-making (Malek, 2017; Hawley & Morris, 2017). Additionally, there is the question if informed choice is possible for any woman when this implies an overload of information. How to tailor the amount and level of information to the needs of the woman?

Finally, a person's values influence their choices; models of shared decision-making recognise their importance in the decision-making process (Légaré et al., 2011; Elwyn et al., 2017). Values are explicit or implicit ideals or beliefs that are personally meaningful. They direct how we understand our lives, interact with other people, and determine our preferences. Values are the standards against which we measure our choices. Consciously or unconsciously, values influence the way we look at the other, the conversations in care, the decision-making process, the final choice, and the care provided. From an ethical perspective, paying attention to values is part of offering 'good' care. How do we bring values into the conversation and gain the right understanding of someone's values? Midwives experience these dilemmas as an increasing reality in the complexity of modern healthcare. In finding the best approach, ethical reflection on these issues may provide a deeper understanding.

Ethical perspectives on dilemmas

Dilemmas in healthcare are often addressed with the four principles of biomedical ethics: respect for autonomy, beneficence, non-maleficence and justice (Beauchamp & Childress, 2013). These principles serve as a guide to healthcare professionals on what needs consideration when facing a complex decision, but they do not give answers as to how to handle a particular situation. Additionally, the principles sometimes conflict with each other and there is no precedence for one above the other. Therefore, dilemmas during pregnancy and childbirth can easily decay to complicated discussion around the rights of the mother and rights of her unborn child (Hollander et al., 2016), or about the beneficence-based obligation of care providers towards the unborn child over the mother making her own choice for herself and her child when she chooses an option that is seen as unreasonable from a medical perspective or outside guidelines (Chervenak et al., 2011).

Newnham and Kirkham (2019) describe how principle-based ethics supports institution-centred care captured in the symbolism of safety, where women, and also midwives, do not have the power to claim personal choices and create opportunities to build relationships that are fundamental for offering 'good' care. This abstract, liberal approach of ethics may mask power relationships and structural inequalities that direct available options and decisions. What is needed is an ethics based on relationship and responsibility that is better aligned with midwifery practice (MacLellan, 2014).

Care ethics

Care ethics offers another perspective on what is morally desirable around dilemmas in midwifery care as it takes into consideration power inequalities; it supports the primacy of the midwife-woman relationship present within midwifery philosophy (ICM, 2014). The fundamentals of care ethics are based on the work of Gilligan (1982) and Tronto (1993). Gilligan, in a critique of Kohlberg's theory of moral development that identified boys as reaching higher levels of moral development than girls, argued that girls solve ethical dilemmas using another perspective. They focus more on responsibilities, relationships and individual circumstances. Gilligan pleaded for an 'ethic of care' that articulates doing good by using moral values as nurturing and caring, next to relying on abstract rules or principles for answering the question of what is right ('ethic of justice').

Tronto presented a political argument for the central role of caring in human life and an 'ethics of care' that is fundamental for thinking about a 'good' society. She identified four elements that are essential for 'good' care: (1) *attentiveness*, or recognising and responding to the needs of others; (2) *responsibility*, or taking on care as a gift and not an obligation; (3) *competence*, or ensuring that care is adequate and safe; and (4) *responsiveness*, or taking care of others in their vulnerability, meeting their needs, without taking over. Care is not just about 'giving care' but also about 'receiving care', making sure that the actual caring needs of the other person are met. In this context, autonomy is seen as 'relational autonomy': the way people realise their autonomy is embedded in their social context and the relations they have with others, including their midwife (Verkerk, 2007). This is particularly true for the perinatal period, where the bond between mother and child and the positive welcoming of the newborn child in the family are basic for a healthy and happy future. A caring relationship between the woman and her midwife is crucial, where the midwife has a genuine sensitivity and attentiveness to the woman's needs and circumstances and that balances the hazards of interfering with a woman's choices against the dangers of abandonment (Verkerk, 2007).

Addressing dilemmas: a relational approach to care

In addressing ethical dilemmas around decision-making, it is wise to realise that forcing one right solution is not the answer. The absence of an absolute right answer that solves the concerns of everybody involved is what makes the issue an ethical dilemma. However, there is the possibility of a 'good' approach with an open dialogue that can attribute to understanding and the right attentiveness. In line with care ethics, addressing or even avoiding the rise of dilemmas in midwifery care starts with the relationship between a woman and midwife.

A good approach for decision-making in midwifery care requires a careful process, where the focus is as much on the dialogue as on the decision made (Edwards, 2004). This process builds on a trustful relationship between the woman and her midwife (Nieuwenhuijze et al., 2014). The midwife is attentive: she recognises and responds to the woman's needs, supports her in identifying her values, exploring options and setting goals, advises her with competence and involves the woman's partner or significant others if the woman agrees. There is an interactive exchange of trustworthy information (options, benefits, harms, uncertainties and professional experiences) and personal information (circumstances, values, preferences and matters important to quality of life), building towards the woman making a well-informed decision (Elwyn et al., 2017; Nieuwenhuijze & Kane Low, 2013).

A trustful relationship implicates trustworthiness, being honest and realistic, promising what can be realised and keeping promises (O'Neill, 2013). A woman's autonomy to make choice for herself and her child is respected but not separated from her social context and the relations she has with others, including midwives. Responsibility is linked to 'attentiveness' and 'responsiveness' of the midwife: making sure that the actual caring needs of the woman are met and given as a gift. A caring relationship is characterised by a genuine sensitivity and attentiveness to the woman's needs and desires. Sensitivity to and respect for other cultures' norms and practices should be part of the core commitments in the care of midwives (Malek, 2017). Even though this shared decision-making process might not be possible in all situations during pregnancy or birth, this is the principle starting point of the decision-making process.

Individual midwives cannot solve all of the problems, as some are inherently structural and part of the way health systems are organised. Midwives will offer woman-centred care to the best of their abilities and the possibilities in the given setting, but they are often restricted by institutional requirements and power imbalances in the system. There is a need to strengthen the strategic and political influence of midwifery in every country to create a midwifery practice built on the ethics of care, as suggested in the paper of Newnham and Kirkham (2019), a political call that provokes a radical change in care, focusing on relationships and enabling continuity of midwifery care for women in all settings.

Conclusion

Irrespective of time and place, 'good' midwifery care (including decision-making) is a relational shared process between a woman and her midwife, where the midwife recognises the mother and her child in their unity when seeking best options in care. Decision-making involves trust, autonomy and caring interactions, integrating a care ethics approach based on Tronto's four elements essential for good care: attentiveness, responsibility, competence and responsiveness.

Care ethics offers a framework for individual midwives to offer *good* midwifery care and decision-making as well as a scope for the political agenda of midwifery.

References

Beauchamp, T. L. and Childress, J. F. (2013) *Principles of biomedical ethics* (7th ed.). Oxford: Oxford University Press.

Chervenak, F., McCullough, L. B. and Brent, R. L. (2011) The professional responsibility model of obstetrical ethics: avoiding the perils of clashing rights. *American Journal of Obstetrics and Gynecology*, 205(315), pp. e1–e5.

Declercq, E. R., Sakala, C., Corry, M. P., Applebaum, S. and Hemlich, A. (2013) *Listening to mothers III: pregnancy and birth*. New York: Childbirth Connection.

De Vries, R. G. (2005) *A pleasing birth: midwifery and maternity care in the Netherlands*. Philadelphia, PA: Temple University Press.

Downe, S., Finlayson, K., Oladapo, O., Bonet, M. and Gülmezoglu, A.M. (2018) What matters to women during childbirth: a systematic qualitative review. *PLoS One*, 13(4), p. e0194906.

Downe, S., Finlayson, K., Tunçalp, Ö. and Gülmezoglu, A.M. (2016) What matters to women: a systematic scoping review to identify the processes and outcomes of antenatal care provision that are important to healthy pregnant women. *BJOG: An International Journal of Obstetrics & Gynaecology*, 123(4), pp. 529–539.

Dugas, M., Shorten, A., Dubé, E., Wassef, M., Bujold, E. and Chaillet, N. (2012) Decision aid tools to support women's decision-making in pregnancy and birth: a systematic review and meta-analysis. *Social Science & Medicine*, 74(12), pp. 1968–1978.

Edwards, N. (2004) Why can't women just say no? And does it really matter? In: Kirkham, M. (ed.), *Informed choice in maternity care*. Basingstoke: Palgrave Macmillan.

Elwyn, G., Durand, M.A., Song, J., Aarts, J., Barr, P.J., Berger, Z., Cochran, N., Frosch, D., Galasiński, D., Gulbrandsen, P., Han, P.K.J., Härter, M., Kinnersley, P., Lloyd, A., Mishra, M., Perestelo-Perez, L., Scholl, I., Tomori, K., Trevena, L., Witteman, H.O. and van der Weijden, T. (2017) A three-talk model for shared decision making: multistage consultation process. *British Medical Journal*, 359, p. j4891.

Elwyn, G., Laitner, S., Coulter, A., Walker, E., Watson, P. and Thomson, R. (2010) Implementing shared decision making in the NHS. *British Medical Journal*, 341, pp. 971–973.

Gilligan, C. (1982/2016) *In a different voice: psychological theory and women's development*. Cambridge, MA: Harvard University Press.

Hawley, S.T. and Morris, A.M. (2017) Cultural challenges to engaging patients in shared decision making. *Patient Education and Counseling*, 100, pp. 18–24.

Hendrix, M., Van Horck, M., Moreta, D., Nieman, F., Nieuwenhuijze, M., Severens, J. and Nijhuis, J. (2009) Why women do not accept randomisation for place of birth: feasibility of a RCT in the Netherlands. *BJOG: An International Journal of Obstetrics & Gynaecology*, 116, pp. 537–542.

Hollander, M., van Dillen, J., Lagro-Janssen T, van Leeuwen, E. and Vandenbussche, F. (2016) Women refusing standard obstetric care: maternal fetal conflict or doctor-patient conflict? *Journal of Pregnancy and Child Health*, 3(2), pp. 1–4.

ICM. (2014) *ICM core document philosophy and model of midwifery care*. The Hague. Accessed on 20 January 2019: www.internationalmidwives.org/assets/files/definitions-files/2018/06/eng-philosophy-and-model-of-midwifery-care.pdf.

Koch, E.J. (2014) How does anticipated regret influence health and safety decisions? A literature review. *Basic and Applied Social Psychology*, 36, pp. 397–412.

Légaré, F., Stacey, D., Pouliot, S., Gauvin, F.P., Desroches, S., Kryworuchko, J., Dunn, S., Elwyn, G., Frosch, D., Gagnon, M.P., Harrison, M.B., Pluye, P. and Graham, I.D. (2011) Interprofessionalism and shared decision-making in primary care: a stepwise approach towards a new model. *Journal of Interprofessional Care*, 25(1), pp. 18–25.

MacLellan, J. (2014) Claiming an ethic of care for midwifery. *Nursing Ethics*, 21(7), pp. 803–811.

Malek, J. (2017) Maternal decision-making during pregnancy: parental obligations and cultural differences. *Best Practice & Research Clinical Obstetrics and Gynecology*, 43, pp. 10–20.

Newnham, E. and Kirkham, M. (2019) Beyond autonomy: care ethics for midwifery and the humanization of birth. *Nursing Ethics*, pp. 1–11. https://doi.org/10.1177/0969733018819119.

Nieuwenhuijze, M.J. and Kane Low, L. (2013) Facilitating women's choice in maternity care. *The Journal of Clinical Ethics*, 24, pp. 276–282.

Nieuwenhuijze, M.J., Korstjens, I., de Jonge, A., de Vries, R. and Lagro-Janssen, T. (2014) On speaking terms: a Delphi study on shared decision-making in maternity care. *BMC Pregnancy and Childbirth*, 14, p. 223. https://doi.org/10.1186/1471-2393-14-223.

Noseworthy, D., Phibbs, S. and Benn, C. (2013) Towards a relational model of decision-making in midwifery care. *Midwifery*, 29, pp. e42–e48.

O'Neill, O. (2013) *What we don't understand about trust. TED talk*. Accessed on 20 January 2019: www.youtube.com/watch?v=1PNX6M_dVsk.

Oxford English Dictionary. Accessed on 1 February 2019: www.oed.com/view/Entry/64756?rskey=
1tpDwx&result=2&isAdvanced=true#firstMatch.

Seefat-van Teeffelen, A., Nieuwenhuijze, M. and Korstjens, I. (2011) Women want proactive psychosocial support from midwives during transition to motherhood: a qualitative study. *Midwifery*, 27,
pp. e122–e127.

Tronto, J. (1993/2009) *Moral boundaries: a political argument for an ethic of care*. New York: Routledge.

Verkerk, M. (2007) Care ethics as a feminist perspective on bioethics. In: Gastmans, C., Dierickx, K., Nys,
H. and Schotmans, P. (eds.), *New pathways to European ethics*. Antwerp: Intersentia.

5

RISK WITHIN MATERNITY AND HOW THIS IMPACTS MIDWIVES' DECISION-MAKING

Mandie Scamell

Chapter overview

This chapter provides readers with the opportunity to scrutinise midwifery decision-making from a critical risk analysis perspective. Drawing from the social theory of risk – particularly the seminal cultural theory of risk proposed by risk theorist Mary Douglas – the contestable nature of the meaning of risk in midwifery practice will be introduced. The chapter begins by presenting a case study in the form of a story. The case is taken from an ethnographic investigation into midwifery practice in the UK and has been used previously in a publication in the *British Medical Journal*, where ethical and research design considerations of the study can be found (Scamell, 2014). Using this story, the links between perceptions of risk and safety and midwifery decision-making will be explored.

Introduction

The aim of this book is to critically review a range of decision-making theories and their relevance to midwifery practice. Through this aim, the links between midwifery governance, risk and safety are explored to encourage critical thinking and reflection as an essential element of clinical decision-making. The contribution this chapter will make to this debate is to demonstrate the impact of the socio/policy context of risk on midwifery clinical decision-making. To achieve this, the chapter introduces two propositions. The first is that sensitivity to risk is not only omnipresent in maternity care across the world; its meaning is not self-evident and therefore deserves critical scrutiny. Despite risk management being a central tenet in health policy in both the Southern and Northern Hemispheres of our world (Daemers et al., 2017; Mander and Murphy-Lawless, 2013; McIntyre et al., 2011; Miller and Shriver, 2012; Skinner, 2008), the precise meaning of risk within the contemporary maternity care setting is taken as a given and has rarely been subjected to sustained analysis (MacKenzie Bryers and van Teijlingen, 2010; Scamell and Alaszewski, 2012). Furthermore, as Lee (2017) has demonstrated, understandings of risk tend to be complicated by a false-consensus effect (Ross et al., 1977).

Although maternity care professionals may believe that a common understanding of risk prevails across the multidisciplinary team, the consensus of opinion is in fact overestimated.

The second proposition to be introduced in this chapter is simply that midwifery decision-making does not take place within a cultural vacuum. That is to say, each clinical decision, in every birthing environment – be it in a home, hospital or birth centre – in low-, medium- and high-income countries across the world, can be thought of as being shaped by international, national and local ideas on the nature of childbirth, the meaning of risk and the role and capacity of women's birthing bodies.

By exploring these two propositions, this chapter provides readers with the opportunity to engage with some of the key debates within the risk analysis literature to understand how risk theory can be usefully applied to critically evaluate midwifery decision-making. The complexities of the meaning making of risk, the maternity care professionals' reactive and proactive responses to an imagination where the future is colonised with poor outcomes and how to mediate against such overreactions to risks that are identified in the present will be considered.

BOX 5.1 JOSEPHINE'S STORY

Meet Josephine (pseudonym), a well-educated, healthy first-time mother who, having read a broad selection of both lay and professional literature, decided that having her baby in a low-risk birth centre – staffed exclusively by midwives – was the safest option for her and her baby. Josephine made this decision knowing that the nearest high-risk obstetric unit was in the next town some 20 km away.

Despite being healthy, Josephine (along with approximately 30% of the general population) was colonised for group B streptococcus (GBS). As a result of her positive colonisation, Mandy, her midwife, made the clinical decision to advise Josephine to have her baby in a high-risk obstetric unit where she could access the appropriate antibiotic treatment for her colonisation. The rationale for Mandy's recommendation was her professional understanding that if untreated, GBS could have a negative impact on the wellbeing of Josephine's baby.

Being a resourceful and articulate woman, Josephine took it upon herself to research the risks associated with GBS, for her baby. Having conducted this search, she made the informed decision that the potential risks did not warrant a change in her original plan to have her baby in a low-risk birth centre.

In an effort to dissuade Josephine and convince her of the seriousness of the risks to her baby, Mandy decided to enrol the support of a more senior consultant midwife, Martha.

A joint decision was made to offer Josephine additional antenatal care where Martha could counsel her about her birth plan preferences in relation to place of birth. During this counselling appointment Martha attempted to dissuade Josephine from what she considered to be uninformed choice about her preferred place of birth by warning: 'You know your baby could die'.

Risk – probability calculation

This story describes the practice of two midwives – a community midwife and a consultant midwife – both working for a state-run maternity service in a high-income country where the maternity services are free at the point of access to all documented residents. To interrogate Mandy's and Martha's decisions, the probability calculations and evidence base driving their rationale first needs to be explored. This approach to risk management is described in the risk literature as the rational, technico-scientific approach to risk (Lupton, 2013a), where risk is considered to be an impartially calculated probability of harm that emerges out of reliable statistical evidence.

What are the mathematical probabilities of harm to Josephine's baby that result from her GBS colonisation? GBS infection can be fatal for a new-born baby; this fact is not being challenged in this analysis. Martha's warning that Josephine's baby may die as a direct result of her GBS colonisation was correct. The risk of perinatal fatality, however, is influenced by a range of clinical features including the gestation and size of the baby, prolonged rupture of membranes and any signs or symptoms of disease in the mother, in particular raised maternal temperature or signs of sepsis (Hughes et al., 2017). In Josephine's case, the pregnancy had already reached full term (beyond 37 weeks' gestation) and the baby was considered to be 'a good size' (not presenting with any indicators to suggest intra-uterine growth restriction). Moreover, Josephine was known to be in good health.

In developed countries it is estimated that around 1% of babies born of pregnant women with GBS colonisation develop symptoms of the disease (Le Doare and Heath, 2013). Although the evidence for low-income countries is less reliable, current estimates suggest a global infection rate of 0.53 per 1,000 live births (Edmond et al., 2012). More recent research undertaken in the UK indicates a new-born GBS infection rate of just under 1:1,000 (O'Sullivan et al., 2016). The O'Sullivan study is one of the most recent, large-scale analyses of GBS that has been published and therefore, for the purposes of this chapter, it is their risk ratio that will be used to illustrate the meaning making of risk in Josephine's story. It should be noted that although inferences taken from this research should be made with caution, the authors findings are consistent with previous international research meta-synthesis.

According to the evidence, the highest overall new-born infection risk of GBS is 0.1%. The mortality rate for those babies who contract the disease is around 4.7%, giving an overall risk of mortality of 0.000047% (O'Sullivan et al., 2016). It should be noted that these calculations are per live birth and are not adjusted for maternal GBS burden, the rate of which is widely contested in the literature but estimated in developed countries to be anything between 20% and 30% of the population (Edmond et al., 2012; Hughes et al., 2017; Le Doare and Heath, 2013). If this rate is used to calculate Josephine's baby's risk of disease and dying, the probabilities come out to around 0.36% and 0.00017%, respectively. Granted, the risks are increased for Josephine's baby, but the question is, do these probabilities justify the midwives' decision-making described in the story?

To put Josephine's baby's risks into perspective, the overall global neonatal mortality rate, according to the United Nations Inter-agency Group for Child Mortality Estimation, was 18:1,000 births (Alkema et al., 2014) – just under a 2% mortality risk. This is five times Josephine's baby's GBS infection risk and more than 10,000 times higher than the child's GBS fatality risk. Despite this, however, midwives working across the world routinely provide out-of-hospital intra-partum care on the basis that the neonatal mortality risk is low enough to justify this clinical decision. The question from a critical analysis perspective is, why did the midwives described in this story choose to select the relatively low probabilities associated with GBS as a legitimate rationale for one decision when, at the same time, they actively choose to ignore the higher overall mortality risks when making decisions about other women's place of birth? To try to make sense of the midwifery decision-making in Josephine's story, the remainder of the chapter will draw from the social theory of risk to critically evaluate the meaning making of risk that takes place through midwifery talk and practice and illuminate the nature of the cultural context in which midwifery decision-making is suspended in different geographical settings in high-, middle- and low-income countries.

Social theory of risk

Taken-for-granted understanding of risk in midwifery practice might assume that risk calculations (and consequently decision-making in risk counselling) are made out of impartial probability calculations – a techno-rational approach to risk (Skinner, 2008). The cultural analysis of risk carried out by anthropologist Mary Douglas, however, suggests the way risk operates in society is more complex (Douglas, 1985). This kind of risk analysis emerges from an understanding that all decision-making about risk is best understood as shaped by institutions and culture rather than directed by impartial, scientifically based calculations.

Risks are infinite, as Douglas points out. The precise nature of the risks a particular group chooses to select, amplify as important and manage, by contrast, is limited and socially negotiated. How a social group is organised inevitably influences which risks are selected and which are ignored. This decision-making process is not only linked to material considerations such as resource availability – as is the case in low-income countries – but also to more obtuse cultural drivers inherent in the technologies of risk management, such as clinical protocols, that are often assumed to be benign in their efforts to attain safety. Furthermore, risk selection, amplification, taking and management is far from impartial; instead it is closely linked to emotions, or as Lupton (2013b) puts it: 'both emotion and risk are inevitably and always configured via social and cultural processes and through interaction with others' bodies, material objects, space and place' (p. 624).

In Josephine's story, Martha provides an important clue as to the nature of the institution in which she and Mandy work. Martha explains that Josephine's choice of birthplace could not be tolerated because it did not fit within the organisation's protocol. The expansion of such risk management in the form of technologies such as practice protocols, guidelines and algorithms is, according to risk theorists, a defining feature of our contemporary society. As Power (2004) points out: 'Not only private sector companies, but hospitals, schools, universities and many other public organisations, including the very highest levels of central government, have been invaded to varying degrees by ideas about risk and its management' (p. 8).

Various metaphors have been used in the risk literature to describe this activity. Taylor-Gooby (2002) describes it as a 'mushrooming'; Skolbekken (1995) as a 'risk epidemic'; and Gabe (2005) calls it 'an explosion'. Beck (1992) goes so far as to suggest that our contemporary society is suspended within a historical epoch of risk, and that we live in what he calls a 'risk society'. Regardless of which description is used, the message is clear: risk and its management prevail, and therefore we cannot afford to ignore how these impact upon midwifery decision-making.

By scrutinising the decision-making of these two midwives using this understanding of how risk operates in society, we can begin to make sense of why these midwives were so keen to select one low probability risk while actively ignoring another. Martha's and Mandy's decision-making is closely aligned to their institutional technologies of risk management. In their efforts to comply with the institution's protocol – where the low-probability, high-impact risk of GBS perinatal fatality is picked out as demanding robust management – the actual probability calculation that has informed Josephine's choice becomes irrelevant. As Douglas (1992) points out: 'The reality of dangers is not at issue. The dangers are only too horribly real. . . . This argument is not about the reality of dangers, but about how they are politicised' (p. 29). What matters to these midwives is that their decision-making reflects the standardised clinical protocol regardless of Josephine's preferences.

The story in this chapter describes the collision of two interpretations of risk and the impact these incompatible interpretations have on decision-making. Ironically, both interpretations can be said to arise out of a commitment to a rational technico-scientific understanding of risk. Josephine's decisions about where to give birth were based upon her understanding of the very low, evidence-based statistical risk her GBS colonisation posed to her baby (infection rate below 1%). Mandy and Martha's decisions, by contrast, arose out of their professional commitment to the standardisation of care prescribed in their maternity service clinical protocol. Such protocols form part of the robust and seemingly ever-growing technology of risk management that prevails within maternity services across the world – and, in this story, operates to constitute a midwifery practice that is alienated from women-centred decision-making.

The moral nature of risk

A further observation of note in the story is the emotive nature of Martha's counselling. In an effort to gain Josephine's compliance and align her informed choice with Mandy's clinical decision-making about place of birth, Martha chose language which aimed not only to alienate but also to frighten Josephine. Martha's decision to 'shroud wave' (Dagustun, 2012), amplifying the low probability of a high-impact outcome – namely the death of Josephine's baby – can be explained according to Douglas by risk being understood as a moral discourse of social control (Douglas, 1992). Once a social group or society has chosen to amplify a particular risk and develop rules for managing that risk, individuals who choose to defy these rules will be relegated to being undesirable or even deviant. 'The concept of risk emerges as a key idea', argues Douglas (1992, p. 24), 'because of its uses as a forensic resource'. From Mandy and Martha's point of view, Josephine's choice of place of birth threatens the social fabric of their practice. Josephine's refusal to recognise the GBS risk as relevant to her choice of place of birth defied the clinical protocol that both midwives were both so desperate to preserve. Given such an assault, Martha and Mandie decided to draw from the forensic resource of risk management and used frightening language and an authoritative approach to practice, regaining a social order where compliance to the clinical protocol could be guaranteed.

Conclusion

In this chapter a rather unexceptional clinical scenario, in the form of Josephine's story, was used to explore how midwifery clinical decision-making is shaped by the omnipresence of risk and risk management within contemporary maternity services. Through the application of risk theory, it is possible to unpick how midwives' understanding of risk may not be as self-evident or as politically neutral as they may appear at face value. This critical scrutiny provides insight into how risk operates in clinical decision-making, exposing a disturbing consequence of our risk society which permeates high-, medium- and low-income countries alike.

The exploration of Josephine's story revealed a tension within midwifery clinical decision-making. This tension arises out of the cultural context in which midwifery decision-making is suspended. On the one hand, midwives are committed to women-centred, evidence-based decision-making. On the other, they are professionally responsible for the management of risk within a culture of strict adherence to organisational risk technology. Should midwives choose to prioritise women-centred decision-making over and above the management of risks that are selected and amplified within institutional protocols, they face the forensic nature of risk which can threaten their professional identity. Given this threat, it is not surprising that both the midwives in Josephine's story concentrated their efforts on ensuring that the institutional protocol prevailed over Josephine's birth choices.

References

Alkema, L., Chao, F., You, D., Pedersen, J., & Sawyer, C.C. (2014). National, regional, and global sex ratios of infant, child, and under-5 mortality and identification of countries with outlying ratios: a systematic assessment. *The Lancet Global Health, 2*, e521–e530. https://doi.org/10.1016/S2214-109X(14)70280-3

Beck, U. (1992). *Risk society*. Newbury Park, CA: Sage.

Daemers, D.O.A., van Limbeek, E.B.M., Wijnen, H.A.A., Nieuwenhuijze, M.J., & de Vries, R.G. (2017). Factors influencing the clinical decision-making of midwives: a qualitative study. *BMC Pregnancy Childbirth, 17*, 345. https://doi.org/10.1186/s12884-017-1511-5

Dagustun, J. (2012). *Beware the dead baby card . . . . AIMS Journal, 24*(3).

Douglas, M. (1985). *Risk acceptability according to the social sciences*. New York: Russell Sage Foundation.

Douglas, M. (Ed.). (1992). *Risk and blame: Essays in cultural theory*. London: Routledge.

Edmond, K., Kortsalloudaki, C., Scotte, S., Schrag, S., Zaidi, A., & Heath, P. (2012). Group B Strepococcal disease in infants aged younger than 3 months: systematic review and meta-analysis. *The Lancet, 379*, 548–556.

Hughes, R.G., Brocklehurst, P., Steer, P.J., Heath, P., & Stenson, B.M. (2017). Prevention of early-onset neonatal group B Streptococcal disease. *BJOG: An International Journal of Obstetrics and Gynaecology, 124*, e280–e305. https://doi.org/10.1111/1471-0528.14821

Le Doare, K. & Heath, P.T. (2013). An overview of global GBS epidemiology. *Vaccine, 31*, D7–D12. https://doi.org/10.1016/J.VACCINE.2013.01.009

Lee, S., Penny, J., & Holden, D. (2017). *Pregnancy related risk perception in pregnant women, midwives & obstetricians*. Society for Reproductive and Infant Psychology (SRIP) 37th Annual Conference.

Lupton, D. (2013a). *Risk*. Oxon: Routledge.

Lupton, D. (2013b). Risk and emotion: Towards an alternative theoretical perspective. *Health, Risk and Society, 15*(8), 634–647. https://doi.org/10.1080/13698575.2013.848847

MacKenzie Bryers, H. & van Teijlingen, E. (2010). Risk, theory, social and medical models: A critical analysis of the concept of risk in maternity care. *Midwifery, 26*, 488–496. https://doi.org/10.1016/J.MIDW.2010.07.003

Mander, R. & Murphy-Lawless, J. (2013). *The politics of maternity*. London: Routledge.

McIntyre, M.J., Chapman, Y., & Francis, K. (2011). Hidden costs associated with the universal application of risk management in maternity care. *Australian Health Review, 35*, 211. https://doi.org/10.1071/AH10919

Miller, A.C. & Shriver, T.E., 2012. Women's childbirth preferences and practices in the United States. *Social Science and Medicine*, 75, 709–716. https://doi.org/10.1016/J.SOCSCIMED.2012.03.051

O'Sullivan, C., Lamagni, T., Efstratiou, A., Patel, D., Cunney, R., Meehan, M., . . ., Heath, P., 2016. P3 group B Streptococcal (GBS) disease in UK and Irish infants younger than 90 days, 2014–2015. *Archives of Disease in Childhood*, 101, A2.1–A2. https://doi.org/10.1136/archdischild-2016-310863.3

Power, M. (2004). The risk management of everything: Rethinking the politics of uncertainty. London: Demos.

Ross, L., Greene, D., & House, P. (1977). The "false consensus effect": An egocentric bias in social perception and attribution processes. *Journal of Experimental Social Psychology*, 13(3), pp. 279–301.

Scamell, M. (2014). "She can't come here!" Ethics and the case of birth centre admission policy in the UK. *Journal of Medical Ethics*, 40. https://doi.org/10.1136/medethics-2013-101847

Scamell, M. & Alaszewski, A. (2012). Fateful moments and the categorisation of risk: Midwifery practice and the ever-narrowing window of normality during childbirth. *Health, Risk and Society*, 14. https://doi.org/10.1080/13698575.2012.661041

Skinner, J. (2008). Risk: Let's look at the bigger picture. *Women and Birth*, 21, 53–54. https://doi.org/10.1016/j.wombi.2008.03.007

Skolbekken, J.-A. (1995). The risk epidemic in medical journals. *Social Science and Medicine*, 40, 291–305.

Taylor-Gooby, P. (2002). Varieties of risk. *Health, Risk and Society*, 4, 109–111.

6

MIDWIFERY ABDICATION

Elaine Jefford and Julie Jomeen

Chapter overview

The concept of 'midwifery abdication' is provocative and may be regarded as somewhat unpalatable. The term is not intended to criticise or attack midwives, rather to foster explicit recognition so that the construct can facilitate authentic challenge to the complex context within which midwives work. The first part of this chapter presents the theoretical constructs and influencing variables identified within midwifery abdication. Using a clinical narrative from a practising midwife, the second part provides evidence of how midwifery abdication was enacted when a practising midwife was caring for a woman.

Midwifery abdication

Internationally, midwives are governed by profession-specific regulatory and legal obligations, as discussed in Chapters 2 and 3. The regulatory framework for midwifery ensures midwives are educated and trained to clearly defined standards of practice in which they are expected to demonstrate competence. Midwives ensure public safety by conducting themselves in a professional manner and practice ethically within a defined scope of practice. In other words, the midwife must provide safe, effective, high-quality care whilst honouring the woman's right to make decisions about her care (International Confederation of Midwives, 2008a, 2017; Nursing and Midwifery Board of Australia, 2008, 2011, 2018; Nursing and Midwifery Council, 2012).

The midwife becomes accountable to legal, professional and regulatory frameworks but also to a woman from the point at which a midwife undertakes the care of a woman in childbirth. Being accountable to both the woman and the legal, professional and regulatory frameworks is complex yet must be navigated. Such a situation may position the midwife in a contested space. Attempts to successfully navigate this contested space may inadvertently result in a midwife abdicating her professional responsibilities (Jefford and Jomeen, 2015). This situation was first described and defined by Jefford (2012) applying the term 'midwifery abdication', which is where:

a midwife surrenders one's voice and/or forsakes one's midwifery skills and/or knowledge, consciously or unconsciously, failing to fulfil and be accountable for one's own professional behaviour in accordance with professional frameworks as (primary) maternity care provider for the woman.

(Jefford, 2012, p. 14)

Initial exploration of midwifery abdication identified three influencing interrelated variables: (1) 'internalized perceptions of midwifery practice'; (2) 'knowing but failing to act'; and (3) 'prioritization of the woman's needs' (Jefford and Jomeen, 2015).

- **'Internalized perceptions of midwifery practice'** relates to a midwife's personal philosophy and the unquestionable need to give a woman an optimum birth. Interlinked with this is the necessity for the midwife to be perceived as a 'good' midwife, by those within and external to the childbearing environment.
- **'Knowing but failing to act'** is when a midwife feels disempowered through experiencing a fear of conflict with either the woman, her family, peers, and colleagues and/or the environment (organisation) within which she practices. This disempowerment results in the midwife remaining silent despite having the knowledge and skills to effectively communicate opinions and options or to act as the woman's advocate.
- **'Prioritization of the woman's needs'** is when the midwife honours the woman as the final decision-maker within her own care. This can be honouring needs, wishes and decisions made in the antenatal period. While honourable, it becomes problematic when a midwife gate-keeps information irrespective of a changing clinical picture, thus failing to give the woman the option to re-evaluate her original needs, wishes or decisions.

Further work sought to determine the international validity of the term midwifery abdication. This work has served to confirm two of the existing variables ('knowing but failing to act', and 'prioritization of the woman's needs') and developed the construct further by identifying an extension of the 'internalized perceptions of midwifery practice' variable to include 'external perceptions of midwifery practice' (Jefford, Jomeen and Wallin, 2018).

Knowing but failing to act

The international validation of this influencing variable identified midwives feeling 'powerless' and 'intimidated' as a result of the medicalisation of childbirth, often characterised by frequent interventions. Internally, midwives disagree with the technocratic (medicalised) model of intervention. Externally most midwives stay silent, witnessing or reluctantly becoming a part of the technocratic model. Hierarchical and imbalanced power are reasons for inaction, loss of professional voice and cultural acceptance of the woman 'belonging' to a medical professional.

The acceptance of the medical presumption that a woman's body will fail so intervention is necessary juxtaposes the midwifery philosophy of trusting the woman's body to birth. Midwives are therefore forced into a vulnerable position as they try to navigate the contested space between midwifery and medical philosophy. Internationally, within the variable, midwives feel challenged and at times fearful to voice their own professional perspective. Examples of this in the literature include a midwife who was 'dragged' by a fellow midwife from the birthing room, to re-enforce acceptance of the norm of the birth suite stating 'this is what happens . . . we all know what he does . . . they're his clients and there is nothing you can do about it' (Rice and Warland, 2013, p. 1059).

We acknowledge in such an environment that a midwife might consciously or unconsciously feel her ability to have a voice or to advocate for woman-centred care is overridden by hierarchical and imbalanced cultural power. The need to belong, to fit in and to be connected and accepted is natural (Baumeister, 2011). Yet to belong, some midwives choose to conform, failing to apply professional knowledge, skills and expertise to question unnecessary interventions and in doing so abdicate their professional accountability and responsibility. There may be a numbers of reasons for this. It has been documented by other authors that (senior) midwives endeavour to influence a subservient reaction of obedience to a decision or behaviour (Hollins Martin and Bull, 2005). This particularly applies to junior midwives, who find it difficult to step outside the imposed hierarchy and hence are obedient even if they are not in agreement with what they are observing or being asked to participate in (Hollins Martin and Bull, 2006), thus placing the midwife in the tenuous position of powerlessness.

Prioritisation of the women's needs

This variable, as described earlier, manifests itself differently when explored through the international literature. Rather than referring to how a midwife sets out to achieve a woman's wishes for her ideal birth, ignoring anything or anyone internal or external to the environment that might derail it (Jefford and Jomeen, 2015); the international context highlights how midwives often do not feel able to facilitate prioritisation of the women's needs. Instead midwives were placed in a vulnerable position trying to balance the women's wishes with those situational factors such as technocratic environment, risk philosophy and a need to conform. The findings do not appear to be dependent on traditional maternity settings as the literature drawn upon highlights this occurring in midwives from diverse practice settings such as the community, midwifery group practice, birth centres and hospitals (Rice and Warland, 2013).

External perceptions of midwifery practice

This new extended construct links with the initial variable of 'internalized perceptions of midwifery practice' of midwifery abdication. Externalised perceptions contribute to or influence internalised perceptions. In other words, a midwife may well internalise what she perceives to be 'good' midwifery and adapt her own social identity within midwifery to align with the external perceptions of 'good' midwifery. A reason for this is to facilitate her place within such a midwifery environment.

One antecedent of externalised perceptions may be the environment within which a midwife undertook her midwifery education. In many midwifery educational programmes the ethos is one of being woman-centred and the belief that childbirth is a natural healthy phenomena which women intrinsically know how to perform (Australian College of Midwives, 2017; International Confederation of Midwives, 2008b). Such educational programs seek to develop midwives who can work autonomously and to their full scope of practice (International Confederation of Midwives, 2005 (revised 2011 and 2017)). When internationally validating the concept of midwifery abdication, it was evident that some midwifery education programmes remain grounded in a technocratic (medical) philosophy (Davis-Floyd, 2004). This model of education focuses on the perception that risk is inherent in childbirth and medical interventions are needed to limit or manage this risk (Davis-Floyd, 2004). Mitigating potential risk is symbiotic with control and belongs within the medical hierarchy and not midwifery. Educational programmes based within the midwifery philosophy teach midwives the knowledge and skills to assess risk whilst remaining focused on 'normal', as Fahy and Hastie (2008) term it, midwives are the guardians of normal. This type of midwifery education embraces a midwife-woman reciprocal partnership relationship. Within this relationship, the midwife acknowledges and respects the woman as the final decision-maker irrespective of the perception of risk (Leap and Pairman, 2006; Pairman, 2010; Miller and Wilkes, 2014; Pairman and McAra-Couper, 2014). Ultimately such educational programmes aim to develop midwives who are accountable practitioners which is incumbent with being an autonomous practitioner. This is discussed in the last chapter of this book.

The technocratic (medical) educational programmes are the opposite. Students are taught to be subservient, thus when entering the workforce as midwives they have often not learnt how to be autonomous practitioners. Rather, what they have learnt in the classroom is reinforced within the clinical working environment, leaving them disempowered within a midwifery role. In other words the insidious risk philosophy of the technocratic (medicalised) model of education pervades the clinical environment promoting obedience and fostering a continued censorship of midwives and midwifery knowledge (Hollins Martin and Bull, 2006) irrespective of setting or geographical location around the world. If the external environment has a risk philosophy and therefore does not support or erodes normality, a midwife may or may not adapt to 'fit' in. This may interrelate with the social hierarchy and/or seniority that can result in a culture of obedience.

It could be postulated that a lack of professional recognition, within some contexts, by fellow health practitioners and ultimately the woman, is inevitable when midwives have been educated within a technocratic discourse of childbirth. The impact of this contested space between two philosophies, technocratic and midwifery, is unbalanced power. This can restrict one's ability to maintain a midwife's full scope of practice within a woman-centred philosophy. As a result, this can influence a midwife's identity and where this positions her within the midwifery profession.

How can reflection facilitate change?

This variable is a consequence of midwifery abdication rather than a contributing variable.

Within oneself is the need to ensure our actions or inaction align with ethical principles of non-maleficence and beneficence (Beauchamp and Childress, 1994). To act in such a way, one must have a moral compass of right and wrong. Intrinsically interwoven in this are feelings of 'regret', 'guilt', a 'sense of failure' and a 'sense of responsibility' that can arise if we believe harm has been caused to someone through our actions or failure to act. Further, international validation found, some midwives feel traumatised on behalf of the woman when forced to stay silent, to be a witness or a participant in the technocratic model of care. In such situations, the midwife does not feel able to prioritise the women's needs, which further fuels their feelings of guilt.

Reflection is useful tool for professional development and can be transformative. It can provide a framework to explore clinical situations and why one feels certain emotions or reacts in a specific way (for reflective tools, see Chapter 8). A key element of being a reflective practitioner is critical thinking. Critical thinking, as described in Chapter 7, can facilitate knowledge development and assist in becoming an accountable and autonomous practitioner as well as refine a midwife's decision-making. Within midwifery abdication, reflection is therefore useful.

Enactment of midwifery abdication

The Enhancing Decision-making and Assessment in Midwifery (EDAM) tool, as discussed in Chapter 1, has been applied to the following clinical narrative, where EDAM's two domains (clinical reasoning and midwifery practice) and the two distinct subscales under each respectively (clinical reasoning process and integration and intervention; women's relationship with the midwife and general midwifery practice) are noted. The variables under each sub-scales are denoted in parentheses, bold and italicised ((*MP – WRM – stays in room & – CR – CRP – Cue)*). Pseudonyms have been used to provide anonymity for the midwife and the woman.

BOX 6.1   HELEN'S STORY

Background to Helen's story

Helen has been a midwife for 24 years. She is currently practising midwifery in a consultant-led public hospital in a regional city. Helen highlighted there is not always respectful collaboration between medicine and midwifery within her working environment. Helen's story starts when she arrived on a morning shift to care for Jacqui whose first birth was by emergency caesarean section during the second stage of labour. Jacqui had been labouring for the majority of the night and was draining meconium-stained liquor. Jacqui's birth plan was to have no intervention apart from intermittent auscultation of the fetal heart rate (FHR) and a vaginal birth. The night staff had minimal contact with Jacqui, only entering the birthing room to intermittently listen to the FHR, due to the busy state of the birth suite.

Helen's story and analysis

I introduced myself to Jacqui and she made it clear that she was annoyed she had been left alone most of the night and now there was another new person involved in her care *(MP – WRM – Stays in room)*. I felt there was animosity towards me *(CR – I & I – Intuition)*. I certainly didn't want to do anything that was in contravention to her birth plan *(MP – WRM – common goal:)*, so I retreated into my little cupboard *(MP – GMP – Accountability & Negotiation)* where I made sure I had everything ready in case something didn't go quite right *(CR – I & I – Treatment options)*.

    While I was hiding in the cupboard trying to work out how I was going to find some common ground with this girl *(MP – GMP – Reflexive)*, Jacqui went and sat in the dark on the toilet so I stood in the dark. I asked Jacqui if I could assess her progress by performing a vaginal examination and listen to the fetal heart rate as I was new on the scene and really needed to know what was happening *(CR – CRP – Cue – Hypothesis and CRP – I & I – Treatment options & MP – WRM – Trust)*.

Jacqui returned to the bed. The fetal heart rate was normal *(CR – CRP – Cue)*, but I had concerns as I could not determine on VE whether she was fully dilated or not *(CR – CRP – Cue Interpretation)*, so I left the [birthing room] to report my findings to my colleagues and the registrar *(MP – GMP – Consultation)*. As I walked out the birthing room I noticed that the bath was full *(CR – CRP – Cue)*. At our hospital, the policy states if you are a 'VBAC' [vaginal birth after caesarean section], you are not allowed to have a water birth.

I came back into the room, a few minutes later, and Jacqui was in the bath with the lights turned off. Jacqui had a contraction *(CR – CRP – Cue)*, she wasn't expulsive *(CR – CRP – Cue)*, but her breathing had changed *(Cue)* and I thought we're going to have a baby *(CR – CRP – Focused Cue, Ruling in hypothesis)*. She had another [contraction] *(CR – CRP – Cue)*; it was a little bit more expulsive *(CR – CRP – Cue)*. When the contraction was over, I put my hand on her shoulder and asked, 'Would you like to get out the bath?' Jacqui answered, 'No, I'm quite comfortable here thank-you'.

There was nothing else I could say *(CR – CRP – Reaches decision & MP – WRM – Trust – GMP – Honest information)* but I was squirming inside as I am not water-birth accredited *(MP – GMP – Accountability – Responsibility)*.

I knew I had a mother who had a previous caesarean section *(CR – CRP – Cue)*, there was meconium-stained liquor *(CR – CRP – Cue)*, which requires continuous fetal monitoring as per policy *(CR – CRP – Cue)*, and she was in the bath *(CR – CRP – (Cue)*. I was thinking there had been no deviations in the FHRs; Jacqui had no analgesic on board *(CR – CRP – Cue)*. I decided I was just going to go with it [Jacqui having a water birth] *(CR – CRP – focused cue, ruling in, making a decision & MP – GMP – Accountability & Responsibility)*. I just thought [if] it [the birth] goes well all well and good, if it [the birth] goes pear-shaped I have to wear it, I could even lose my registration over this, I honestly thought about it in those seconds I had to make a decision *(MP – GMP – Reflexive & CR – I & I Evaluation of treatment options and outcomes)*.

Outcome

Jacqui gave birth in the water.

Helen's reflection

My decision was made in that I was doing something that was against hospital policy. I know I did the wrong thing *(MP – GMP – Accountability & Responsibility)*, but I very much did the right thing as I wanted the best thing for Jacqui *(MP – GMP – Accountability & Responsibility)*.

Discussion on this narrative

Globally, many midwives and the women they work with experience a fragmented model of care, sometimes meeting each other for the first time during the birth. At this crucial time, the midwife has to establish some form of midwife-woman reciprocal partnership relationship. Despite such an environment, many midwives do this well, whilst others, as demonstrated in Helen's (midwife) narrative, find this more challenging. Being unknown to each other, whilst trying to create an environment whereby a meaningful and respectful relationship can develop, in Helen's narrative, was further hindered as tension already existed in the birthing environment when she entered. Feeling disempowered, Helen chooses to do nothing that might upset Jacqui further, such as discussing openly and honestly with Jacqui about her goals, rather she finds sanctuary in the 'little cupboard'. As a result, Helen consciously relinquishes her professional accountability which is embedded in regulatory, professional and legal documents of the country within which she practices. Further, she relinquishes her professional responsibility and accountability as defined by the International Confederation of Midwives (International Confederation of Midwives, 2014a, 2014b, 2017, 2018). In other words, within moments of entering the birthing environment, Helen is enacting 'midwifery abdication', specifically the construct of 'knowing but failing to act'.

Helen has her own 'internalised perceptions of midwifery practice' and what constitutes a 'good' midwife. In the clinical narrative this is evidenced when Helen requests to perform an invasive vaginal examination to gain empirical data rather than reading non-invasive signs of labour progression. She fails to see childbirth as a natural healthy phenomena, intrinsically trusting Jacqui and her body's ability to birth. Further, Helen feels the need to inform a senior midwife and medical colleagues. In other words, Helen's social identity as a 'good' midwife is to conform to the technocratic 'surveillance' model of care within the hospital environment she is working in.

When Helen re-enters the birthing room, she find Jacqui in the bath. Helen knows the potential implications of both meconium-stained liquor and a trial of vaginal birth following a previous caesarean section. She is also aware of the hospital policies around these two aspects and the water birth criteria. Further, Helen knows her professional responsibilities and accountability around the need to be accredited to conduct a water-birth, which she was not. Yet Helen fails to communicate any of this to Jacqui, thus enacting the 'knowing and failing to act' sub-scale of midwifery abdication. Helen's silence renders Jacqui powerless to make an informed decision and places her and her baby into a vulnerable and potentially unsafe situation. Nevertheless, Helen believes prioritising Jacqui's need to have a water birth is more important than protecting Jacqui or her baby, thus enacting another sub-scale of midwifery abdication.

When Helen reflected upon this clinical narrative, she is aware her decision-making and subsequent care provision are based upon her internalised perceptions of a what a 'good' midwife does, which is to provide an optimal birth experience for Jacqui. Further, she prioritises Jacqui's needs, wishes and decisions even though she is working outside her professional scope of practice. In doing so Helen consciously surrenders her midwifery voice, and her professional midwifery skills and knowledge. Yet interestingly Helen feels no feelings of regret or guilt or sense of responsibility normally interwoven with the ethical principles of non-maleficence, thus her reflection will not become transformative or facilitate a change in behaviour. In other words, Helen fails to fulfil and be accountable for her professional behaviour in accordance with regulatory, professional and legal documents, and therefore midwifery abdication occurs.

BOX 6.2 HELEN'S STORY – LINKED ACTIVITY 1

Activity

Using another clinical narrative from a practising midwife, apply to the following clinical narrative EDAM's two domains (clinical reasoning and midwifery practice) and the two distinct subscales under each respectively (clinical reasoning process and integration and intervention; women's relationship with the midwife and general midwifery practice), as discussed in Chapter 1.

Background to Henri's Story

Henri has been a midwife for 16 years but works primarily in administration. Henri was primary carer for Lyn, a primigravida, but a colleague [Lillian] had cared for Lyn for approximately 12 hours. During this time Lyn had been transferred to the local consultant-led delivery suite because she was draining meconium-stained liquor. A vaginal examination (done by medical staff) had determined Lyn's cervix was fully dilated. When Henri and Amy entered the birthing room, Lyn had continuous fetal monitoring (CTG) in situ and was being actively coached to push on the bed by Lillian. Amy was a new doula and a personal friend of Henri's.

Henri's story and analysis

We re-introduced ourselves to Lyn and Tom (her partner) and Lillian left. The atmosphere in the birthing room was like a train wreck because labour hadn't been going as Lyn wanted. Lyn and Tom were obviously fed up and it was almost like (*hesitation*) they had given up fighting for what they wanted. Approximately an hour after we arrived Lyn felt the natural urge to push and was pushing really well. There's a hospital policy which states that following an hour of active pushing, if there is no progress, medical assessment and possible intervention is required.

I saw Lyn's labia and vagina were becoming more oedematous as time as passing and she had been fully dilated and pushing for well over an hour and half and there seemed to be little visible evidence of fetal descent. Lyn was really tired and had really low energy reserves. But she was having [intravenous] fluids and was moving around and changing positions. Meconium-stained liquor was still draining but the CTG was good. Despite these things, I knew from when I saw her antenatally that first and foremost Lyn didn't want any intervention or any drugs. I thought, we can really push the hospital policy time limits further to achieve this for Lyn. I was being sensitive around what Lyn wanted. I also knew there is some research around the benefits for both mother and baby in a birth that had no intervention and is drug-free. These benefits include both short and long term and avoidance of postnatal depression.

I decided to try and collaborate with the doctor and get them to agree to do what Lyn wanted: wait longer. My communication style with the doctor and midwifery staff was pushy. I was telling them what I wanted: for Lyn to birth without any help or intervention. The [midwife/doctor] collaboration went downhill from that. The doctor said he wanted to come in to the birthing room to assess Lyn's situation. I refused, verbally preventing him from entering the room. I also made the decision to ignore the policy, the time limits, the doctor and the midwives and get Lyn to push the baby out in her own time The doctor and the labour midwifery staff were unhappy with my decision and I was [verbally] fighting everyone not to intervene because I knew Lyn wanted a drug and intervention-free birth (*silence*). I was also conscious that I felt pressure to make that decision because I had Amy with me. She was a new doula and very excited as it was our first birth together and it was all going to crap (*laughs*). I was thinking how come I'm not showing myself as a good midwife here at all? (*laughs*)

As I had stopped the doctor and midwifery staff coming in the birthing room by my [verbal] interaction, I went back into the birthing room. By the time three hours had passed, post the diagnosis of full dilation, Lyn's labia and vagina became more oedematous than I've ever seen before or since. It was like all the intravenous fluid had just gone straight to her perineum. It was horrible. By this time Lyn had become bothered and very distressed, although the fetal heart rate remained normal.

Outcome

I talked with Lyn and we agreed that we needed medical help now as the baby was not birthing. I then had had to ask the same doctors who I had been fighting with for over three hours for help. Lyn had a drug-free ventouse delivery.

Henri's reflection

It was just a really awful situation that I couldn't rescue and Lyn was really traumatised by her birth.

What did you find? Does Henri make good clinical decisions? Is this another case of midwifery abdication?

Conclusion

There do seem to be clear circumstances where midwives consciously abdicate their professional role. This does not and cannot support informed decision-making if, for example, a midwife's assessment of a changing clinical situation is unshared. Often in these circumstances midwives will experience feelings of regret and guilt. The explicit naming of the construct 'midwifery abdication' seems to be a first step in raising a challenge to midwifery at a professional and systemic level. Reflection appears to be a key element. When reflection becomes reflexive, it can have transformative personal and professional consequences and facilitate change for both midwives and women. There are legitimate reasons why some midwives do not engage in reflection and reflexivity in that it becomes too challenging and even potentially traumatic, something of which we must remain mindful. As a result, however, this can impact further upon current and future interactions and a negative cycle emerges. Education can play a key role in supporting student midwives to become empowered practitioners. Midwives, in addition, need to be given the support and time to reflect safely and meaningfully and to develop skills which allow them to feel empowered to challenge appropriately and lead practice and culture changes. In addition, the continued generation of evidence related to the benefits of an effective midwife-woman relationship on women's satisfaction and psychological health outcomes is critical as a counterbalance to the risk-focused evidence base.

References

Australian College of Midwives. 2017. *Australian College of Midwives: Philosophy Statement for Midwifery* [Online]. Canberra: Australian College of Midwives. Available: www.midwives.org.au [Accessed 27 November 2017].

Baumeister, R. 2011. Need-to-Belong Theory. *In:* van Lange, P., Kruglanski, A. & Higgins, T. (eds.) *Handbook of Theories of Social Psychology: Volume 2.* Sage.

Beauchamp, T. & Childress, J. 1994. *Principles of Biomedical Ethics.* Oxford: Oxford University Press.

Davis-Floyd, R. 2004. The Technocratic Model. *In:* Davis-Floyd, R. (ed.) *Birth as an American Rite of Passage.* London: University of California Press.

Fahy, K. & Hastie, C. 2008. Midwifery Guardianship: Reclaiming the Sacred in Birth. *In:* Fahy, K., Foureur, M. & Hastie, C. (eds.) *Birth Territory and Midwifery Guardianship.* Glasgow: Elsevier Science.

Hollins Martin, C. & Bull, P. 2005. Measuring Social Influence of a Senior Midwife on Decision-Making in Maternity Care: An Experimental Study. *Community Applied Social Psychology*, 15, 120–126.

Hollins Martin, C. & Bull, P. 2006. What Features of the Maternity Unit Promote Obedient Behaviour from Midwives. *Clinical Effectiveness in Nursing*, 9, e221–e231.

International Confederation of Midwives. 2005 (revised 2011 and 2017). *Definition of the Midwife.* The Hague: International Confederation of Midwives. Available: www.medicalknowledgeinstitute.com/files/ICM%20Definition%20of%20the%20Midwife%202005.pdf [Accessed 27 November 2017].

International Confederation of Midwives. 2008a. *ICM International Code of Ethics for Midwives* [Online]. The Hague: International Confederation of Midwives. Available: www.internationalmidwives.org [Accessed 10 February 2010].

International Confederation of Midwives. 2008b. *Keeping Birth Normal* [Online]. The Netherlands: International Confederation of Midwives. Available: www.internationalmidwives.org [Accessed 9 February 2010].

International Confederation of Midwives. 2014a. *Philosophy and Model of Midwifery Care.* International Confederation of Midwives.

International Confederation of Midwives. 2014b. *Professional Accountability of the Midwife.* Geneva: International Confederation of Midwives.

International Confederation of Midwives. 2017. *Definition of the Midwife* [Online]. Brisbane: International Confederation of Midwives. Available: www.internationalmidwives.org [Accessed 4 September 2015].

International Confederation of Midwives. 2018. *Essential Competencies for Basic Midwifery Practice* [Online]. International Confederation of Midwives. Available: www.internationalmidwives.org [Accessed 17 December 2018].

Jefford, E. 2012. *Optimal Midwifery Decision-Making During 2nd Stage Labour: The Integration of Clinical Reasoning into Practice.* PhD Research. NSW: Southern Cross University.

Jefford, E. & Jomeen, J. 2015. 'Midwifery Abdication': A Finding From an Interpretive Study. *International Journal of Childbirth*, 5, 116–125.

Leap, N. & Pairman, S. 2006. Working in Partnership. *In:* Pairman, S., Pincombe, J., Thorogood, C. & Tracy, S. (eds.) *Midwifery: Preparation for Practice.* NSW: Elsevier.

Miller, S. & Wilkes, L. 2014. Working in Partnership. *In:* Pairman, S., Pincombe, J., Thorogood, C. & Tracy, S. (eds.) *Midwifery: Preparation for Practice.* 3rd ed. Sydney: Churchill Livingstone -Elsevier.

Nursing and Midwifery Board of Australia. 2008. *Code of Ethics for Midwives in Australia.* Canberra: Nursing and Midwifery Board of Australia.

Nursing and Midwifery Board of Australia. 2011. Safety and Quality Framework for Privately Practicing Midwives Attending Homebirths. *In: The Framework*. Canberra: Nursing and Midwifery Board of Australia.

Nursing and Midwifery Board of Australia. 2018. *Code of Conduct for Midwives*. Canberra: Nursing and Midwifery Board of Australia.

Nursing and Midwifery Council 2012. *Midwives Rules and Standards*. London: Nursing and Midwifery Council.

Pairman, S. 2010. Midwifery Partnership: A Professionalizing Strategy for Midwives. *In:* Kirkham, M. (ed.) *The Midwife-Mother Relationship*. New York: Palgrave Macmillan.

Pairman, S. & Mcara-Couper, J. 2014. Theoretical Frameworks for Midwifery Practice. *In:* Pairman, S., Pincombe, J., Thorogood, C. & Tracy, M. (eds.) *Midwifery: Preparation for Practice*. NSW: Churchill Livingstone Elsevier.

Rice, H. & Warland, J. 2013. Bearing Witness: Midwives Experiences of Witnessing Traumatic Birth. *Midwifery*, 29, 1056–1063.

7

CRITICAL THINKING

Amanda Carter

Chapter overview

This chapter will provide an in-depth discussion and analysis of critical thinking in midwifery practice. Initially the concept of critical thinking will be defined. The distinction between decision-making and critical thinking will then be explored, outlining how critical thinking underpins decision-making. The application of critical thinking and how it aligns with the provision of safe autonomous midwifery practice will be explored, justifying the importance of midwives developing this vital cognitive skill. A conceptual model for critical thinking in midwifery will then be presented utilising a case study approach. Finally, a multi-method approach to the measurement of critical thinking will be discussed.

What is critical thinking?

The importance of developing critical thinking skills has been a well-established priority in tertiary education for many decades. This type of cognitive thinking facilitates deep learning through critical analysis of new ideas, facts and information. Learning is greatly improved when critical thinking is applied, as new knowledge is interpreted, analysed and applied to complex situations (Facione, 2013).

However, the need for well-developed critical thinking skills is not confined to academic study. Critical thinking skills are essential to guide and assist in decision-making in everyday life. Consider the choice of which telephone company you would like to use for your mobile phone. To make this decision you will evaluate the different plans that are on offer, perhaps talk to a few other people to obtain their experience, compare prices and inclusions and then make a judgement on which company to choose, all of which engage critical thinking skills. In an academic context, critical thinking moves beyond merely retrieving information; critical thinking involves the ability to reason, process and evaluate information, using it to problem-solve, reach accurate conclusions and inform action.

A pioneering Delphi study by the American Philosophical Association (APA) produced an international expert consensus definition of critical thinking. This consensus definition describes critical thinking as a process of purposeful, self-regulatory thinking using the cognitive skills of interpretation, analysis, evaluation and inference (Facione, 1990). When critical thinking is applied to events or problems, they are considered and deliberated using a controlled, purposeful, focused and conscious approach (Mong-Chue, 2000). Paul (1993) suggests that critical thinking is the art of thinking about your thinking while you are thinking, in order to make your thinking better. This type of meta-cognition enhances decision-making and judgement. The word 'critical' is a Greek derivative and signifies the ability to discern, to choose, evaluate and make a judgement (Mong-Chue, 2000). In summary, critical thinking is essentially a tool of inquiry that informs professional judgement and decision-making.

What is the relationship between critical thinking and decision-making?

Critical thinking underpins independent and interdependent decision-making. It is considered the 'cognitive engine' informing professional judgement and skilled decision-making (Facione & Facione, 1996). Effective decision-making is not possible without the application of critical thinking to the nature of a problem and potential solutions (Paul et al., 1995). The higher-order thinking used in critical thinking facilitates knowledge development informing contextualised decision-making and problem-solving, analysing the situation from different perspectives (Facione & Facione, 1996).

Within the context of healthcare, irrespective of where in the world it is located, the use of critical thinking is particularly important where regular clinical decision-making occurs and sound judgement is crucial for the provision of safe and effective care. Critical thinking facilitates the careful definition and analysis of problems, promoting inquisitiveness and questioning of information and decisions (Castledine, 2010). This in-depth type of cognitive thinking allows for deep exploration of the situation and possible solutions, which informs decision-making. This is in direct contrast to the rote learning of facts, rules or ritualistic behaviour and routines where tasks are performed with minimal understanding and evaluation.

To ensure care is safe, clinical decisions need to be based on the best available evidence. Rather than simply retrieving information, critical thinking is required to reason, process, analyse, critique and evaluate the evidence for the current context and the needs of those in your care. The application of critical thinking ensures evidence is not blindly applied to practice but that a process of critical analysis is utilised to reach conclusions about the quality of evidence and applicability in each clinical situation.

In 2000 Scheffer and Rubenfeld undertook an international Delphi study with recognised nursing experts in research, education and practice from diverse cultures and geography. The group developed a discipline specific consensus definition of critical thinking for nursing. The study also identified and defined ten habits of mind (affective elements) and seven skills (cognitive elements) for critical thinking in nursing, which are outlined in Table 7.1 (Scheffer & Rubenfeld, 2000).

To assist readers in understanding the habits of mind and skills in critical thinking in nursing (as noted in Table 7.1) and how these may apply to midwifery practice in any midwifery setting around the globe, please undertake the following activity.

TABLE 7.1 Habits of mind and skills in critical thinking in nursing

	Definition
Habit	
Confidence	Self-assurance of reasoning capabilities
Contextual perspective	Considers the whole situation, including relationships, background and environment, pertinent to a set of circumstances
Creativity	Uses intellectual ingenuity to generate, discover or restructure ideas, devising alternatives
Flexibility	Able to adapt, accommodate, modify or change thoughts, ideas and behaviours
Inquisitiveness	A zeal to learn, seeking knowledge and understanding through observation and considered questioning to explore possibilities and options
Intellectual integrity	Seeks the truth through sincere, honest processes, even when the results conflict with own assumptions, values and beliefs
Intuition	Rapid and unconscious sense of knowing and judgement
Open-mindedness	Is receptive differing opinions and interpretation and aware of own biases
Perseverance	Determined to overcome obstacles
Reflection	Uses contemplation of thoughts, feelings and experiences related to a specific event to enhance understanding and self-evaluation
Skill	
Analysing	Separates or breaks an issue into its constituent parts to discover their nature, function and relationships
Applying standards	Makes judgements according to established personal reasoning, professional or social rules or criteria
Discriminating	Recognises differences and connections in situations and uses careful consideration to categorise or rank
Information seeking	Searches for evidence, facts and knowledge through identification of relevant sources and gathering objective, subjective, historical and current data
Logical reasoning	Draws inferences or conclusions that are supported and validated by evidence
Predicting	Can envisage a plan and its outcomes
Transforming knowledge	Changes or converts the condition, nature, form or function of concepts among contexts

Source: Adapted from Scheffer and Rubenfeld (2000, p. 358)

BOX 7.1 REFLECTIVE EXERCISE

Choose a recent clinical experience where you were required to make a complex clinical judgement and decision. Using the elements outlined in Table 7.1, rate the thinking processes that you utilised within your midwifery decision-making. According to each of the 17 criteria, give yourself a score out of 5 per criterion assessing how well you utilised each critical habit or skill during the decision-making process (5 being the highest, 1 being the lowest).

Following this exercise, consider the following questions:

1 Was this an easy exercise to undertake?
2 What areas have you identified you need to develop further?
3 Did these criteria cover all aspects of thinking undertaken in midwifery decision-making?

Given the unique and complex nature of midwifery practice, it is surprising that to date a consensus definition of critical thinking in midwifery has not been developed.

Is critical thinking in midwifery unique?

Midwifery is often characterised as comprising both 'science' and 'art'. This presents challenges in midwifery clinical decision-making. In isolation, the 'science' component of midwifery allows for straightforward, uncomplicated decision-making. Using an analytical or rational approach, the woman's clinical information could simply be combined with the evidence to inform decision-making. It is the 'art' of midwifery that makes midwifery practice unique and complex and presents more challenges in decision-making.

The philosophy of midwifery practice views and acknowledges pregnancy and birth as normal physiological events and premises midwifery care within a primary, social healthcare model (International Confederation of Midwives, 2014). Midwifery care utilises holistic decision-making which values diverse ways of knowing, including the woman's own knowledge of her body and decision-making abilities (Siddiqui, 2005). Decision-making occurs in a relationship between the woman and the midwife and is based on a partnership model underpinned by trust, respect, equity and shared decision-making (Pairman & McAra-Couper, 2015). The midwife and the woman, therefore, base decisions related to the provision of care on the woman's preferences and values in combination with the best available evidence (Noseworthy et al., 2013). Providing holistic individualised midwifery care involves a highly developed cognitive ability to critically analyse the individual woman's circumstances in combination with the evidence and her preferences or wishes for care (Gilkison et al., 2016). There is an increasing wealth of literature and clinical practice guidelines in maternity care. However, evidence that is congruent with the woman's unique situation is often absent. An essential skill in contextualised evidence-informed decision-making in midwifery is the use of critical thinking skills to evaluate the evidence in terms of quality and applicability to the individual woman's unique circumstances.

A high degree of cognitive skill is required to balance midwifery decision-making that is inclusive of the holistic philosophical foundations of midwifery care, contextualised evidence, and the woman's individual preferences and choices (Carter et al., 2018a). Due to this distinctive nature of midwifery decision-making, all midwives need to utilise unique and deliberate cognitive skills. Given the unique and multidimensional nature of midwifery decision-making and hence critical thinking skills required, it is surprising that there is little published literature on thinking processes in midwifery.

Conceptual model of critical thinking in midwifery practice

To promote greater understanding of the uniqueness and complexity of critical thinking in midwifery practice, a conceptual model was developed. Elements and concepts that shape critical thinking in midwifery practice emerged from (1) the review of literature on critical thinking and midwifery, (2) systematic reviews of the literature evaluating current available tools used to measure critical thinking, (3) development of survey items and expert review of these, and (4) testing of tools that aim to measure critical thinking in midwifery practice from different perspectives. The conceptual model of critical thinking in midwifery practice offers new knowledge and a framework about the application of this vital cognitive skill to practice (Carter et al., 2018a). The conceptual model represents the holistic philosophical underpinnings of midwifery care, irrespective of model of care or geographical location around the world, whilst also incorporating the constructs of critical thinking.

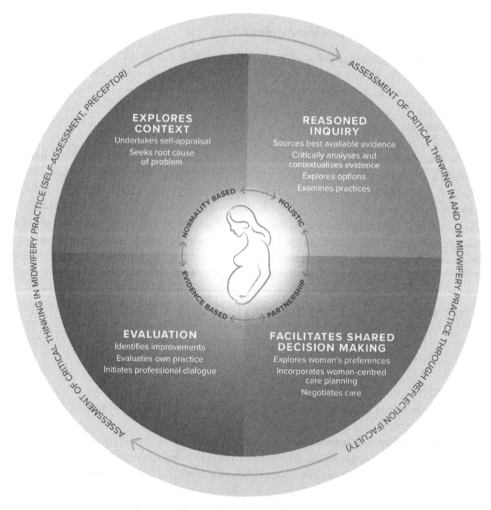

FIGURE 7.1 Conceptual model of critical thinking in midwifery practice

Source: Carter et al. (2018a, p. 117; reproduced with permission of Elsevier).

The conceptual model of critical thinking in midwifery practice is rooted within a framework of woman-centred care. The conceptual model is underpinned by the philosophical beliefs that:

- Pregnancy and birth are normal physiological events
- Midwifery care and decision-making are based on the best available evidence
- Midwifery care involves the development of a partnership relationship between the woman and midwife of equal power and mutual respect
- Midwifery care is holistic and individualised (Carter et al., 2018a, p. 116).

The conceptual model of critical thinking in midwifery comprises four phases and 12 elements within these four phases. There is no particular sequencing to the conceptual model; dependent on the situation, the phases may be used in any order. To explain the conceptual model of critical thinking in midwifery practice, a case study approach will be utilised. Following a short description of the case, an explanation of how the model could be utilised to apply critical thinking skills to midwifery practice and thereby inform midwifery decision-making is provided. To facilitate understanding of the conceptual model, a relatively uncomplicated case study has been chosen to illustrate application of the model rather than the complexity of the case and decision-making.

BOX 7.2 SALLY'S STORY

Sally is a primigravida and accessing a midwifery-led model of care. Sally is a healthy 31-year-old woman with no medical conditions and is experiencing an uncomplicated pregnancy. Sally's membranes ruptured at term + 2 days with clear liquor present. Sally contacts her midwife Angela and they agree to meet at the local birth centre. It is now ten hours since rupture of the membranes and Sally has not yet experienced any contractions. Angela needs to undertake midwifery decision-making related to care.

Phase 1: explores context

Undertakes self-appraisal

In accordance with this element, Angela would undertake a critical self-assessment of her skills and knowledge in relation to Sally's situation and determine whether she requires additional resources or consultation with another midwife or her obstetric colleagues. Depending on Angela's experience in caring for women with term pre-labour rupture of the membranes, she may need to access specific information regarding management, for example, local clinical guidelines of the birthing environment where she works. She may seek advice from a more senior midwifery colleague and/or discuss Sally's care with the obstetric team. This stage of self-appraisal may prompt Angela at a later time to undertake professional development or further learning to address any identified gaps.

Seeks root cause of a problem

Although term pre-labour rupture of the membranes is not normally considered a 'problem' but rather a variance, Angela would still need to consider whether there are any underlying causes for this occurrence, adding additional information to guide decision-making. For example, has a malpresentation or position caused the membranes to rupture? Is polyhydramnios present? Are there any signs of chorioamnionitis? This element encourages deeper cognitive thinking instead of simply reacting and responding to the symptoms or presentation.

Phase 2: reasoned inquiry

Sources best available evidence

Within this element Angela would source the best available evidence relating to term pre-labour rupture of the membranes. This would include the prioritisation of high-level evidence and seeking relevant clinical guidelines or policies.

Critically analyses and contextualises evidence

Within this element Angela would utilise critical thinking skills to critically analyse literature or evidence pertaining to this situation, making judgements about the quality of the evidence and its relevance to Sally's individual set of circumstances. The contextualisation of the evidence would involve Angela considering Sally's situation and knowledge of her as a woman and her pregnancy and current clinical cues. For example, Angela would consider whether Sally has previously experienced any other pre-labour signs such as strong Braxton Hicks contractions (and consider the likelihood of spontaneous labour commencing). She would also consider whether Sally has any identified factors that would increase her risk of chorioamnionitis (e.g. positive group B streptococcus). Equally, Angela would need to consider the contextual appropriateness of care recommended, for example, Sally's home situation and whether her environment is conducive to home monitoring.

During this stage Angela would also critically analyse any available clinical guidelines. Although clinical guidelines generally provide guidance for best practice, not all are based on the best available evidence, and are often out of date (Ménage, 2016; Prusova et al., 2014). An evaluation of the Green-top Guidelines (produced by the Royal College of Obstetricians and Gynaecologists in the United Kingdom) revealed that only 9%–12% were founded on the best quality evidence (Prusova et al., 2014).

Explores options

This element encourages the explorations of a range of options for Sally's individual situation. Angela would use a variety of strategies within this type of critical thinking to devise alternatives, including consideration of the evidence, Sally's preferences and individual circumstances. Angela may also utilise midwifery intuition and creativity to generate options of care. Utilising intuition to guide decision-making relies on an exquisite sensitivity to pattern recognition where unconscious judgements are made based on a variety of cues and past experiences (Steinhauer, 2015; Geraghty, 2015).

Examines practices

Critical thinking within this element involves examination of others' practices. In this specific case study where Angela is the lead carer, it would involve observing others' practices, interventions, recommendations or care provided to Sally, evaluating whether they are evidence informed and/or woman-centred and seek clarification around these. It may also involve recognising and addressing 'unwritten rules' within the organisation. Unwritten rules are based on tradition and institutional etiquette rather than evidence and can quickly become the cultural norm of an organisation (Hunter, 2005). An example of 'unwritten rules' relevant to this case study may be the recommendation of active management approach to term prelabour rupture of membranes, 'because it's what we always do here'.

Phase 3: facilitates shared decision-making

Explores woman's preferences

Within this element Angela would explore Sally's preferences for care. This may include an exploration of Sally's thoughts and knowledge around induction of labour, her perception of risk and her knowledge of her own body and what is right for her. This element of critical thinking acknowledges Sally's right to autonomy in decision-making. As mentioned previously, elements of the model can be used flexibly. In this case, Angela may have had several previous conversations with Sally about her preferences and have an agreed birth plan in place.

Incorporates woman-centred care planning

Once Sally's preferences of care are established, Angela would ensure that any care planning is centred around Sally's needs and preferences. Using critical thinking and judgement, Angela would share with Sally her interpretation and contextualisation of the best available evidence. Individualised planning of care and sequencing of care would then occur.

Negotiates care

Within this element critical thinking skills are utilised in gathering and synthesising information from all of the other elements and discussing these with Sally and other health professionals. In this case study, this would most likely involve discussing with obstetric colleagues an individualised plan of care for Sally and advocating for Sally's choices.

Phase 4: evaluation

Identifies improvements

This component of critical thinking would involve Angela taking a proactive stance and addressing any deficits in policies/guidelines, practices or the environment that hinder care (Carter et al., 2018a). In this case it may involve updating current policies or guidelines related to term pre-labour rupture of membranes or information brochures/literature provided to women. It is acknowledged in some environments around the globe that resources such as equipment, policies and access to healthcare staff may be limited, thereby restricting implementation of identified improvements. This element of critical thinking requires the midwife to contextualise improvements within the limitations of their maternity service providers.

Evaluates own practice

In recognition that critical thinking and reflection are intrinsically linked (Carter et al., 2017b), this phase of self-evaluation is a vital element of critical thinking. To assist in this self-evaluation Angela would seek feedback on the care provided from Sally, her family and others involved in her care. This type of reflection informed by critical thinking may identify parts of Angela's practice that could be improved.

Initiates professional dialogue

This element of critical thinking is motivated by the generation of new knowledge (Carter et al., 2018a). This would involve Angela discussing options and care related to Sally's situation with colleagues; this discussion may occur during or following the care provided. It also may involve debriefing with colleagues following Sally's care if complexities or unexpected events arose.

BOX 7.3 *REFLECTIVE EXERCISE*

It is now time to revisit the reflective exercise you undertook earlier in this chapter. Using the same clinical experience you chose previously, use the 12 elements of the Conceptual Model of Critical Thinking in Midwifery Practice to rate the thinking processes that you used during this decision-making. For each criterion, give yourself a score out of 5 assessing how well you utilised each of the elements during the decision-making process (5 being the highest, 1 being the lowest).

Following this exercise, consider the following questions:

1   Was this an easy exercise to undertake?
2   What areas have you identified you need to develop further?
3   Did these criteria cover all aspects of thinking undertaken in midwifery decision-making?
4   How did this exercise and your results compare to the one you completed earlier using the habits of mind and skills in critical thinking in nursing?

Although the Conceptual Model of Critical Thinking in Midwifery Practice aims to provide a greater understanding of the elements and concepts that encompass critical thinking in midwifery practice, tools and processes to measure these elements are necessary to further improve practice. These tools were required to evaluate the development of critical thinking and provide enhanced knowledge of the practical application of critical thinking to midwifery practice. Due to the unique and complex nature of critical thinking in midwifery and the lack of specific discipline measurement tools available, three tools were developed to measure the application of critical thinking to midwifery practice. The following section describes these three tools, which were originally developed to assess critical thinking in Australian midwifery students, however they are also relevant for use in assessing critical thinking of newly qualified midwives and experienced midwives around the globe.

Measuring and developing critical thinking skills in midwifery

Three tools were piloted and psychometrically tested with Australian undergraduate midwifery students, their clinical preceptors (mentors) and academic faculty. The three tools were specially designed to measure the application of critical thinking in midwifery practice, through preceptor rating, student self-assessment and evaluation of reflective writing on midwifery practice by academic faculty. The tools were called the Carter Assessment of Critical Thinking in Midwifery (CACTiM) (Preceptor/Mentor, Student, and Reflection versions). Through psychometric testing of each individual tool, all three were found to be reliable and valid measures of critical thinking skills in midwifery practice (Carter et al., 2016a, 2017a, 2017b). A longitudinal study using another cohort of midwifery students further established concurrent validity and reliability. Positive associations were found between the three scales and student characteristics, including grade point average, year level and previous qualifications (Carter et al., 2018b).

A comprehensive process was undertaken to develop items for the three CACTiM tools guided by an eight-stage developed approach advocated by DeVellis (2017). Steps undertaken included the following:

1   Systematic reviews of the literature and examination of items within other critical thinking measurement tools (Carter et al., 2015, 2016b).
2   A review of Australian National Competency Standards for the Midwife (Nursing and Midwifery Board of Australia, 2010) to ensure congruency with the core competencies and conceptual framework of midwifery practice.
3   Draft items were generated that represented the skills and habits of mind of critical thinking but also assimilated holistic philosophical foundations of midwifery care. Draft items reflected elements of the conceptual model where woman-centred care, the midwifery-woman partnership and the promotion of informed choice were signified. (4) Mapping of draft items to the consensus definition of critical thinking in nursing (Scheffer & Rubenfeld, 2000) was conducted to ensure conceptual congruence between items and critical thinking attributes.
5   The draft items were then reviewed by a panel of expert midwifery lecturers and clinicians.
6   Each draft tool was then completed by samples of students, clinical preceptors and midwifery lecturers.
7   Items were then statistically assessed for performance, dimensionality (factor analysis) and reliability.
8   Finally, the length of each tool was considered and any poor performing items were removed.

The items of each tool require respondents to evaluate the student's or midwife's application of critical thinking to midwifery practice on a Likert scale (such as 1 = strongly disagree to 5 = strongly agree). To ascertain a comprehensive evaluation of the application of

TABLE 7.2 Examples of items from CACTiM tools

Name of Tool	Item
CACTiM – Student (self-assessment)	I choose relevant literature and education strategies to facilitate the woman's decision-making
	I often instinctively know what type of care is right for the woman
	If problems arise when caring for the woman, I try to seek the root cause
	I can provide the rationale for following (or departing from) established guidelines and policies
CACTiM – preceptor/ mentor	The student . . .
	effectively explores multiple solutions to a given situation
	identifies organisational/service improvement opportunities
	questions the 'unwritten rules' in midwifery practice that are not evidence-based
	initiates professional dialogue around midwifery practice
CACTiM – reflection	The student . . .
	demonstrates insight into the need to provide individualised care to the woman
	critically analyses the quality of the literature and its relevance to the individual woman's situation
	identifies and examines appropriateness of clinical procedures and practice
	evaluates own practice and its effect on the woman and others

this complex cognitive skill, it is recommended that the student or midwife completes the CACTiM self-assessment tool, their preceptor or mentor completes the CACTiM preceptor/ mentor tool and a piece of reflective writing on midwifery practice is also assessed (usually by faculty). The qualified midwife could still seek feedback from a mentor and also seek feedback on their reflective writing from a midwifery colleague, educator or manager. Such reflections could be added to the midwife's professional portfolio which, in some countries (e.g. Australia and New Zealand), is undertaken regularly as part of a midwifery practice review process to assist midwives to identify improvements to practice and professional development needs.

Using the three tools to evaluate critical thinking skills provides the student or midwife with useful and objective feedback from multiple sources and provides holistic real-world assessment on the application of critical thinking skills in practice. This multi-method approach also provides the student or midwife with opportunities to explore and compare their perceptions of their own practice with others' perceptions. Examples of items from each of the tools are provided in Table 7.2.

Conclusion

The provision of autonomous, safe, evidence-informed, woman-centred midwifery care requires technical expertise and highly developed critical thinking skills that inform midwifery decision-making. Due to the distinct nature of midwifery decision-making, all midwives need to utilise unique and deliberate cognitive skills to balance philosophical underpinnings of midwifery care with contextualised evidence whilst honouring the woman's individual preferences and choices. A greater understanding of how critical thinking informs midwifery decision-making and measurement of this vital skill to promote continual development will ultimately result in improvements in practice and midwifery care provided to women and their families.

References

Carter, A. G., Creedy, D. K. & Sidebotham, M. 2015. Evaluation of Tools Used to Measure Critical Thinking Development in Nursing and Midwifery Undergraduate Students: A Systematic Review. *Nurse Education Today*, 35, 864–874.

Carter, A. G., Creedy, D. K. & Sidebotham, M. 2016a. Development and Psychometric Testing of the Carter Assessment of Critical Thinking in Midwifery (Preceptor/Mentor version). *Midwifery*, 34, 141–149.

Carter, A. G., Creedy, D. K. & Sidebotham, M. 2016b. Efficacy of Teaching Methods Used to Develop Critical Thinking in Nursing and Midwifery Undergraduate Students: A Systematic Review of the Literature. *Nurse Education Today*, 40, 209–218.

Carter, A. G., Creedy, D. K. & Sidebotham, M. 2017a. Critical Thinking Skills in Midwifery Practice: Development of a Self-Assessment Tool for Students. *Midwifery*, 50, 184–192.

Carter, A. G., Creedy, D. K. & Sidebotham, M. 2017b. Critical Thinking Evaluation in Reflective Writing: Development and Testing of Carter Assessment of Critical Thinking in Midwifery (Reflection). *Midwifery*, 54, 73–80.

Carter, A. G., Creedy, D. K. & Sidebotham, M. 2018a. Critical Thinking in Midwifery Practice: A Conceptual Model. *Nurse Education in Practice*, 33, 114–120.

Carter, A. G., Creedy, D. K. & Sidebotham, M. 2018b. Measuring Critical Thinking in Pre-Registration Midwifery Students: A Multi-Method Approach. *Nurse Education Today*, 61, 169–174.

Castledine, G. 2010. Castledine Column: Critical Thinking Is Crucial. *British Journal of Nursing*, 19, 271–271.

DeVellis, R. F. 2017. *Scale Development: Theory and Applications* (4th ed.). Sage, Thousand Oaks, CA.

Facione, N. C. 2013. *The California Critical Thinking Skills Test: CCTST Test Manual*. California Academic Press, Millbrae, CA.

Facione, N. C. & Facione, P. A. 1996. Externalizing the Critical Thinking in Knowledge Development and Clinical Judgment. *Nursing Outlook*, 44, 129–136.

Facione, P. A. 1990. *Critical Thinking: A Statement of Expert Consensus for Purposes of Educational Assessment and Instruction, Executive Summary: 'The Delphi Report'*. The Californian Academic Press, CA. Viewed January 2019. www.insightassessment.com/Resources/Importance-of-Critical-Thinking/Expert-Consensus-on-Critical-Thinking/Delphi-Consensus-Report-Executive-Summary-PDF.

Geraghty, S. 2015. Keeping the Shining Roads Open: Intuition in Midwifery Practice. *The Practising Midwife*, 18, 42–45.

Gilkison, A., Giddings, L. & Smythe, L. 2016. Real Life Narratives Enhance Learning About the 'Art and Science' of Midwifery Practice. *Advances in Health Sciences Education: Theory and Practice*, 21, 19–32.

Hunter, B. 2005. Emotion Work and Boundary Maintenance in Hospital-Based Midwifery. *Midwifery*, 21, 253–266.

International Confederation of Midwives. 2014. *Philosophy and Model of Midwifery Care*. The Hague. Viewed February 2019. www.internationalmidwives.org/assets/uploads/documents/CoreDocuments/CD2005_001%20V2014%20ENG%20Philosophy%20and%20model%20of%20midwifery%20care.pdf.

Ménage, D. 2016. Part 2: A Model for Evidence-Based Decision-Making in Midwifery Care. *British Journal of Midwifery*, 24, 137–143.

Mong-Chue, C. 2000. Professional Issues: The Challenges of Midwifery Practice for Critical Thinking. *British Journal of Midwifery*, 8, 179–183.

Noseworthy, D. A., Phibbs, S. R. & Benn, C. A. 2013. Towards a Relational Model of Decision-Making in Midwifery Care. *Midwifery*, 29, e42–e48.

Nursing and Midwifery Board of Australia. 2010. *National Competency Standards for the Midwife*. Viewed January 2019. www.nursingmidwiferyboard.gov.au/Codes-Guidelines-Statements/Professional-standards.aspx.

Pairman, S., & McAra-Couper, J. 2015. Theoretical Frameworks for Midwifery Practice. In S. Pairman, S.K., Tracy, C. Thorogood & J. Pincombe (eds.), *Midwifery: Preparation for Practice* (3rd ed.). Churchill Livingstone, Chatswood, NSW, pp. 383–411.

Paul, R.W. 1993. *Critical Thinking: What Every Person Needs to Survive in a Rapidly Changing World* (2nd ed.). Foundation for Critical Thinking, Santa Rosa, CA.

Paul, R.W., Binker, A.J.A. & Willsen, J. 1995. *Critical Thinking: How to Prepare Students for a Rapidly Changing World*. Foundation for Critical Thinking, Santa Rosa, CA.

Prusova, K., Churcher, L., Tyler, A. & Lokugamage, A.U. 2014. Royal College of Obstetricians and Gynaecologists Guidelines: How Evidence-Based Are They? *Journal of Obstetrics and Gynaecology*, 34, 706–711.

Scheffer, B.K. & Rubenfeld, M.G. 2000. A Consensus Statement on Critical Thinking in Nursing. *Journal of Nursing Education*, 39, 352–359.

Siddiqui, J. 2005. The Role of Knowledge in Midwifery Decision-Making. In M.D. Raynor, J.E. Marshall & A. Sullivan (eds.), *Decision-Making in Midwifery Practice*. Churchill Livingstone, London, pp. 23–36.

Steinhauer, S. 2015. Decision-Making in Midwifery: Rationality and Intuition. *The Practising Midwife*, 18, 14–18.

8

THE USE OF REFLECTION IN MIDWIFERY PRACTICE TO INFORM CLINICAL DECISION-MAKING

Amanda Wain

Overview

This chapter will evaluate how encouraging the use of critical reflection within a contemporary midwifery practice setting can influence a midwife's ability to make important clinical decisions. Models of reflection will be considered which can enhance self-awareness and insight and empower midwives' decision-making skills to influence their practice irrespective of the type of maternity setting they work in throughout the world. The chapter will also consider international concepts surrounding how the use of reflection is used to support midwives and student midwives through a continuous improvement process which aims to build personal and professional resilience, enhance quality of care and support preparedness for professional revalidation (Nursing and Midwifery Council, NMC 2015).

Introduction

An essential element of continual, evolving midwifery practice is the need for midwives to critically reflect on their practice in order to support them to make clinical decisions and judgements, which inform and improve care for childbearing women and their families. Reflection is a function that allows us to appraise former beliefs and assumptions and their implications, and transform a situation where there was uncertainty and ambiguity into one that is comprehensible, clear and logical (Dewey 1933).

What is reflection?

Reflection is an everyday human activity that is essential to cognitive development and personal growth and lies between the concept of learning and thinking. Reflection occurs either during a particular activity, or afterwards when we have more time or better opportunity to think over what happened. We reflect on the bus, at work, over meals or during and after our general conversations – basically whenever we have the thinking space to contemplate events (Howatson-Jones 2013). Reflection is a process of learning through our everyday experiences whereby a person will appraise a situation or incident in order to consider what happened. People, in this case midwives, will weigh up their individual feelings about the events, evaluate how particular actions were influenced and then deliberate how they would respond if the situation were to arise again. We reflect in order to learn, but equally, we learn as a result of reflection creating a partnership between clinical experiences and education (Armstrong et al. 2017).

The concept of reflective thinking as an aspect of learning was initiated by the American philosopher and educationalist, John Dewey (1859–1952), who claimed we learn by doing and by realising what becomes of what we do (Dewey 1938). Central to his theory is that reflection should include recalling the event and then posing questions to explore why things turned out the way they did, before evaluating what possible actions could have given a different outcome. Reflective learning is based on the assumption that all human beings learn by reflecting on both positive and negative real-life experiences. Put simply, reflection allows us to make sense of events by considering the who, what, where, how and why (Wain 2017). Dewey's concept of reflective thinking is mainly placed within the wider context of education, however the philosophy underpinning his model has been replicated in many definitions and models for reflective practice.

Within the context of midwifery, reflection is a principal learning strategy advocated by many regulatory authorities, non-governmental organisations (NGOs) and higher education institutions across the world. Reflective practice is a recent paradigm for midwifery education and fosters a systematic way of thinking about actions and responses to inform learning and decision-making, and if necessary change future actions and responses. As a learning approach, reflection increases awareness of perceptions and is an essential element of knowledge and skill acquisition and development (Horton-Deutsch and Sherwood 2017). It provides opportunity to evaluate our midwifery clinical practice experiences and apply existing knowledge to gain new insight and understanding to inform and change our future practice (Bass et al. 2017). Reflection is known to be beneficial in experiential learning and for the development of critical thinking skills to facilitate the application between theory and practice. Reflection also increases self-awareness and allows for deeper understanding of analysis and evaluation to therefore strengthen critical thinking and influence decision-making. Developing the ability to think critically is also an essential constituent of midwifery higher education programmes and can be defined as 'the process of purposeful, self-regulatory judgement: an interactive reflective, reasoning process' (Facione et al. 1994:345). Critical thinking and decision-making utilises reflection skills, as it requires the practitioner to problem-solve by considering opposing viewpoints or theories to weigh up the possibilities for actions in order to make reasoned and rational choices to inform professional practice.

Within contemporary midwifery practice, midwives are increasingly faced with a need to make challenging, complex decisions and clinical judgements, often in unpredictable situations which need intuitive reflective and reflexive processes. Reflexivity is the process of questioning and comprehending our prejudices, values, assumptions and attitudes to help us understand our roles in relation to others (Bolton 2014). It enables conscientious and ethical action and develops self-awareness of how our views are determined depending on cultural or social norms. Being able to critically reflect on our experiences allows us to explore and express difficult situations and enables enquiry into what we think, feel, believe, value and understand about our role (Bolton 2014). It is the critical thinking that provides us the knowledge and understanding that allows us to draw our conclusions about an experience, to learn from the event and form an action plan for our future practice (Nicol and Dosser 2016). To do this, midwives need to be able to reflect both in and on actions to develop the tacit and practical knowledge required to learn from the experience and therefore inform and influence clinical decisions and actions (Horton-Deutsch and Sherwood 2017).

Models of reflection

There are many different models of reflection which provide a structured framework in which to evaluate learning and foster continual thought and innovation and allow for concepts and theories to become embedded into clinical practice (Heyer 2015). The models of Gibbs (1988), Schon (1991), Kolb (1984), and Bass et al. (2017) are popular within midwifery practice and education as the different stages lend themselves well when considering professional issues and allow for a logical, sequential approach on which to structure the reflection.

Gibbs (1988)

One of the most commonly used models of reflection is that of the educational researcher Graham Gibbs, who developed the idea of a reflective cycle to encourage learners to systematically think about the different phases of an activity or an experience (Heyer 2015). The model is prescriptive and focuses usually on a singular event. Gibbs perceived the process of reflection to be a cyclical pattern of behaviour which allows the reflector to focus on three particular aspects of a situation, that of description and feelings, evaluation and analysis, and how someone would act if the events were to happen again. This process sits well with the andragogy teaching and learning strategy of higher education midwifery programmes, which allows the student midwife to cultivate pre-existing knowledge and understanding and correlate this to their developing clinical skills (Walsh 2014). An example of this may be whereby a student midwife considers her own personal experiences of childbirth as she develops new knowledge and understanding. Doing this allows for the student midwife to develop a deeper comprehension of factors, which she as a mother she may not have been fully aware of.

Andragogy was derived by the humanist educator Malcolm Knowles (1990) and falls within the humanistic pedagogy, which centres around lifelong learning, self-motivation and self-actualisation, whereby the student has the desire to learn to fulfil their own potential (Rogers 2002). Knowles identified the following four themes which make up the principle components of andragogy:

1 *Self-concept* – The student takes responsibility for their own learning and is more involved with the planning and evaluation of their own goals and objectives.
2 *Experience* – Adults have a wealth of knowledge and experiences which can be used as a resource to direct their learning.
3 *Orientation to learning* – Adults relate learning to their real-life situations, so learning becomes more problem-focused and motivated.
4 *Readiness to learn* – Adult learners are voluntary with a motivation and willingness to learn (Knowles 1990).

The process of reflection within the clinical setting endorses the values of adult lifelong learning and education as it fosters insight into professional practice. Therefore it is an essential element for the continued development of personal accountability and professional growth (Kirkham 1997; Bass et al. 2017), both of which are key elements of being part of the midwifery profession.

BOX 8.1   CASE SCENARIO 1

Let's consider how Gibbs's (1988) model can be used by means of an example where a midwife has made an error with drug administration.

- The main priority is for the midwife to describe what happened, drawing on powers of observation and the ability to recall salient points with accuracy and impartiality.
- Second, there is acknowledgement of feelings at the time of the event, and what the reactions were to them.
- Was the midwife distracted, or was it a drug she was unfamiliar with?

Asking such reflective questions helps the midwife to consider processes and understand any challenging emotions, which can be associated with issues experienced in clinical practice, especially in this case where there could be an adverse reaction to the error. Evaluation begins by the weighing up of positive and negative aspects of the experience and a consideration of the main issues:

- What did the midwife do well or not so well? Was the error immediately recognised and the appropriate action taken?

These can be further analysed by benchmarking personal interactions against available knowledge, literature and research. It allows for the consideration of choices available and what the potential consequences may have been had one of those choices been chosen instead (Howatson-Jones 2013). The conclusion provides a summary of the midwife's response to the events, what has been learnt and how one might react or respond in the future.

The most important factor of this cycle is the ability to form an action plan to formalise the outcome of the reflection and take learning forward to inform future practice. Gibbs's cycle was later amended by Reid (2000), who portrayed reflection as learning from practice, and a process of reviewing an experience of practice in order to describe, analyse and evaluate and thus inform (Reid 2000).

Schon (1991)

One of the most influential interpretations of reflective practice is the approach of Donald Schon (1991), who described professional practice as 'being in a flat place where we can't see very far' (Bolton and Delderfield 2014:3). His evocative image of the swampy lowlands of professional practice, where theories are not always clearly expressed, suggests we often learn by our mistakes or by trial and error. Schon introduced the concepts of 'reflection-in-action' and 'reflection-on-action'. Reflection-in-action refers to the process of observing our thinking and actions as they occur in order to make adjustments in the moment, and is what we do when we perform on-the-spot testing of the situation based on experience, knowledge and skills. It requires the individual to think on their feet to decide what to do next. This is particularly important within a midwifery setting where midwives need to respond to rapidly changing events during any part of the childbearing journey.

Using Schon's theory, when faced with a new situation a midwife may often feel confused or surprised, and thus will reflect on both the current circumstances and on former understanding. We act immediately, drawing on our knowledge and experience as we go along (Bolton 2014). An illustration of this may be how a midwife responds to an emergency situation. This of course depends on where it takes place. A midwife's actions when responding to a postpartum haemorrhage (PPH) occurring in a tertiary hospital, where there is clear guidance and protocols and a responsive multi-professional team, may greatly differ from a midwife working in a poorer socioeconomic country, perhaps in a remote setting or in a country with limited staff or resources. Irrespective of whether a midwife practices in a high-, middle- or low-income country or within a tertiary maternity service or a remote village, midwives develop and adapt their knowledge, skills and values to reflect-in-action more quickly and use these skills to inform our decision-making relevant to our practice setting.

Schon's model was later developed by Killion and Todnem (1991) to include 'reflection-for-action' to guide future action based on past thoughts and actions (Thomas 2008). Reflection-on-action is the process of looking back on and learning from some of those 'in the moment' actions in order to gain clarity and insight and therefore consider how our choices and ways of thinking might shape and determine future actions and clinical decision-making. Using the same example of a PPH, a midwife would look back on how she responded to the event in her own particular circumstances and therefore base subsequent practice on this deliberation and thinking.

Kolb (1984)

A third model of reflection is that of Kolb (1984), who attempted to integrate thinking and practice into a single act (Rolfe et al. 2011). Kolb proposed that a person learns through discovery and experience, and produced his Experiential Learning Cycle (1984) to demonstrate that effective learning takes place as people move through a four-stage cycle. Kolb extends the reflective process beyond observation and reflection on past events by encouraging practitioners, in this case midwives, to theorise on these reflections and then consider new approaches based on those theories and beliefs. This leads to new experiences, and thus the cycle is repeated (Rolfe et al. 2011). Incorporating active experimentation into the model integrates thought and action. Reflection allows for the formulation of concepts and theories. Theories in turn generate hypotheses that can be tested once the midwife is back in the clinical practice setting. The framework provides a holistic model of the learning process and is called 'experimental learning' to emphasise the pivotal role that experience plays in the learning process.

The four-stage model is utilised well within midwifery education and practice and demonstrates learning and reflection in the clinical setting, an example of which is the teaching of female catheterisation.

1 *Concrete experience* – The assignment of a task whereby active involvement is key to learning. Being guided through the stages of catheterisation and given the opportunity to practice the skill in a safe environment.

2   *Reflective observation* – Taking time out from the 'doing' to reflect on what has been done and experienced.

3   *Abstract conceptualisation* – The process of making sense of what has occurred, including consideration of values and attitudes, and interpreting the events to promote understanding and deep learning. The student may consider situations where a woman may need catheterisation and the rationale or implications of this, and reflect on issues such as informed consent and choice or protocols.

4   *Active experimentation* – The student midwife considers how to apply this new knowledge to contemporary midwifery practice. This will include generating new hypotheses, so in this case it could include correlation of the midwife's role to promote accurate fluid balance in order to identify and prevent acute kidney injury and thus reduce potential for long-term maternal morbidity.

The framework can be described as a cycle of experiencing, reflecting, thinking and acting, however from this Kolb identified different learning styles which he subsequently termed diverging, assimilating, converging and accommodating. A diverting learning style allows the learner or midwife to reflect on what has been observed, allowing for the ability to analyse tasks from different viewpoints, and develop new ideas. An assimilating learning style merges the ability to conceptualise abstract ideas and reflective observation. Such midwives are often good problem-solvers and tend to be very structured in their thinking. Converging learning styles combine experimentation and abstract concepts. This leads to learning from experience and applying this new knowledge to future actions. Finally, accommodating learning styles are grounded by concrete experiences and being able to experiment, allowing for the learner to demonstrate a practical approach to problem-solving (Hinchcliff 2009). All these stages are essential for developing the critical thinking skills of inquiry, consideration of differing viewpoints and theories and problem-solving, which allow practitioners to make reasoned and rational clinical judgements and decisions.

Bass et al. (2017)

The Holistic Reflective Model (Bass et al. 2017) was developed by midwives for midwives as an educational resource tool for midwifery educators to facilitate the development of reflective and critical thinking skills of Australian midwifery students, on which to foster reflexivity and reflection in practice. The model was designed to reflect the holistic ethos of women-centred midwifery care and is similar to that of Gibbs in that it allows for six phases of reflection through a continual learning cycle, which are:

1   Self-awareness
2   Description
3   Reflection
4   Influences
5   Evaluation
6   Learning.

The model embeds a conceptual continuum of reflection, critical reflection and reflexivity which is integral for the development of holistic reflective practice throughout the learning cycle.

Activity 1

Using the following scenario, how can this six-phase model of reflection be utilised in global midwifery practice?

BOX 8.2   ANITA'S STORY – LINKED ACTIVITY 1

Anita is a second-year student midwife and is currently working within a midwifery-led model (e.g. birth-centre, or home). She has seen a lot of women supported to have a physiological third stage of labour by her midwives. Anita has not practiced within an obstetric-led maternity service (hospital), so has not witnessed an active (medicalised) third stage of labour. How can the use of reflection inform Anita's decision-making regarding women's choice for the third stage of labour?

- *Self-awareness* – Anita is encouraged to maintain an open mind to consider her thoughts, responses and emotions during the experience.
- *Description* – Anita recalls a factual description of events, highlighting any significant or important aspects. In this instance, the women are all experiencing normal childbirth cared for by midwives who are experienced in facilitating a physiological third stage of labour.
- *Reflection* – Internal thoughts and feeling are explored, including underpinning values, assumptions and beliefs to develop critical thinking skills and deeper understanding. Again the concept of informed choice may be considered: are midwives in the obstetric-led maternity service following a medicalised social norm? As a result, have the midwives become disempowered or are they less confident to support women with a physiological third stage of labour, especially within a midwifery-led service where medical support is not available should an emergency arise?
- *Influences* – Anita draws on her existing knowledge and experience from her educational midwifery training and ongoing professional development learning: what does the evidence say, and how does this influence clinical practice? Anita then draws on her develop and adapt their knowledge, skills and values from practising in her specific maternity service to holistically examine what occurred using a diverse range of evidence on which to apply her knowledge and develop critical thinking skills.
- *Evaluation* – The events are objectively and critically analysed to consider how a similar situation may be handled differently in the future utilising critical reflection. How can Anita use her new knowledge to inform her management of the third stage of labour? Could this new understanding influence a change in her or other midwives' practice?
- *Learning* – The final phase encompasses transformational learning, allowing for Anita to synthesise and integrate the evidence reviewed during the reflection. This enables her to consider what she has learned from the event and identify any changes in perspective that may have transpired. The key message from this stage is to consider how Anita can apply this transformative leaning to inform her future practice and enable her to continue to develop the skills of a reflective practitioner.

Reflection within midwifery regulation

The International Confederation of Midwives (ICM) acknowledged the variation and quality of international midwifery regulation and education programmes, and took measures to clearly define standards and essential competencies in the ICM Global Standards for Midwifery Education (2013) in order to significantly reduce global maternal and perinatal mortality. These standards recommend a curriculum based on the principles of adult education, which as previously discussed encompasses a variety of teaching and learning strategies, including the use of reflection to promote the development of midwifery competencies. In many areas of the developed world, reflection is also a key concept used by midwives to demonstrate the requirements of their professional regulator. For example, in the United Kingdom, revalidation is the process by which all registered nurses and midwives must follow in order to demonstrate safe and effective practice to maintain their professional registration with the Nursing and Midwifery Council (NMC 2012). One of the key aspects of revalidation is that midwives are required to demonstrate their fitness to practice every three years through evidence of five written reflections either on clinical practice or professional development to support their continuous, lifelong learning (NMC 2015).

Globally, the impact that regulated, competent midwives make to positive maternal and infant health is paramount. However, it must be acknowledged that midwives working in some middle- and low-income countries may lack access to continued education and professional development, which is essential to improve retention and motivation. Midwives in these areas need resilience and courage and would particularly benefit from a mechanism of supportive supervision, which would allow for the safe, open discussion and opportunity to reflect upon the challenges they may face in practice (Brodie 2013). Restorative Clinical Supervision (RSC) is a support tool being used to support British midwives with their practice and aims to support clear thinking and decision-making through a process of reflection so that stress and anxiety about work-related challenges can be overcome (Wallbank 2012). RCS is concerned with how staff respond emotionally to the challenges of care, and is particularly beneficial to midwives working within contemporary midwifery practice. It fosters resilience through nurturing supportive relationships that offer motivation and encouragement and that can also be drawn upon in times of stress. It offers this by means of elements such as resilience training, stress inoculation and coaching, with the opportunity to use approaches such as appreciative inquiry, emotional containment and motivational interviewing. RCS is concerned with addressing the emotional needs of staff and supporting the development of resilience, allowing for the creation of thinking space through discussion, reflective conversation, supportive challenge and open and honest feedback (NHS England 2017). The process allows the midwife to elicit learning from the event in order to reach their own decisions and conclusions and form an action plan for future practice. Studies have demonstrated that in those professions where a restorative model is aligned to education and leadership, there is potential for improvements in staff engagement, compassion satisfaction and ultimately service provision (Wain et al. 2018). However, the inequalities of global midwifery provision means that those midwives who would particularly benefit from the supportive function of RCS are working in countries which neither have the resources or social and economic infrastructure to provide such support. Midwives from every country, nevertheless, need the practical, organisational and professional support to enable them to fulfil the requirements of their role in order to strengthen the sustainability of the midwifery profession (Brodie 2013).

Conclusion

This chapter has examined how reflection within global midwifery practice can influence a midwife's ability to make critical decisions which can inform future practice. Current maternity care encompasses political and socioeconomic challenges that students and midwives face when meeting the demands of contemporary practice. Continuous learning and professional development is required to enable professionals to adapt to the changing landscape of maternity care, and reflection and the development of reflective skills forms part of this progression to demonstrate lifelong learning. The use of reflection fosters critical thinking and can empower midwives to make decisions as a reflective practitioner. This ultimately increases self-awareness, resilience and personal growth, thus leading to greater job satisfaction, professional fulfilment and overall improved quality of care for the childbearing public.

References

Armstrong, G, Horton-Deutsch, S, Sherwood, G (2017) Reflection in clinical contexts: Learning, collaboration, and evaluation. In Horton-Deutsch, S, Sherwood, G (Eds) *Reflective Practice. Transforming Education and Improving Outcomes.* (2nd Edition). Sigma Theta Tau International. Indianapolis. pp. 214–238

Bass, J, Fenwick, J, Sidebotham, M (2017) Development of a model of holistic reflection to facilitate transformative learning in student midwives. *Women and Birth.* June 30:3:227–235

Bolton, G (2014) *Reflective Practice – Writing and Professional Development.* Sage. London

Bolton, G, Delderfield, R (2014) *Reflective Practice. Writing and Professional Development.* (5th Edition). Sage. London

Brodie, P (2013) 'Midwifing the midwives': Addressing the empowerment, safety of, and respect for, the world's midwives. *Midwifery.* 29:10:1075–1076

Dewey, J (1933) *How We Think: A Restatement of the Relation of Reflective Thinking to the Educative Process.* Health and Co. Boston

Dewey, J (1938) Experience and education. Macmillan. New York. In Rolfe, G, Jasper, M, Freshwater, D. (2011) *Critical Reflection in Practice. Generating Knowledge for Care.* (2nd Edition). Palgrave Macmillan. Basingstoke

Facione, P, Facione, N, Sanchez, C (1994) Critical thinking disposition as a measure of competent clinical judgment. The development of the California critical thinking disposition inventory. *Journal of Nursing Education.* 33:345

Gibbs, G (1988) *Learning by Doing: A Guide to Teaching and Learning Methods.* Further Education Unit Oxford Polytechnic. Oxford

Heyer, R (2015) Learning through reflection: The critical role of reflection in work-based learning. *Journal of Work-Applied Management.* 7:1:15–27

Hinchcliff, S (2009) *The Practitioner as Teacher.* Elsevier. Edinburgh

Horton-Deutsch, S, Sherwood, G (2017) *Reflective Practice. Transforming Education and Improving Outcomes.* (2nd Edition). Sigma Theta Tau International. Indianapolis.

Howatson-Jones, L (2013) *Reflective Practice in Nursing.* (2nd Edition). Los Angeles. CA: Sage Publications.

International Confederation of Midwives (ICM) (2013) *International Confederation of Midwives' Model Curriculum Outlines for Professional Midwifery Education.* ICM. The Hague

Killion, J, Todnem, G (1991) A process of personal theory building. *Educational Leadership.* 48:6:14–17

Kirkham, M (1997) Reflection in midwifery: Professional narcissism or seeing with women. *The British Journal of Midwifery.* 5:5:259–262

Knowles, M (1990) *The Adult Learner.* (4th Edition). Gulf. Houston

Kolb, D (1984) Experiential Learning Cycle. In Hinchcliff. S (Ed.) *The Practitioner as Teacher.* Elsevier. Edinburgh, 2009

NHS England (2017) *A-Equip – A Model of Clinical Supervision. NHS. London*

Nicol, J, Dosser, I (2016) Understanding reflective practice. *Nursing Standard*. 30:36:34–40

Nursing and Midwifery Council (2012) *Midwives Rules and Standards*. NMC. London

Nursing and Midwifery Council (2015) *The Code*. NMC. London

Reid, B (2000) The role of the mentor to aid reflective practice. In Burns. S, Bulman. C (Eds.) *Reflective Practice in Nursing: The Growth of the Professional Practitioner*. (2nd Edition). Blackwell Scientific Publications, London

Rogers, A (2002) *Teaching Adults*. (3rd Edition) Open University Press. Maidenhead

Rolfe, G, Jasper, M, Freshwater, D (2011). *Critical Reflection in Practice: Generating Knowledge for Care*. (2nd Edition). Palgrave Macmillan. Basingstoke

Schon, D (1991) *The Reflective Practitioner: How Professional Think in Action*. Basic Books. New York

Thomas, L (2008) *Reflecting on Practice: An Exploration of the Impact of Targeted Professional Development on Teacher Action*. Penn Libraries. University of Pennsylvania. Pennsylvania

Wain, A (2017) Learning through reflection. *The British Journal of Midwifery*. 25:10:662–666

Wain, A, Britt, S, Divall, B (2018) Development of the bridging programme for the role of the professional midwifery advocate to support quality improvement. *MIDIRS Midwifery Digest*. 28:3:285–289

Wallbank, S (2012) Effectiveness of individual clinical supervision for midwives and doctors in stress reduction: Findings from a pilot study. *Evidence-Based Midwifery*. 8:65–70

Walsh, D (2014) Teaching and learning theory. In *The Nurse Mentor's Handbook*. (2nd Edition). McGraw Hill. Maidenhead. pp. 159–198

PART II
Translating theory into practice

9

DECISION-MAKING IN PERINATAL MENTAL HEALTH

What are the challenges?

Claire Marshall, Catriona Jones and Julie Jomeen

Chapter overview

All aspects of a woman's health must be considered during the maternity episode, and in recent years there has been a growing acknowledgement of the importance of a woman's mental health and its profound impact on outcomes for the mother, the baby and the wider family. This chapter will focus on the importance of the relationship between the midwife and other professionals in the context of perinatal mental health and associated decision-making. The woman's journey through maternity care will be discussed and the essential function of screening and detection will be explored alongside critical decision-making in relation to high-risk groups. Recognition of the complexities of supporting women with mental health conditions will be acknowledged alongside the social factors that impact upon their care and choices.

This chapter will use a clinical case study approach to highlight other pertinent aspects of decision-making, including the need for psychiatric birth planning and the challenges that mothers face when making decisions about medication when pregnant and breastfeeding.

PMH and decision-making: the importance of relationships

It is widely accepted that women affected by perinatal mental illness (PMI) prefer to be actively engaged in decisions about the treatment of their mental health concerns (Patel and Wisner, 2011; Price and Bentley, 2013). Globally, there will be different service models for the provision of perinatal mental health care, and on a global level, different models will involve different practitioners, however, in the United Kingdom (UK), midwives are identified as a workforce that plays a significant role in the promotion of emotional well-being of pregnant women. However, the importance of a universal workforce in the perinatal period cannot be overlooked, including but not exclusive to health visitors, family practitioners, community health nurses and general practitioners. Health professionals and practitioners, working collaboratively as multidisciplinary teams within a shared decision-making (SDM) framework, are key to ensuring the best outcomes are achieved for the mother, child and wider family, even within the context of low- and middle-income countries where the infrastructure may be less well resourced, a joined-up integrated approach to care, potentially within primary healthcare settings (Tsai and Tomlinson, 2012) can be significant for women with PMI.

Shared decision-making within the provider and woman encounter is frequently advocated at the policy level and is an indicator of quality of care in maternity (Molenaar et al., 2018). The intermediate position of SDM is said to involve collaboration (Slade, 2017). Chong, Aslani and Chen (2013) identified that recently the concept has been extended beyond provider and patient (woman) to include the interprofessional team. Research advocates that positive relationships are key to the success of SDM. The relationship should facilitate the sharing of knowledge and expertise on an equal basis in order for informed decisions about care and treatment to be made (Coultier, 2010). A recent integrative review presents SDM as a 'comprehensive process that takes place between the nurse and the patient' (Truglio-Londrigan and Slyer, 2018, p. 9).

Tomlinson (2018) stresses the need for a paradigm shift for SDM to be achieved, from 'care that is centred on biology, diseases, patients, or doctors to one that is centred on human relationships with an understanding of how power operates' (Tomlinson, 2018, p. 1). There is an extensive body of literature on SDM, with numerous attempts to define, conceptualise (Park and Cho, 2018) and operationalise SDM. Elwyn et al. (2017) propose that there are varying views on what SDM is and how it can be done – giving rise to a lack of an agreed set of steps or guidance of how it can be achieved, and an absence of literature which describes the process (Rosenbaum, 2015; Legare and Thompson-Leduc, 2014). A model of SDM based on choice, option and decision talk by Elwyn (2012) is described in Chapter 1.

SDM in the context of perinatal mental illness

There is limited research available, which explores SDM in the context of perinatal mental illness. In the broader literature on adult mental health, Bradley and Green (2018) emphasise the importance of the family in the context of SDM, illustrating that healthcare staff in particular value the contextual information that family members can provide. In the UK, the National Institute of Clinical Excellence (NICE) (2014) identify that the active involvement of mental health patients in shared decision-making with respect to screening, treatment, and care is key to improving the overall patient experience. Research by Bradley and Green (2018) suggest that family involvement should be more considered, with respect to seeking service user permission and the timely sharing of information, and this may be particularly pertinent to SDM in the context of perinatal mental health where pregnancy and childbirth is a time of intense family involvement.

Midwives/relationships with others and decision-making

Perinatal mental healthcare in the UK (at its most basic) is characterised by close cooperation between midwives, obstetricians, perinatal mental health nurses, psychiatrists, health visitors, and general practitioners. The level of conflict or cooperation between these depends on the organisations and the culture of the working environment. Research from other areas of midwifery care demonstrate that where collaboration is effective, women feel confident about the decisions they make and consequently are more likely to be happier with their overall experience of maternity care (Freeman and Griew, 2007). Furthermore, collaboration and respectful team working are likely to influence staff satisfaction. It is widely accepted that philosophical differences over childbirth practice can generate tension – equally this tension exists when philosophical differences about mental illness exist. Some of these differences between health professionals and practitioners are rooted in assumptions and beliefs – and these differences can impact upon health professional's decision-making and subsequent care/treatment. Whilst models of care for PMH care vary across the world, and there are variations in the rates of common mental health problems, such as perinatal anxiety and depression between low- and middle-income countries compared to high-income countries, cooperation is the key for successful shared decision-making, and one of the challenges being faced on a global level is how it can be achieved in countries where the infrastructure for care delivery is less well developed.

The complexities of supporting women with perinatal mental health conditions

Women with mental health problems frequently have a number of issues in their lives which impact upon their interaction, uptake and decision-making about their health. Understanding these complexities is critical for the informed healthcare provider to make compassionate and insightful decisions and plans when engaging this patient group.

Women with mental health problems are likely to have more complicated pregnancies (Judd, 2014), with higher rates of pre-eclampsia and gestational diabetes (Nguyen et al., 2013); their babies are at risk of poor outcomes, such as preterm delivery (Pare Miron et al., 2016) and low birth weight (Kitai et al., 2014); and these outcomes are influenced by social economic determinants common in this population, such as higher rates of smoking (Prochaska, Das and Young-Wolff, 2017), lack of social support (Hetherington et al., 2017), lack of maternity care and poor nutrition.

Poverty is one of the most significant determinants of health, including mental health. Experiencing poverty in childhood is associated with global poor outcomes in adulthood and significantly higher rates of every mental illness (Sylvestyre et al., 2018). Families living in poverty frequently have problems with debt and poor housing and other limits to their finances and time. These factors are likely to lead to pressing priorities in terms of the woman's ability to engage with antenatal care, including perinatal mental health care. A UK study found that only 24.8% of women offered specialist perinatal mental health support were attending their appointments (Jones et al., 2017), with a global acknowledgement that perinatal mental health issues often go undetected and untreated (Vivieros and Darling, 2018).

Substance misuse and mental illness have higher incidence through the childbearing years (Hamilton and Campbell, 2013). Women with mental health problems are at increased risk of domestic violence (Khalifeh et al., 2015). There is significant evidence suggesting that domestic violence increases risk for the pregnant woman and baby across a number of issues, including low birth weight and preterm labour (Ferraro et al., 2017, Hamilton and Campbell, 2013). Research suggests that women are fearful of disclosing issues relating to their mental health problems due to concerns about stigma and judgement from professionals, peers or family members (Dolman et al., 2013). Women frequently feel ashamed about their condition and are concerned that others may make assumptions about their ability to parent based upon their diagnosis of mental health problems (Engqvist et al., 2009). This problem can be compounded by the fact that in some non-Westernised countries, there is a cultural unacceptability of mental health, leading to an attitude of cultural stoicism in the face of adversity (Edge, 2006), which was identified in research focused on the absence of perinatal depression in Black Caribbean women.

Mothers are also concerned that their baby and children may be removed from their care as a result of child protection proceedings if they experience mental health issues. This will impact upon their ability to engage with services (Khalifeh et al., 2009).

Identifying women with or at risk of developing mental health problems within the perinatal period is therefore key in order that timely management and support strategies using a biopsychosocial model of care can be put in place. Receiving individualised care from a known identified person is likely to increase engagement with the healthcare professional (Perriman and Davies, 2018). Therefore understanding and conceptualising the competing factors that woman who are pregnant and have a mental health problem face is critical in embracing a true collaboration, in order to inform and undertake SDM. Critically women are more likely to follow a healthcare plan if they feel collaborated with in the decision-making process (Joosten et al., 2008).

Determining the treatment and support needs for women in high-risk groups is essential in order to identify and intervene in a holistic way for women with mental illness and their families. Mental health problems have been identified as a leading cause of perinatal maternal mortality and morbidity (Knight et al., 2015, 2018). There are particular clinical scenarios that should identify women as at particularly high risk; these scenarios are called 'Red Flag' presentations, which include:

- Recent significant change in mental state or emergence of new symptoms
- New thoughts or acts of violent self-harm
- New and persistent expressions of incompetency as a mother or estrangement from the infant (Knight et al., 2018).

There is a lack of evidence regarding the impact of perinatal mental illness in low- to middle-income countries. Yet, it is clear that rates of mental illness are significantly higher in the most socially and economically deprived communities, particularly where families in rural areas are living in crowded households. Gender-based factors are important and include bias against female babies, role restriction regarding childcare and domestic duties, and domestic abuse have a significant impact upon a woman's mental health (Fisher et al., 2012). Some of these relationships are bidirectional, suggesting that developing or scaling up interventions to improve mental health may support efforts to achieve improved health outcomes more broadly, for example, adherence to HIV antiretroviral therapy and improved growth in newborn infants (Tsai and Tomlinson, 2012). Simply adding to the responsibilities of medical officers working within already overburdened primary healthcare systems, however, is probably a non-starter. Interventions using lay health workers in community-based perinatal care interventions is showing some promise (Tsai and Tomlinson 2012), where SDM could play a critical part.

Women with a diagnosis of bipolar disorder and women with a previous diagnosis of post-partum psychosis require particular care and planning when pregnant due to the significant risk of relapse in the perinatal period. The perinatal period is a unique period in an individual's life, where a risk of relapse of a mental illness can be predicted and managed in advance (Salim, Sharma and Anderson, 2018), and this should provide opportunity to intervene and support decision-making for the woman, her family and caregiver, irrespective of who that caregiver is.

Decision-making in high-risk groups

Women with a diagnosis of bipolar disorder have a 37% risk of relapse in the postpartum period, and women with a previous history of postpartum psychosis have a 31% risk of relapse in the postpartum period (Wesseloo et al., 2016). Women with bipolar disorder who discontinue medication during pregnancy can have a 71% risk of relapse (Viguera et al., 2007). Identifying and supporting women with these conditions during pregnancy and in the postpartum and understanding the key decisions regarding their treatment is critical. There are challenging treatment decisions for women and the health professional, as the main treatment for these conditions is a medication that may bring risk to the developing foetus. Decisions about treatment are best made prior to pregnancy, and ideally at least six months prior to a pregnancy, so that any changes to a woman's medication can be made and stabilisation can occur following medication changes, or cessation can take place. Decisions about medication should only take place after careful reviewing of the risks and benefits of starting, changing or ceasing treatment (Knight et al., 2018). The risks of fetal medication exposure needs to be balanced with the risk of maternal mental illness during pregnancy, breastfeeding and the postnatal period and the impact that this may have on the baby and the wider family.

Women sometimes feel that they haven't been given enough information; they want to understand the short- and long-term risks to themselves and their babies and be actively involved in decision-making (Santuki et al., 2010). Aspects of the course and treatment of the illness should be discussed with all women and their partners/families, taking into account heritability; this information should be discussed at regular points prior to pregnancy, taking into account the impact on pregnancy and the postnatal period (Stevens et al., 2018). A collaborative care approach should be offered so that information provided between the health professionals is not conflicting. Providing information to women and their families may be difficult due to the lack of consensus in a number of areas relating to the safety and efficacy of medication for bipolar disorder in pregnancy and breastfeeding (Parker, Graham and Tavella, 2017).

Decisions about medications are recognised as being fundamental to both clinicians and patients, and this is also one of the areas where there is likely to be conflict regarding the ultimate decision that is made (Hamman et al., 2008). It has been suggested that in this situation, particularly where conflict may occur, that what may appear to be a paternalistic intervention by the healthcare professional, such as stopping a medication in pregnancy or not starting a medication, may in fact be some form of advocating role for a secondary patient (i.e. the baby/foetus) (Macfarlane and Greenhalgh, 2018). The legal rights of the foetus will differ globally, and this has to be taken into consideration within the broader context of decision-making and medication.

But by placing the patient at the centre of the decision-making role, it is possible to maximise individual autonomy, promote a person-centred recovery and instil hope, and these themes have been central to individual's personal recovery narratives (Deegan, 1996).

BOX 9.1   CASE EXAMPLE 1

Jenny is 28 years old and pregnant with her first child. She lives with her partner of two years and works full time in a shop. Jenny has experienced problems with her mental health for a number of years and first became unwell at age 19 when she was at university. She was admitted to a mental health unit and detained under the Mental Health Act. She experienced a period of elated mood and experienced delusional beliefs. Jenny has experienced symptoms of depression at times. Jenny has been well over the last couple of years and is prescribed quetiapine, which she continues to take daily. Jenny attends her booking-in appointment with her partner and has a number of questions about her medication; she wonders whether she should stop taking it and is concerned about how it might affect the baby's development. She has a diagnosis of bipolar disorder.

Healthcare providers are ideally placed to help a woman and her partner/family make decisions about medication, both in pregnancy and breastfeeding. Discussions about medications choices are unlikely to be static and will vary dependent on mental health issues, concerns about current or relapsing mental health problems and the woman's thoughts and any concerns that she may have about the medication impacting on the foetus/baby. Research suggest that women also rely on their own experiences and cultural understandings and can be influenced by their families, their partners and societal norms (McDonald, Amir and Davey, 2012). Many women in these situations are conflicted as they navigate the competing priorities of their own health and those of their developing child. These conflicts are compounded for women with mental health problems due to their inherent and complex challenges and adversities.

Discussions about treatments should take place ideally in the preconception period and continue throughout the pregnancy and into the postpartum period, when any concerns about relapsing mental health issues can be identified and managed in a collaborative and proactive manner. Despite increasing advice to women regarding the need for preconception care, Jenny's situation is common. She is pregnant, has a long-term condition, and requires medication treatment. Yet, she does not have a predetermined and collaborative plan for her treatment in pregnancy, for breastfeeding and beyond. Evidence suggests this may be a familiar scenario: in the UK, around half of pregnancies are unplanned (Wellings et al., 2013). In France, a third of pregnancies may be unplanned (Bajos et al., 2003), 40% in Spain (Font-Ribera et al., 2008) almost half in Japan (Goto et al., 2002), and over a third in the United States (Mosher, Jones and Abma, 2012), indicating that the midwife, or the first-line healthcare provider, needs to have confidence in opening a dialogue with women about their mental health needs in the context of family planning.

In the UK there has been significant investment in the development of Specialist Perinatal Mental Health Services with national priorities to expand services to reduce access problems and develop informed care pathways across cultural and social groups (NHS England, 2016). However, globally there is a large treatment gap, particularly in low- to middle-income countries (Eaton et al., 2011). The midwife or nurse is often faced with how to advise the woman in the first instance and determine whether referral to specialist services should take place, if they are available. In the absence of specialist services, the midwife may be best placed to liaise with other healthcare professionals and commence a dialogue with the woman and her family. We propose the midwife (or any healthcare provider) can offer information and advice based on the readily available internet resources. Indeed, evidence suggests that healthcare professionals with no formal training in mental health can effectively deliver mental health services in low-resource settings in low- and middle-income countries (Singla et al., 2017; Van Ginneken et al., 2013), as well as lay community workers (Tsai and Tomlinson, 2012).

Use of technology in decision-making

The internet is an easy to access resource for patients wishing to access health information and has become widely used (Kummervold et al., 2008). There are a number of online resources available for patients and health professionals to use in order to gain current and accurate information about medication in relation to pregnancy and breastfeeding. Encouraging and supporting patients to access these resources will improve the shared element of decision-making and shift the weight of responsibility from the health professional to a more mutual standpoint, improving both communication and the therapeutic alliance (Gerber and Eiser, 2001). This will also improve participation around informed decision-making, optimising the patient's compliance with the treatment plan (Magnavita, 2016). However there are a number of factors that may impede on an individual's ability to make use of the electronic resources, with economic issues being a key factor (Gilmour, 2007). Individuals and families may not own a computer or have access to the internet. This is more common in low-income families and countries; it is termed 'the digital divide'. In addition, patients may not have the required information technology (IT) skills that are required to access the resources (Latulippe, Hamel and Giroux, 2017).

Services providing information about the risk of exposure of a foetus to medications during pregnancy and breastfeeding have developed internationally, including in North America (Organization of Teratology Information Specialists (OTIS)) and Europe and South America (European Network of Teratology Information Services (ENTIS)). These services also operate in Asia and Australia (Hancock et al., 2010).

Detailed evidence-based information regarding fetal risk following medication exposure is available from the UK Teratology Information Service (UKTIS). This organisation also provides information for patients on the patient-focused website Bumps (Best Use of Medicines in Pregnancy).

The LactMed database and app provides free access to a peer-reviewed database of medications and supplements and their impact on breast milk. Drug levels in infant blood and breast milk are reported along with potential adverse effects in the nursing infant. Alternatives for medications are also provided (Fitzpatrick, 2007; Krauscopf, 2018).

In addition to these resources, Table 9.1, adapted for SDM from Macfarlane and Greenhalgh (2018), can facilitate decision-making about taking a medication whilst breastfeeding. We have used Jenny's case to illuminate how a health professional may navigate the information required and present the information to a patient in order for enhance evidence based shared decision-making.

It is the role of health professionals and care providers to assist the patient in navigating the uncertainties in this kind of decision-making. Uncertainties will always be present where there is a lack of empirical evidence; however, having confidence in where and how to access information to share with the patient is likely to improve the confidence of the clinician. What is key here is that the health professional offers consistent, educated professional guidance and support in the difficult process of reaching a decision.

TABLE 9.1 Decision-making plan (Macfarlane and Greenhalgh, 2018)

Frequently asked questions	Continuing the current dose of quetiapine	Lowering the current dose of quetiapine	Stopping taking quetiapine	Changing to another medication
What does it involve?	No change to medication or dose	Over a period of weeks to months, decreasing the amount of quetiapine	Over a period of weeks to months, gradually stopping quetiapine	Switching to a different medication (e.g. lamotrigine or an antipsychotic)
What are the risks to me?	Usual side effects of quetiapine Increased risk of gestational diabetes	Usual side effects of quetiapine, potential for relapse	Higher risk of relapse (depends on a variety of factors – discuss with your clinician), increased risk of puerperal psychosis	Risk of relapse if the other medication is not as effective as quetiapine; risk of new side effects
What are the risks to my baby?	Withdrawal symptoms in the newborn Neonatal adaptation syndrome Risks if mother develops gestational diabetes	Reduced risk of withdrawal symptoms in the newborn Reduced risk of neonatal adaptation syndrome (risk depends on the dose – discuss with your clinician)	Indirect risks, e.g. disinhibition from poorly controlled bipolar disorder (discuss with your clinician)	Some medications are more harmful for your unborn baby
What are the benefits?	You are less likely to relapse or suffer from puerperal psychosis	Your unborn baby will have a lower risk of neonatal adaptation syndrome than if you continue the full dose	Your unborn baby will have the same risk as the general population	If you can tolerate the new drug, you are less likely to relapse or suffer from puerperal psychosis; the other medication could have adverse effects
Who would benefit most from this?	People with bipolar disorder who have been on the medication for some time and remained well who are not controlled on other medication or lower doses of quetiapine	People with bipolar disorder who are well controlled on quetiapine and have not had a relapse for some time	People who have been stable off quetiapine and do not wish to take other medications during pregnancy	People who are not stable on quetiapine, but have been well on alternatives to quetiapine

How will the medicine affect my baby if I breastfeed?	Low levels of the drug transferred to the baby, if under 400 mg daily. Monitor baby for feeding and drowsiness. Exercise further caution if baby is premature, small for gestational date, or has other health complications	Lower level of the drug transferred to the baby. Monitor baby for feeding and drowsiness. Exercise further caution if baby is premature, small for gestational date, or has other health complications	Effect not known	Dependent on choice of medication
How will this affect lactation?	Minimal effect	Minimal effect	Minimal effect	Dependent on medication of choice

Note: The guidance on the use of this drug has been taken from UKTIS and LactMed

Training and support for midwifery and maternity staff

As we have previously identified in this chapter, midwifery and maternity staff as decision-makers can be faced with very difficult choices when it comes to addressing issues of perinatal mental health and illness. Improving the quality of these decisions is of great consequence to perinatal well-being. In the UK, there is a firm policy remit for PMI in its broadest sense and across the maternity spectrum. Maternity health professionals have had a traditional remit to identify and manage perinatal depression, but not the broader spectrum of PMI. Healthcare practitioners caring for pregnant and postnatal women are therefore challenged with identifying both those women who present with a pre-existing mental illness and those for whom childbearing results in some level of PMI. Training has shown to positively impact the ability of health professionals to identify and support women with PMI and to facilitate the process of decision-making within that context (Jomeen et al., 2013; Jones et al., 2015). Developing the skills of maternity professionals to support women and their families in need of PMI support has become key to the achievement of the Governments ambition to reduce the number of stillbirths, neonatal deaths, maternal deaths and brain injuries that occur during or soon after birth by 20% by 2020, and by 50% by 2030 (HEE, 2010a). The Perinatal Mental Health Care Skills Competency Framework (HEE, 2010b) is just one resource available for professionals who work with mothers and families from preconception until one year postnatal to identify required skills and assess team training needs for identifying and supporting women with perinatal mental illness. Research by Jones et al. (2015) exploring the impact of PMH training on health visitor's knowledge and confidence highlighted the ways in which a brief training package facilitates not only improved knowledge but also the ability to apply that knowledge to clinical identification and decision-making, referral decisions and care pathways, resulting in far more person-centred care. It should be noted that whilst training plays a significant part in improving confidence and decision-making, a lack of confidence to identify and manage women can be inherently linked to a perceived lack of availability and access to any specialised PMH services, which potentially may underpin a fear to identify a problem (Jones et al., 2015). Training to enhance decision-making in this context may only be effective if there are appropriate PMH pathways and services in place.

Conclusion

Most women will experience pregnancy, birth and the postpartum period without any need for perinatal mental health support. However, about 10% of pregnant women and 13% of women who have just given birth experience a mental disorder (WHO, 2019). For women and health professionals who require to make decisions about support and treatment when perinatal mental illness, or this risk of/potential for PMI is identified, this can be challenging, and may involve a 'mind shift' from the process of uncomplicated 'normal' pregnancy, birth and postpartum, to having to consider the possibility of a different pregnancy trajectory. This chapter outlines some of the existing decision-making theory that can be applied to cases where PMI is identified. In addition, we provide some strategies and resources for making these practice decisions.

Women with PMI will enter the maternity episode with a set of aspirations for pregnancy and birth. They will be capable of synthesising complicated information in the face of their diagnosis. Their experience of their care, their health and their adherence/compliance with treatment can be enhanced by healthcare professionals embracing shared decision-making and having a considered, nuanced understanding of perinatal mental illness. There are a number of evidence-based decision-making tools that can be used by healthcare providers, depending on where they live, though it is acknowledged that infrastructure and resource issues remain in many parts of the world.

References

Bajos, N., Leridon, H., Goulard, H., Oustry, P. and Job-Spira, N. (2003) The COCON group contraception: from accessibility to efficiency. *Human Reproduction*, 18, 994–999.

Bradley, E. and Green, D. (2018) Involved, inputting or informing: 'Shared' decision making in adult mental health care. *Health Expectations*, 21 (1), 192–200.

Chong, W., Aslani, P. and Chen, T. (2013) Shared decision making and interprofessional collaboration in mental healthcare: a qualitative study exploring perceptions of barriers and facilitators. *Journal of Interprofessional Care*, 27 (5), 373–379.

Coultier, A. (2010) *Implementing Shared Decision Making in the UK*. A Report for the Health Foundation. London: The Health Foundation.

Deegan, P. E. (1996) Recovery as a journey of the heart. *Psychiatric Rehabilitation Journal* 19 (3), 91–97.

Dolman, C., Jones, I. and Howard, L. (2013) Preconception to parenting: a systematic review and meta-synthesis of the qualitative literature on motherhood for women with severe mental illness. *Archives of Women's Mental Health*, 16 (3), 173–196.

Eaton, J., McCay, L., Semrau, M., Chattergee, S., Bainjana, F., Araya, R., Ntulo, C., Thornicroft, J. and Saxena, S. (2011) Scale up services for mental health in low income and middle income countries. *The Lancet*, 378, 1592–1603.

Edge, D. (2006) Perinatal depression in black Caribbean women: lessons for primary care. *Primary Health Care*, 17 (2), 32–35.

Elwyn, G., Durand, M., Song, J., Aarts, J., Barr, P., Berger, Z., Cochran, N., Frosch, D., Galansinki, D., Guldbrandsen, P., Han, P., Harter, M., Klinnersley, P., Lloyd, A., Mischra, M., Perestelo-Perez, L., Scholl, I., Tomori, K., Trevena, L., Wittemann, H. and Van Der Weijden, T. (2017) A three talk model for shared decision making: multistage consultation process. *British Medical Journal*, 359, 4891.

Elwyn, G., Frosch, D., Thompson, R., Joseph-Williams, N., Lloyd, A., Kinnersley, P., Cording, E., Tomson, D., Dodd, C., Rollnick, S., Edwards, A. and Barry, M. (2012) Shared decision making a model for clinical practice. *Journal of General Internal Medicine*, 27 (10), 1361–1367.

Engqvist, I., Ferszt, A., Ahlin, A. and Nilsson, K. (2009) Psychiatric nurses descriptions of women with postpartum psychosis and nurses responses – an exploratory study in Sweden. *Issues in Mental Health Nursing*, 30 (1), 23–30.

Ferraro, A. A., Rohde, L. A., Polanczyk, G. V., Argeu, A., Miguel, E. C., Grisi A and Fleitlich-Bilyk, B. (2017). The specific and combined role of domestic violence and mental health disorders during pregnancy on new-born health. *BMC Pregnancy and Childbirth*. https://doi.org/10.1186/s12884-017-1438-x

Fisher, J., Cabral de Mello, M., Patel, V., Rahman, A., Tran, T., Hilton, S. and Holmes, W. (2012) Prevalence and determinants of common perinatal mental health disorder in women in low and lower-middle income countries: a systematic review. *Bulletin of the World Health Organization*, 90, 139–149.

Fitzpatrick, R. B. (2007) Information Rx. LactMed: drugs and lactation database. *Journal of Electronic Resources in Medical Libraries*, 4 (1), 155–166.

Font-Ribera, L., Pérez, G., Salvador, J. and Borrell, C. (2008) Socioeconomic inequalities in unintended pregnancy and abortion decision. *Journal of Urban Health: Bulletin of the New York Academy of Medicine*, 85 (1), 125–135. doi:10.1007/s11524-007-9233-z

Freeman, L. M. & Griew, K. (2007) Enhancing the midwife–woman relationship through shared decision making and clinical guidelines. *Women and Birth*, 20 (1), 11–15.

Gerber, G. B. and Eiser, A. R. (2001) The patient physician relationship in the internet age: future prospects and the research agenda. *Journal of Medical Internet Research*, 3 (2), 15.

Gilmour, J. (2007) Reducing disparities in the access and use of internet health information. A discussion paper. *International Journal of Nursing Studies*, 44 (7), 1270–1278.

Goto, A., Yasumura, S., Reich, M.R. and Fukao, A. (2002) Factors associated with unintended pregnancy in Yamagata Japan. *Social Science and Medicine*, 54, 1065–1079.

Hamilton, I. and Campbell, A. (2013) Antenatal comorbidity of mental health and substance use: assessment and engagement. *British Journal of Midwifery*, 21 (11), 768–773.

Hamman, J., Mendel, R.T., Fink, B., Pfeiffer, H., Cohen, R. and Kissling, W. (2008) Patients and psychiatrists perceptions of clinical decision making during schizophrenia treatment. *Journal of Nervous Mental Disorder*, 196, 329–332.

Hancock, R., Ungar, W., Einarson, A. and Koren, G. (2010) International practices in the provision of teratology information: a survey of international teratogen information programmes and comparisons with the North American model. *Journal of Evaluation in Clinical Practice*, 16 (5), 957–963.

Health Education England. (2010a) Perinatal mental health. Available online at www.hee.nhs.uk/our-work/mental-health/perinatal-mental-health (Accessed 21st January 2019).

Health Education England. (2010b) The perinatal mental health care skills competency framework. Available online at https://tavistockandportman.nhs.uk/training/workforce-development/competency-framework-perinatal-mental-health/ (Accessed 21st January 2019).

Hetherington, E., McDonald, S., Williamson, T., Pathen, S. and Tough, S. (2017) Social support and maternal mental health at 4 months and 1 year postpartum: analysis from the all our families cohort. *Journal of Epidemiology and Community Health*, 72, 10.

Jomeen, J., Glover, L., Jones, C., Garg, D. and Marshall, C. (2013) Identifying and assessing women's perinatal psychological health: exploring the experiences of health visitors. *Journal of Reproductive and Infant Psychology*, 31.

Jones, C., Jomeen, J., Glover, L., Gardiner, E., Garg, D. and Marshall, C. (2015) Exploring changes in health visitor's knowledge, confidence, and decision making for women with perinatal mental health difficulties following a brief training package. *European Journal for Person Centred Healthcare*, 3 (3), 384–389.

Jones, C., Wadephul, F., Jomeen, J. and Marshall, C. (2017) *Non-attendance and attendance in perinatal mental health care*. Report submitted to Hull Clinical Commissioning Group. Hull: University of Hull.

Joosten, E., DeFuentes-Merillas, G., de Wert, T., Sensky, C., van der Staak, C. and De Jong, C. (2008) Systematic reviews of the effects of shared decision making on patient satisfaction, treatment adherence and health status. *Psychotherapy and Psychosomatics*, 77 (4), 219–226.

Judd, F., Komiti, A., Sheehan, P., Newman, L., Castle, D. and Everall, I. (2014) Adverse obstetric and neonatal outcomes in women with severe mental illness: to what extent can they be prevented? *Schizophrenia Research*, 157 (1–3), 305–309.

Khalifeh, H., Moran, P., Borschmann, R. and Dean, K. (2015) Domestic and sexual violence against patients with severe mental illness. *Psychological Medicine*, 45 (4), 875–886.

Khalifeh, H., Murgatroyd, M., Freeman, S., Johnson, H. and Killaspy, H. (2009) Home treatment as an alternative to hospital admission for mothers in a mental health crisis: a qualitative study. *Psychiatric Services*, 60 (5), 634–639.

Kitai, T., Komoto, Y., Kagubari, R., Konishi, H., Tanaka, E., Nakajima, S., Muraji, M., Ugaki, H., Matsunaga, H. and Takemura, M. (2014) A comparison of maternal and neonatal outcomes of pregnancy with mental disorders: results of an analysis with propensity score-based weighting. *Archives of Gynaecology and Obstetrics*, 290 (5), 883–889.

Knight, M., Bunch, K., Tuffnell, D., Jayakody, H., Shakespeare, J., Kotnis, R., Kenyon, S., Kurinczuk, J.J. (Eds.) (2018) On Behalf of Mbrrace-UK. *Saving lives, improving mothers' care – lessons learned to inform maternity care from the UK and Ireland confidential enquiries into maternal deaths and morbidity 2014–16*. Oxford: National Perinatal Epidemiology Unit, University of Oxford.

Knight, M., Tuffnell, D., Kenyon, S., Shakespeare, J., Gray, R., Kurinczuk, J.J. Eds. (2015) On Behalf of Mbrrace-UK. *Saving lives, improving mothers' care – surveillance of maternal deaths in the UK 2011–13 and lessons learned to inform maternity care from the UK and Ireland confidential enquiries into maternal deaths and morbidity 2009–13*. Oxford: National Perinatal Epidemiology Unit, University of Oxford.

Krauscopf, P. (2018) LactMed and heads up apps. *Journal for Nurse Practitioners*, 14 (6), e134.

Kummervold, P. E., Chronaki, C. E., Lausen, B., Prokosch, H., Rasmussen, J., Santana, S., Staniszewski, A. and Wangberg, S. C. (2008) eHealth trends in Europe 2005–2007: a population-based survey. *Journal of Medical Internet Research*, 10(4), e42.

Latulippe, K., Hamel, C. and Giroux, D. (2017). Social health inequalities and eHealth: a literature review with qualitative synthesis of theoretical and empirical studies. *Journal of Medical Internet Research*, 19 (4), e136.

Legare, F. and Thompson-Leduc, P. (2014) Twelve myths about shared decision making. *Patient Education and Counselling*, 96, 281–286.

Macfarlane, A. and Greenhalgh, T. (2018) Sodium valproate in pregnancy: what are the risks and should we use a shared decision making approach? *BMC Pregnancy and Childbirth*, 18 (1), 200.

Magnavita, J. (2016) *Clinical decision making in mental health practice*. First edition. Washington, DC: American Psychiatric Association. 189.

McDonald, K., Amir, L. and Davey, M. (2012) Maternal bodies and medicines: a commentary on risk and decision making of pregnant and breastfeeding women and health professionals. *Neonatal Intensive Care*, 25 (2), 38–55.

Molenaar, J., Korstjens, I., Hendrix, M., DeVries, R. and Nieuwenhuijze, M. (2018) Needs of parents and professionals to improve shared decision making in interprofessional maternity practice: a qualitative study. *Birth Issues in Perinatal Care*, 45, 245–254.

Mosher, W. D., Jones, J. and Abma, J.C. (2012) Intended and unintended births in the United States: 1982–2010. *National Health Statistics Report*, 55, July 24.

Nguyen, T., Faulkner, J., Frayne, S., Allen, Y., Hauck, D., Rock, D. and Rampono, J. (2013) Obstetric and neonatal outcomes of pregnant women with severe mental illness at a specialist antenatal clinic. *Medical Journal of Australia*, 199 (3), 26.

NHS England. (2016) The five year forward view for mental health. A Report from the Mental Health Taskforce to the NHS in England. NHS England.

NICE. (2014) Antenatal and postnatal mental health: clinical management and service guidance. Available at www.nice.org.uk/guidance/cg192/.

Pare Miron, V., Czuzoj-Schilman, N., Oddy, L., Spence, A. & Abenhaim, H. (2016) Effect of borderline personality disorder on obstetrical and neonatal outcomes. *Women's Health Issues*, 26 (6), 190–195.

Park, E. and Cho, I. (2018) Shared decision making in the paediatric field: a literature review and concept analysis. *Scandinavian Journal of Caring Sciences*, 32 (2), 478–489.

Parker, G., Graham, R. and Tavella, G. 2017. Is there a consensus across international evidence based guidelines for the management of bipolar disorder? *Acta Psychiatrica Scandinavica*, 135 (6), 515–526.

Patel, S. and Wisner, K. (2011) Decision making for depression treatment during pregnancy and the postpartum period. *Depression and Anxiety*, 28 (7), 589–595.

Perriman, N. and Davies, D. (2018) What women value in the midwifery continuity of care model: a systematic review with meta-synthesis. *Midwifery*, 62, 220–229.

Price, S. & Bentley, K. (2013) Psychopharmacology decision making among pregnant and postpartum women and health providers. *Women and Health*, 53 (2), 154–172.

Prochaska, J., Das, S. and Young-Wolff, K. (2017) Smoking, mental illness and public health. *Annual Review of Public Health*, 38, 165–185.

Remenick, A., Whitfield, T., Zurick, A., Stowe, Z., Newport, D., Viguera, A., Cohen, L. and Baldessarini, R. (2007) Risk of recurrence in women with bipolar disorder during pregnancy: prospective study of mood stabiliser discontinuation. *American Journal of Psychiatry*, 164 (12), 1817–1824.

Rosenbaum, L. (2015) The paternalism preference: choosing unshared decision making. *New England Journal of Medicine*, 373, 589–592.

Salim, M., Sharma, V. and Anderson, K. (2018) Recurrence of bipolar disorder during pregnancy: a systematic review. *Archives of Women's Mental Health*, 21, 475–479.

Santuki, A., Gold, M., Akers, A., Borrero, S. and Schwatz, E. (2010) Women's perspectives on counselling about risks for medication induced birth defects. *Birth Defects Research*, 88 64–69.

Singla, D., Kohrt, B., Murray, L., Anand, A., Chorpita, B. and Patel, V. (2017) Psychological treatments for the world: lessons from low and middle income countries. *Annual Review of Clinical Psychology*, 8 (13), 149–181.

Slade, M. (2017) Implementing shared decision making in routine mental healthcare. *World Psychiatry*, 1, 146–153.

Stevens, A., Daggenvoorde, T., van der Klis, S., Kupta, R. and Goosens, P. (2018) Thoughts and considerations of women with bipolar disorder about family planning and pregnancy: a qualitative study. *Journal of the American Nurses Association*, 24 (2), 118.

Sylvestyre, J., Notten, N., Kerman, A., Pollilo, K. and Czechowki, K. (2018) Poverty and serious mental illness: Towards action on a seemingly intractable problem. *American Journal of Community Psychology*, 61 (1–2), 153–165.

Tomlinson, J. (2018) Letters. *British Medical Journal*. 360, k53.

Truglio-Londrigan, M. and Slyer, J. (2018) Shared decision making for nursing practice: an integrative review. *The Open Nursing Journal*, 12, 1–14.

Tsai, A.C. and Tomlinson, M. (2012). Mental health spill overs and the millennium development goals: the case of perinatal depression in Khayelitsha, South Africa. *Journal of Global Health*, 2 (1), 010302.

Van Ginneken, N., Tharyan, P., Lewin, S., Rao, G.N., Meera, S., Pian, J., Chandrashekar, S. and Patel, V. (2013) Non-specialist health worker interventions for the care of mental, neurological and substance-abuse disorders in low-and middle-income countries. *The Cochrane Database of Systematic Reviews*, Nov 19 (11), CD009149.

Viguera, A.C., Whitfield, T., Baldessarini, R.J., Newport, D.L., Stowe, Z., Reminick, A., Zurick, A. & Cohen, L.S. (2007) Risk of recurrence in women with bipolar disorder during pregnancy: prospective study of mood stabilizer discontinuation. *American Journal of Psychiatry*, 164 (12), 1817–1824.

Vivieros, C. and Darling, E. (2018) Barriers and facilitators of accessing perinatal mental health services: the perspectives of women receiving continuity of care midwifery. *Midwifery*, 65, 81.

Wellings, K., Jones, K., Mercer, C., Tanton, C., Clifton, S., Datta, J., Copas, A., Erens, B., Gibson, L., Macdowall, W., Sonnenburg, P., Phelps, A. and Johnson, A. (2013) The prevalence of unplanned pregnancy and associated factors in Britain: findings from the third national survey of sexual attitudes and lifestyles (Natsal-3). *The Lancet: North American Edition*, 383 (9907).

Wesseloo, R., Kamperman, A., Munk-Olsen, T., Pop, V., Kushner, S. and Bergink, V. (2016) Risk of postpartum relapse in bipolar disorder and postpartum psychosis: a systematic review and meta-analysis. *American Journal of Psychiatry*, 173, 117–127.

World Health Organization (WHO). (2019) Maternal mental health. Available online at www.who.int/mental_health/maternal-child/maternal_mental_health/en/.

10

STRESS URINARY INCONTINENCE IN PREGNANCY AND COLLABORATIVE DECISION-MAKING

Jinguo Helen Zhai and Elaine Jefford

Chapter overview

Stress urinary incontinence (SUI) is defined as the involuntary loss of urine on effort or physical exertion, or on sneezing or coughing. This can occur anytime during the childbearing journey, although it is more prevalent in the last trimester. For midwives to support women who experience SUI, it is imperative they are aware of the possible reasons it occurs, what treatments might be offered and how SUI can impact a woman's quality of life. These aspects are explored within this chapter with the aim of facilitating the midwife to provide information when engaging in a shared decision-making approach with women.

Introduction

Approximately 80% of pregnant women, both primigravidae and multigravidae, experience increased micturition frequency at some time during pregnancy (Sangsawang & Sangsawang 2013). The first trimester is the most common time of onset (DeLancey 2010). The increasing weight of the uterus is the most common factor affecting micturition frequency throughout the pregnancy, as the growing uterus not only exerts pressure on the bladder but also irritates it. Compounding this bladder irritation during late pregnancy is the descent of the presenting part of the foetus. During the postnatal period, as women's hormone levels return to their pre-pregnancy levels, and pressure of the enlarged uterus on the bladder and pelvic floor muscles resolves, in most cases so does micturition frequency (King et al. 2019).

Stress urinary incontinence in childbirth

In general, incontinence in women is typically related to dysfunction of the bladder or pelvic floor muscles. Such dysfunction often arises during pregnancy or childbirth, or during menopause. Most early epidemiological studies did not, however, differentiate between stress and urgency of urinary incontinence. For women around the world, Stress urinary incontinence (SUI) is more common than urgency incontinence. According to the International

Urogynecological Association (IUGA) and the International Continence Society (ICS), the standard definition of SUI is the complaint of urine leakage in association with coughing, sneezing or physical exertion. Despite the International Classification of Diseases (ICD) categorisation, some policymakers, members of the medical profession and the general public remain unaware that SUI is a disease.

Although not life-threatening, SUI can certainly prove to be life-changing and is a contributing risk factor for poor quality of life (QOL). For example, SUI has been noted to have a negative effect on one's mental health as well as impact upon engagement and enjoyment in social activities (Aoki et al. 2017). In pregnant women, approximately 54.3% report their QOL was affected by SUI across four domains: physical activity, travel, social relationships and emotional health. In a comparative study (Zhai et al. 2017) between Chinese and American women, it was found there were significant differences related to the influence of urine leakage within the Chinese women, on their QOL (IIQ-SF). This was specifically related to physical activity, travel, social relationships and emotional health ($p < 0.001$) (Zhai et al. 2017). Interlinked with these multifarious elements of SUI and the impact on a woman's QOL is that it is considered a stigmatising condition in most cultures. This latter point has been noted to contribute to low rates of women seeking help or treatment (Heesakkers & deVries 2018).

Risk factors and common reasons for SUI in childbirth

It is imperative that midwives understand the risk factors and common reasons for SUI in childbirth, as it has implications for midwives and the care they provide as well as influencing their decision-making processes. The main risk factors for development of SUI within childbirth are age, parity, obesity and type of birth. Yet, when focusing on a Chinese cohort of pregnant women, the authors found a new predictive model for SUI (Zhai et al. 2017). They found the predicting risk factors could be categorised in three specific areas: constipation, pre-pregnancy BMI level and a family history of SUI.

Normal bladder capacity in the first trimester is 410 ml and reduces to 272 ml in the third trimester (Sangsawang & Sangsawang 2013). Attributing to this bladder capacity reduction is descent of the presenting part of the foetus. The most common reasons why pregnant women suffer SUI, however, is urethral hypermobility, which may be contributed to hormonal changes during pregnancy that soften and relax muscle tone (King et al. 2019). As a result, there is a loss of support of the bladder neck and urethra, thus enabling the urethra to move downward without any abdominal pressure being exerted. The consequences of this movement is multifactorial, in that is there is lower pressure in the urethra than in the bladder, and there may be an increase in intra-abdominal pressure from coughing, sneezing, laughing, moving or during a contraction, in conjunction with increased irritability of detrusor muscles. The end result is that the pressure inside the bladder becomes greater than the urethral closure pressure and the urethral sphincter is not strong enough to maintain urethral closure, thus there is urine leakage (Aoki et al. 2017).

Genital trauma often associated with vaginal births, such as a third- and fourth-degree perineal tear or a surgical incision (episiotomy), may increase the incidence of SUI (Abdulaziz et al. 2017; Aasheim et al. 2017). Increased intra-rectal pressure during the second stage of labour and/or duration of this stage of labour has also been significantly correlated with some SUI and pelvic floor issues 14 months after spontaneous birth and forceps-assisted delivery in parous women (Meyer et al. 2017). It could therefore be postulated that for parous women, vaginal delivery is a key risk factor for SUI (Waqiah et al. 2019). In an Iranian cohort of primiparae women, vaginal birth was associated with a twofold increased risk of postpartum SUI after one month ($p < 0.001$), six months ($p < 0.001$) and 12 months ($p < 0.001$), along with instrument-assisted vaginal birth ($p < 0.001$) and episiotomy ($p < 0.001$) Kokabi and Yazdanpanah (2017). These findings are challenged, however, by Bo et al. (2016), who found no significant differences in prevalence of SUI (37.5% vs. 46.6%) or UI (23.6% vs. 35.6%), between women with or without episiotomy, respectively at six weeks postpartum in a cohort of 238 Norwegian nulliparous women. Horng et al. (2017), further refute Kokabi and Yazdanpanah's (2017) findings, when no difference in rates of SUI was found in their study comparing postpartum SUI between vaginal delivery and elective caesarean section (Horng et al. 2017). The authors also posed questions related to the instrument chosen for an assisted birth and its application with the risk and benefit ratio of a caesarean section. One also needs to be cautious as to the motive of comparing vaginal birth with planned caesarean and decide if it is an area worthy of study or if it is ethical. For example, the Twin Birth Study (Hutton et al. 2019) randomised women from 25 countries between 32 and 38 weeks of gestation with a twin pregnancy to planned caesarean or planned vaginal birth. The findings showed women who had a vaginal birth had higher SUI issues than those who had elective caesarean section 93/1147 (8.11%) versus 140/1143 (12.25%); odds ratio, 0.63; 95% confidence interval, 0.47–0.83; $p = 0.001$. Further, those women with SUI, their QoL was not different for planned caesarean versus planned vaginal birth groups (mean (SD): 18.4 (21.0) versus 19.1 (21.5); $p = 0.82$) (Hutton et al. 2019).

In a systematic review of the literature, Newton (2018) found that any position that expanded the pelvic outlet and decreased weight on the sacral area, such as kneeling, upright, on hands and knees, squatting and birthing chairs, were associated with increased perineal trauma. Yet, adopting an upright position in second stage of labour in an Italian cohort of women has been linked to lower rates of SUI and UI in women compared to supine birthing (40.5% vs. 48.9%, $p = 0.03$) (Serati et al. 2016) The perineum appeared to be protected in the lateral position (Newton 2018). It is worth noting that women who have experienced female genital mutilation (FGM) suffer with symptom prevalence and QoL impact from lower urinary tract symptoms (Geynisman-Tan et al. 2019). This can be exacerbated during childbirth. It however, beyond the scope of this chapter to explore FGM in depth.

In essence, therefore, pregnancy and birth-related factors/trauma are considered to be the main risk factors for SUI development during pregnancy (Ge et al. 2015; Macarthur et al. 2016; Van der Woude et al. 2015; Waqiah et al. 2019). It would be unethical to restrict a woman's choice of birthing position, or not to apply different perineal techniques to slow down the birth of the baby's head, allowing the perineum to stretch slowly to prevent injury. Prolonged second stage of labour requires midwives to consider the implications this has on the perineum both in the short and long term. It is important, therefore for midwives to discuss these elements with women so that informed choices and decisions can be made.

Midwifery decision-making and interventions/treatments: points to consider

Despite SUI potentially having detrimental effects on a woman's QOL, including but not limited to physical activity, travel, social relationships and emotional health and well-being (Aoki et al. 2017), not all women will seek advice or treatment. The reasons behind this are complex and diverse, which may well be influenced by culture, social norms, values and beliefs. For example, in an Indian study, 15.3% of 500 pregnant women suffering from SUI did not necessarily seek treatment, and it is postulated that this may be due to incontinence being accepted as normal within pregnancy and therefore women lack awareness of the condition being abnormal (Pryria et al. 2017). It is therefore imperative that midwives need to be aware of the sensitive nature of SUI and the potential physiological and personal implications suffering from it has on a woman. The midwife must draw upon her emotional intelligence and communication skills in order to uncover if a woman is suffering from SUI, understand what matters, what is valued and why for each woman. Once the subject of SUI has been raised, the midwife can engage in sharing information and decision-making. A model of decision-making that might help facilitate this is the Three-Talk Model for Shared Decision-Making (Elwyn et al. 2017). This model is discussed in Chapter 1, including its strengths and limitations. This model focuses on what is most important to the woman, and can help facilitate empowering her to engage and negotiate with the midwife and other health professionals. It is from this stance that the woman and midwife can begin to openly and honestly discuss treatment options. This is particularly important in view that SUI during pregnancy might not spontaneously resolve in the postnatal period, rather there may be short- and/or long-term implications for the woman and her QOL.

The most common type and first-line treatment that midwives can offer women who are suffering from SUI is that of Pelvic Floor Muscle Training (PFMT) (Waqiah et al. 2019). The oldest form of PFMT are Kegel exercises, named after the urologist Arnold Kegel who first described these in 1948. They consist of sets of 8–12 contractions of the pelvic floor that have to be sustained for about ten seconds. These exercises require discipline and perseverance as they should be repeated multiple times a day for four to five months. In those who are unable to contract the pelvic floor, biofeedback techniques such as simple manual palpation and/or vaginal cones might be useful. Although short-term efficacy of PFMT is good and there are no harmful effects, evidence of long-term benefit is lacking. Nevertheless, PFMT is a treatment option a midwife can discuss, explain and offer women either face-to-face or by using other means if face-to-face contact is not possible, for example via the internet or smartphone. Self-management of SUI, using a mobile app with a focus on PFMT within a Swedish cohort of women, had significant and clinically relevant long-term effects (Hoffman et al. 2017). Such a method has been successful in Dutch women too (Nyström et al. 2017). A consideration in the decision-making process for a midwife to contemplate is whilst such an app may offer an alternative method to provide this first-line treatment option, an area not explicit in these studies is the level of group support an app offers. To compliment such an app, perhaps a support group or blog would prove beneficial, or exploration of other ways to provide group support in a digital age is required. The midwife should also take into account that PFMT has no financial implications for the woman, and no one would be aware she was doing these exercises. This form of self-management could increase access to care and enable women to seek it who otherwise would not do so. If, however, the woman reports that the PFMT exercises are not reducing or stopping the SUI, it is important the midwife discusses with the woman the need to consult and refer to other health professionals who are specialised in this area. Such health professionals may include a physiotherapist, occupational therapist, gynaecologist or urologist as well as counsellors.

As weight gain is synonymous with pregnancy, it is important the midwife spends time exploring the interventions in lifestyle aimed at weight reduction as well as the woman's thoughts and feelings around this and how it may interlink with SUI. Fluid and/or dietary management in general can be beneficial, as reducing the fluid intake reduces the production of urine. Midwives should, however, be careful to ensure women understand the need to avoid dehydration. It should be note that no clinical trial has confirmed the effect of fluid management on SUI. Ongoing studies aim to test the acceptability of providing pregnant women with tailored risk estimates for incontinence. Such studies will help to provide valuable insights into the efficacy of risk-reducing antenatal and intrapartum SUI as well as interventions that target high-risk women. Thus the role of the midwife in promoting and negotiating lifestyle modifications choices is important. Interconnected with this are modifications to daily activities, which might impact positively or negatively on SUI such as lifting, carrying children, and standing for prolonged periods.

Although outside the scope of the midwife, it is essential that midwives are aware of other treatment options that may be offered by specialists in SUI, so they can help support women in discussing their thoughts and feelings with the choices available. There are medications being used to treat SUI such as duloxetine, yet caution needs to be exercised as further trials are required as the benefits and potential harm of this drug are inconclusive at the present time (Maund et al. 2017). Medication, however, may be a relatively cheap option when compared with other treatments. It is possible that incontinence pessaries and intravaginal devices, which aim to compress the urethra, are options, especially in women wishing to avoid or defer surgery who are unable to adhere to behavioural therapy. Periurethral injection of urethral bulking agents (UBAs) is a simple and cost-effective treatment for SUI and currently shows the greatest benefit in those with severe SUI (de Vries et al. 2018). New options are becoming available, including tampon-like devices licensed for over-the-counter sale, but the effectiveness of these devices is yet to be established. Different types of surgeries are available but only to be proposed when all other options have been exhausted (Aoki et al. 2017).

Learning activity

Now you have read about some of the points to consider around midwifery decision-making and SUI, reflect on your practice within your current location using the following activity.

BOX 10.1 CASE SCENARIO – LINKED ACTIVITY 1

Whilst conducting an antenatal appointment with Mary at her home, your intuition tells you there is something not quite right as when her partner told a funny joke, she just smiled. You have the impression she is not saying or wants to say something but isn't. Mary is currently 33 weeks' gestation, with her third baby. How do you collect cues to substantiate your intuition?

After a little probing, Mary tells you she is experiencing urinary leakage every time she laughs or coughs.

1 How do you explain to Mary the reason(s) this might be happening?
2 What points should you consider around how this might be impacting on Mary's life?

---

3   As a midwife, what might your next step be?

4   When would you consider consulting with another health professional, who would this be and why?

Mary goes into spontaneous labour. When you go to assist at the birth of her baby, Mary is sitting on a birth ball and the primary accoucheur tells you the vertex, although visible has been advancing very slowly for 90 minutes and the fetal heart rate is around 150 bpm. What should you do as a midwife?

Conclusion

Urinary leakage and SUI may be a symptom many women accept as normal within pregnancy. Some midwives may accept it as normal too, especially as it can be related to hormonal changes during childbirth, weight of the uterus and/or fetal descent. Yet the potential detrimental effects on a woman's QOL, including but not limited to physical activity, travel, social relationships and emotional health and well-being, need to be at the forefront of midwives' care provision. Women need to be the final decision-makers in their care, and to enable this midwives need to engage in shared decision-making and provide evidence-informed information so an informed choice can be made.

References

Aasheim, V, Nilsen, ABV, Reinar, LM & Lukasse, M 2017, 'Perineal techniques during the second stage of labour for reducing perineal trauma', *Cochrane Database of Systemic Reviews*, no. 6, doi:10.1002/14651858.CD006672.pub2.

Abdulaziz, M, Deegan, E, Kavanagh, A, Stothers, L, Pugash, D & Macnab, A 2017, 'Advances in basic science methodologies for clinical diagnosis in female stress urinary incontinence', *Canadian Urological Association Journal*, vol. 11, no. 6(S2), pp. 117–120, http://dx.doi.org/10.5489/cuaj.4583.

Aoki, Y, Brown, HW, Brubaker, L, Cornu, JN, Oliver Daly, J & Cartwright, R 2017, 'Urinary incontinence in women', *Nature Reviews Disease Primers*, vol. 3, doi:10.1038/nrdp.2017.97.

Bo, K, Hilde, G, Kolberg Tennfjord, M & Ellstrom Engh, M 2016, 'Does episiotomy influence vaginal resting pressure, pelvic floor muscle strength and endurance, and prevalence of urinary incontinence 6 weeks postpartum?' *Neurology and Urodynamics*, vol. 36, no. 2, pp. 683–686, doi:10.1002/nau.22995 | .

Delancey, JO 2010, 'Why do women have stress urinary incontinence?' *Neurourology Urodynamics*, vol. 29, pp. 13–17, doi:10.1002/nau.20888.

de Vries, AM, Wadhwa, H, Huang, J, Farag, F, Heesakkers, JPFA & Kocjancic, E 2018, 'Complications of urethral bulking agents for stress urinary incontinence: An extensive review including case reports', *Female Pelvic Medicine & Reconstructive Surgery*, vol. 24, no. 6, pp. 392–398, doi:10.1097/SPV.0000000000000495.

Elwyn, G, Durand, MA, Song, J, Aarts, J, Barr, PJ, Berger, Z, Cochran, N, Frosch, D, Galasiński, D, Gulbrandsen, P, Han, PKJ, Härter, M, Kinnersley, P, Lloyd, A, Mishra, M, Perestelo-Perez, L, Scholl, I, Tomori, K, Trevena, L, Witteman, HO & Van der Weijden, T 2017, 'A three-talk model for shared decision making: Multistage consultation process', *The British Medical Journal*, vol. 359, no. 4891, pp. 359–4891, doi:10.1136/bmj.j4891.

Ge, J, Yang, P, Zhang, Y, Li, X, Wang, Q & Lu, Y 2015, 'Prevalence and risk factors of urinary incontinence in Chinese women: A population-based study', *Asia-Pacific Journal of Public Health*, vol. 27, no. 2, pp. 1118–1131, doi:10.1177/1010539511429370.

Geynisman-Tan, J, Milewski, A, Dahl, C, Collins, S, Mueller, M, Kenton, K & Lewicky-Gaupp, C 2019, 'Prevalence and risk factors of urinary incontinence in Chinese women: A population-based study', *Female Pelvic Medicine and Reconstructive Surgery*, vol. 25, no. 2, pp. 157–160, doi:10.1097/SPV.0000000000000649.

Heesakkers, JPFA & de Vries, AM 2018, 'Contemporary diagnostics and treatment options or female stress urinary incontinence', *Asian Journal of Urology*, vol. 5, no. 3, pp. 141–148, http://dx.doi.org/10.1016/j.ajur.2017.09.001.

Hoffman, V, Söderström, L & Samuelsson, E 2017, 'Self-management of stress urinary incontinence via a mobile app: Two-year follow-up of a randomized controlled trial', *Acta Obstetricia et Gynecologica Scandinavica*, vol. 96, no. 10, pp. 1180–1187, doi:10.1111/aogs.13192.

Horng, HC, Chen, YJ & Wang, PH 2017, 'Urinary incontinence: Is vaginal delivery a cause?' *Journal of the Chinese Medical Association*, vol. 80, no. 8, pp. 465–466, doi:10.1016/j.jcma.2016.09.004.

Hutton, EK, Hannah, ME, Willan, A, Ross, S, Armson, A, Gafni, A, Joseph, KS, Mangoff, K, Ohlsson, A, Sanchez, J, Asztalos, E & Barret, J 2019, 'Urinary stress incontinence and other maternal outcomes 2 years after caesarean or vaginal birth for twin pregnancy: A multicentre randomised trial', *BJOG: An International Journal of Obstetrics and Gynaecology*, vol. 125, no. 13, pp. 1682–1690, doi:10.1111/1471-0528.15407.

International Confederation of Midwives 2014, 'Philosophy and model of midwifery care', The Netherlands, www.internationalmidwives.org/assets/files/definitions-files/2018/06/eng-philosophy-and-model-of-midwifery-care.pdf.

King, T, Brucker, M, Osborne, K & Jevitt, C 2019, *Varney's Midwifery*, 6th edn, Jones and Bartlett Publishers, Sudbury, MA.

Kokabi, R & Yazdanpanah, D 2017, 'Effects of delivery mode and sociodemographic factors on postpartum stress urinary incontinency in primipara women: A prospective cohort study', *Journal of the Chinese Medical Association*, vol. 80, no. 8, pp. 498–502, doi:10.1016/j.jcma.2016.06.008.

MacArthur, C, Wilson, D, Herbison P, Lancashire, RJ, Hagen S, Toozs-Hobson P, Dean N & Glazener, C 2016, 'Urinary incontinence persisting after childbirth: Extent, delivery history, and effects in a 21-year longitudinal cohort study', *British Journal of Obstetrics and Gynaecology*, vol. 123, no. 6, pp. 1022–1029, doi: 10.1111/1471-0528.13395.

Maund, E, Schow Guski, L & Gøtzsche, PC 2017, 'Considering benefits and harms of duloxetine for treatment of stress urinary incontinence: A meta-analysis of clinical study reports', *The Canadian Medical Association Journal*, vol. 189, no. 5, pp. 194–230, doi:10.1503/cmaj.151104.

Meyer, S, Salchli, F, Hohlfeld, P, Baud, D, Vial, Y & Achtari, C 2017, 'Continuous recording of intrarectal pressures during the second phase of labour: Correlations with postpartum pelvic floor complaints', *International Urogynecology Journal*, vol. 28, no. 8, pp. 1209–1216, doi:10.1007/s00192-016-3249-4.

Newton, E 2018, 'Birthing positions and perineal trauma: A systematic review of the literature', BSN thesis, Salem State University, Salem, MA.

Nyström, E, Asklund, I, Sjöström, M, Stenlund, H & Samuelsson, E 2017, 'Treatment of stress urinary incontinence with a mobile app: Factors associate with success', *International Urogynecology Journal*, vol. 29, no. 9, pp. 1325–1333, doi:10.1007/s00192-017-3514-1.

Pryria, B, Singh, N & Rajaram, S 2017, 'Prevalence and risk factors of urinary incontinence during antenatal period in women delivering in a tertiary care centre of Northern India', *International Journal of Community Medicine and Public Health*, vol. 4, no. 6, pp. 2071–2074, http://dx.doi.org/10.18203/2394-6040.ijcmph20172179.

Sangsawang, B & Sangsawang, N 2013, 'Stress urinary incontinence in pregnant women: A review of prevalence, pathophysiology, and treatment', *International Urogynecology Journal*, vol. 24, no. 6, pp. 901–912.

Serati, M, DiDedda, M, Bogani, G, Sorice, P, Cromi, A, Uccella, S, Lapenna, M, Soligi, M & Ghezzi, F 2016, 'Position in the second stage of labour and de novo onset of post-partum urinary incontinence', *International Urogynecology Journal*, vol. 27, no. 2, pp. 281–286, doi:10.1007/s00192-015-2829-z.

Van der Woude, DA, Pijnenborg, JM & de Vries, J 2015, 'Health status and quality of life in postpartum women: A systematic review of associated factors', *European Journal of Obstetrics and Gynecology*, vol. 185, pp. 45–42, doi:10.1016/j.ejogrb.2014.11.041.

Waqiah, N, Lotisna, D & Abdullah, N 2019, 'Risk factors for stress urinary incontinence following vaginal and caesarean delivery', *Indonesian Journal of Obstetrics and Gynecology*, vol. 7, no. 1, pp. 49–52, https://doi.org/10.32771/inajog.v7i1.830.

Zhai, J, Tyer-Viola, L & Hagan, J 2017, 'Differences between Chinese and American women and their experience of stress urinary incontinence in pregnancy', presented at the Sigma International Nursing Research Congress, Conference Identifier INRC17R02 Ireland.

11

ENHANCED DECISION-MAKING IN MIDWIFERY

Care for pregnant and parenting adolescents

Samantha Nolan and Joyce Hendricks

This chapter explores the context of caring for pregnant and parenting adolescents and its relevance to decision-making in midwifery care. The focus is to enhance understanding around the global context of adolescent pregnancy and parenting, examine the challenges commonly faced by midwives when providing care to this often vulnerable group and explore ways in which this knowledge can enhance care decisions. Activities will encourage reflexivity and suggestions will be made regarding ways to facilitate shared decision-making, a central tenet of woman-centred care.

Introduction

Becoming pregnant, and subsequently a parent during adolescence (defined as between 10–19 years of age; World Health Organization [WHO], 2014a) presents many challenges, regardless of the global context. Reducing rates of adolescent pregnancy has long been the focus of global strategic plans and interventions (Department of Health, 2010; Department of Health & Human Services & Office of Adolescent Health, 2016; World Health Organization, 2014). Rates of adolescent pregnancy worldwide have reduced significantly (WHO, 2018), and in countries such as the UK (a high-income country) they have nearly halved in some health authorities/districts within the last decade (Skinner & Marino, 2016). Contributors to these rate reductions have been widespread availability of contraception, particularly long-acting reversible contraceptives (LARC), abortion services and improved sexual health education in schools (Narring & Yaron, 2014; Skinner & Marino, 2016). Moreover, Skinner and Marino (2016) highlight collaborative, multi-agency approaches as a successful contributor to improved outcomes.

Despite these overall successes, high-income countries still have large populations of pregnant and parenting adolescents. Further, area-specific availability of and access to tailored services remains inconsistent. However, it should be noted that inconsistent or even lack of adolescent specific services is not only limited to high-income countries (Rukundo, Abaasa, Natukunda, Ashabahebwa, & Allain, 2015). This, therefore, presents a challenge for all midwives working towards outcome improvements for vulnerable women such as adolescent mothers, particularly in underfunded, fragmented public health systems. Moreover, it is rightly questioned whether it is adolescent pregnancy itself or society's construction of it that frames the problem (Best, 2017; Brand, Morrison, & Down, 2014; Cense & Ruard Ganzevoort, 2018; Harrison, Clarkin, Worth, Norris, & Rohde, 2016; Linders & Bogard, 2014; Macvarish, 2010; Moore & Reynolds, 2018). Irrespective of location or cultural influence, all midwives need to be able to offer woman-centred care and facilitate shared decision-making. Ensuring care remains woman-centred and facilitating shared decision-making for women with complex care needs (pregnant and parenting adolescents) often requires special consideration and the provision of tailored midwifery approaches.

The risks associated with adolescent pregnancy and parenting

Adolescent pregnancy remains a major contributor to maternal and infant mortality (World Health Organization [WHO], 2016), particularly in developing countries. In many low- and middle-income countries, this challenge is often compounded by unmet needs for contraception and skilled maternity care attendants and societal pressures to marry early and have children (WHO, 2018; Yakubu & Salisu, 2018). Of the world's 16 million annual births to adolescents, 95% take place in low- and middle-income countries. Further, for approximately nine out of ten of these young women, the birth occurs within the context of a marriage (UNFPA, 2017; WHO, 2018). In high-income countries dominated by Western culture, most adolescent births are unintended and take place outside of marriage (Martin, Hamilton, Osterman, Driscoll, & Drake, 2018; Office for National Statistics [ONS], 2017). Naturally, decision-making may differ according to the context in which adolescent pregnancy occurs, both for the adolescent and for the midwife – this will be further explored in an activity.

In high-income countries, becoming pregnant during adolescence is largely perceived as a societal problem, or 'ill', due to the prevalent, intergenerational cycles of ill-health and poverty that often eventuate (Best, 2017; Duncan, Edwards, & Alexander, 2010; Macvarish, 2010). Equally, within this context, children of adolescent mothers are more likely to experience less favourable outcomes related to long-term health and development, educational attainment and social outcomes such as increased welfare dependence and adolescent parenthood in their own lives (Falster et al., 2018; Jutte et al., 2010). In low- and middle-income countries, it is more common for adolescent girls to enter marital relationships and have children early; it is often culturally and socially acceptable. Irrespective of these cultural differences, the Sustainable Development Goals (SDGs) aim to eradicate child marriage and promote the rights of all adolescents to appropriate health and education services (Every Woman Every Child, 2015; United Nations [UN], 2015). Nonetheless, at present, becoming an adolescent mother in any global context limits educational potential which, in turn, is suggested to negatively affect educational attainment and the long-term prospects of their children (Fall et al., 2015; Jutte et al., 2010; UNFPA, 2013).

Irrespective of the cultural construction of adolescent pregnancy, short- and long-term health and psychosocial outcomes are significantly poorer for adolescent mothers and their children (Australian Institute of Health and Welfare [AIHW], 2018; Fall et al., 2015;

Ganchimeg et al., 2014; WHO, 2018), with younger adolescents (< 16 years) considered most at risk (Althabe et al., 2015; Mombo-Ngoma et al., 2016; Torvie, Callegari, Schiff, & Debiec, 2015). This issue is compounded by evidence of significantly more adolescent pregnancies in rural and indigenous populations that often have limited access to health and maternity care (Australian Institute of Health and Welfare [AIHW], 2018; Every Woman Every Child, 2015; WHO, 2018). Globally, poverty, social disadvantage and marginalisation are viewed as both precursors to and a result of becoming pregnant as an adolescent (Harden, Brunton, Fletcher, & Oakley, 2009; Penman-Aguilar, Carter, Snead, & Kourtis, 2013; UNFPA, 2013). For example, in low- and middle-income countries, of which sub-Saharan Africa and South Asia demonstrate the highest numbers of adolescent pregnancies, early pregnancy is often a consequence of little or no access to education, appropriate information or healthcare (UNFPA, 2013). In high-income countries, pregnancy during adolescence is also linked closely to the social determinants of health such as low socioeconomic status, poor housing and limited educational attainment (Kumar, Raker, Ware, & Phipps, 2017), with the United States consistently demonstrating the highest rate of births to adolescents (Raphael-Leff, 2018; Sedgh, Finer, Bankole, Eilers, & Singh, 2015).

In high-income countries, ongoing maternal risks include depression, rapid repeat pregnancy and difficulties returning to education or employment – issues that often result in long-term financial strain and feelings of isolation for the adolescent mother (Marino, Lewis, Bateson, Hickey, & Skinner, 2016; Siegel & Brandon, 2014; Teenage Pregnancy Independent Advisory Group, 2010; Whitworth, Cockerill, & Lamb, 2017). Consequently, depression is associated with adverse effects on maternal-infant attachment and mother-infant interactions that negatively impact the infants' cognitive, social, and emotional development (Dubber, Reck, Müller, & Gawlik, 2015; Miklush & Connelly, 2013). For infants of adolescent mothers across all-income countries, risks include stillbirth and infant death, prematurity, low birth weight and subsequent cognitive and developmental delay (Fall et al., 2015; Ganchimeg et al., 2014; Jahromi, Umaña-Taylor, Updegraff, & Lara, 2012; Morinis, Carson, & Quigley, 2013; Torvie et al., 2015; Whitworth et al., 2017). Importantly, it must be acknowledged that that many of the identified risks to adolescent mothers and their children can be ameliorated by successful engagement with appropriate health, psychosocial and education services in any global context (Marino et al., 2016; Price-Robertson, 2010; Sagili, Pramya, Prabhu, Mascarenhas, & Reddi Rani, 2012; Smyth & Anderson, 2014). Challenges associated with and strategies to enhance successful engagement with services will now be explored.

Accessing maternity services

In low- and middle-income countries, access to skilled maternity services is often limited. Compounding this, the evidence highlights that for women in these countries pregnancies are often unplanned and unwanted (Nyambe, Lungowe, Musonda, & Michelo, 2016), and antenatal care is often misunderstood as being curative, rather than preventative in nature – meaning many women book late for antenatal services (Ebeigbe, Ndidi, Igberase, & Oseremen, 2010). In high-income countries, problems also exist for adolescents accessing maternity care despite widespread government-funded maternity service availability. For example, in

New Zealand, where midwifery-led care is commonplace, Makowharemahihi et al. (2014) found adolescent mothers received inadequate information and insufficient support to successfully navigate enrolment with ongoing midwifery services despite having engaged early with a general practitioner or school-based health service. In addition, pregnant adolescents in high-income countries also claim that they have difficulty accessing maternity services due to limited finances or transport provision (Ireson, 2015; Whitworth et al., 2017), and that they often encounter inappropriately tailored services (Harrison, Clarkin, Rohde, Worth, & Fleming, 2017; Morris & Rushwan, 2015; Reibel, Morrison, Griffin, Chapman, & Woods, 2015). Consequently, many adolescents across all-income countries present late and irregularly for antenatal care (Baker & Rajasingam, 2012; Department of Health, 2015; Kapaya et al., 2015; Wellings et al., 2016), which in turn contributes to less favourable pregnancy and birth outcomes.

Irrespective of location, pregnant and parenting adolescents tend to prefer services that cater specifically to their needs (Chikalipo, Nyondo-Mipando, Ngalande, Muheriwa, & Kafulafula, 2018; Muzik, Kirk, Alfafara, Jonika, & Waddell, 2016; Romagnoli & Wall, 2012). Despite global inconsistency, a plethora of services, predominately in high- and middle-income countries, have been created to cater for the specific needs of pregnant and parenting adolescents. These include extended parent support programmes (McGeechan, Baldwin, Allan, O'Neill, & Newbury-Birch, 2018), collaborative multidisciplinary team clinics (Ickovics et al., 2016; Robinson, O'Donohue, Drolet, & Di Meglio, 2015) and specialised midwifery liaison roles (Butcher, Williams, & Jones, 2016). All ultimately work to improve outcomes by providing a supportive and collaborative approach to adolescent maternity care. Whilst valued antenatal and parenting support programmes for adolescent mothers have been initiated by many nursing and education providers, they often demonstrate inconsistent results in terms of efficacy and outcome improvement (Hollowell, Oakley, Kurinczuk, Brocklehurst, & Gray, 2011; Robling et al., 2016; SmithBattle, Loman, Chantamit-o-pas, & Schneider, 2017). Hence, access to, attendance to and evaluation of appropriate adolescent maternity services can be problematic in any global context. An understanding of the context and construct of adolescence, adolescent pregnancy and the barriers/enablers that affect engagement with maternity services requires consideration by midwives to ensure appropriate, woman-centred care is delivered. This understanding and its relevance to midwifery decision-making will now be explored.

What is the relevance for midwifery and decision-making?

Irrespective of global location or model of midwifery care, all midwives need to consider the decision-making processes of adolescence and understand what influences this. This consideration will enable midwives to make decisions that enhance the provision of appropriate, woman-centred care and facilitate shared decision-making. It has unfortunately been demonstrated that the attitudes and stereotypical preconceptions of healthcare professionals often affect adolescents' engagement with reproductive and maternity services (Harrison et al., 2017; Norman, Moffatt, & Rankin, 2016; Yakubu & Salisu, 2018). It is therefore imperative when engaged in care provision and decision-making with this often vulnerable group, midwives consider their own biases and reflect on the impact these may have on their practice.

Activity – reflect on your perceptions of and experiences of caring for pregnant and parenting adolescents

BOX 11.1   REFLECT ON YOUR PERCEPTIONS OF AND EXPERIENCES OF CARING FOR PREGNANT AND PARENTING ADOLESCENTS – LINKED ACTIVITY 1

Setting – High-income country such as UK or Australia

You are a midwife in a publicly funded maternity hospital. Working a shift on the postnatal ward, you are asked to care for Ally, a 15-year-old mother who gave birth to a healthy daughter, Mia, yesterday. On entering the room, Ally and her boyfriend, Zane (aged 17 years old), are both engaged in mobile phone use and Mia is asleep in the cot.

Setting – Low- or middle-income country such as Iraq or Somalia

You are a midwife working in a rural community setting. A 14-year-old, Sumaya, presents to the clinic at what appears to be an advanced stage of pregnancy, accompanied by her mother and her aunt. Sumaya is married to Asad, a 30-year-old farmer.

- *What immediate thoughts enter your mind regarding these young women?*
- *Do you have any preconceived ideas or beliefs about Ally and/or Sumaya?*
- *Will your ideas/biases affect your attitude towards or your midwifery care of Ally and/or Sumaya?*
- *How will you ensure your care is culturally appropriate and facilitates both Ally and Sumaya to engage in informed decision-making?*
- *Consider ways in which you may also have ensured culturally competent care was provided to Ally/is provided to Sumaya throughout the childbearing continuum.*

Did you have any images of Ally or Sumaya in your mind? Did you have preconceived ideas about Ally or Sumaya's social, family or educational background?

Were you able to reflect on whether preconceived ideas, judgements or beliefs may impact your decision-making relating to the care of these mothers in each context?

The process of reflection to enhance midwifery decision-making is highlighted further in Chapter 8.

In either context, the following considerations may affect the decision-making processes of the midwife and/or the adolescent. In the first instance, midwives need to fully understand Ally's/Sumaya's perceptions of their situation – their values, concerns, aspirations, significant influences and past experiences. It is unclear from either scenario whether the pregnancy was planned and/or wanted and whether it is viewed as a positive or negative event by those involved.

How may this understanding be facilitated? What decisions need to be considered when organising midwifery care?

Receiving care by a known continuous care provider would likely facilitate this level of understanding, however, particularly in medically dominated maternity systems such as those of the United States and Australia, when pregnancy is classed as 'high-risk' (as is the case for adolescent pregnancy) care often becomes fragmented in large tertiary hospitals. Providing continuity of carer (COC) has been highlighted as a highly successful strategy in facilitating trusting relationships with pregnant adolescents (Allen, Kildea, & Stapleton, 2016; Dahlen, 2016). Moreover, Dahlen (2016) found that pregnant adolescents receiving caseload midwifery care were less likely to have a preterm birth and have their babies admitted to neonatal intensive care. Allen et al. (2016), in addition to these findings, discovered that adolescents decided to engage earlier and more regularly with antenatal care when offered COC. Equally, COC can facilitate adolescents to make appropriately informed decisions about future contraceptive use (Wilson, Samandari, Koo, & Tucker, 2011) – considered important, as the provision of no-cost, immediate contraception has been shown to significantly affect rates of rapid, repeat pregnancy for adolescent mothers (Damle, Gohari, McEvoy, Desale, & Gomez-Lobo, 2015; Secura et al., 2014; Tocce, Sheeder, & Teal, 2012). In low-income countries, where childbearing women are often assisted by traditional birth attendants, receiving care by a known and trusted female from within the local community is more commonplace. In this context, however, continuity of care provider does not necessarily increase safety or improve outcomes for childbearing women unless accompanied by adequate midwifery training, skills and expertise (World Health Organization [WHO], 2014b).

Additional considerations when deciding how to organise care for pregnant and parenting adolescents

- *Consider environment* – providing care in less formal, more welcoming environments promotes trusting partnerships. Consider flexibility in terms of the timing and location of clinics/home visits/parenting classes to minimise barriers relating to schooling/lifestyle/transport/finance and reliance on others. Adolescents often lack housing stability and rely on family members for accommodation; provide extended follow-up/liaison to ensure vulnerable adolescents do not 'fall through the cracks' of care provision. Consider use of young women-specific clinics, parenting classes and support groups.
- *Consider collaborative approaches* – Multidisciplinary, specialised clinics are suggested to produce superior results in terms of engagement and attendance (McCarthy, O'Brien, & Kenny, 2014; National Institute for Health and Care Excellence [NICE], 2010). Moreover, guidance from NICE (2010) highlights the need for specialised midwifery roles for adolescents, with such roles having been shown to improve rates of spontaneous vaginal birth, infant birth weight and intention to breastfeed (Butcher et al., 2016). Specialised liaison midwives may also provide advocacy and support during child safeguarding processes or interactions with other healthcare providers – acting as a known, trusted representative.
- *Develop strong links with and consider referrals* to local supports/agencies to facilitate ongoing support with infant feeding, child health and development, mental and sexual health (including contraception), education and peer engagement opportunities.

It is, however, acknowledged that not all countries have the educational, financial or structural resources to provide specialised roles, tailored programs or agencies of support.

What/who may influence adolescent decision-making?

Adolescents in high-income countries are significantly influenced by their stage of development, their parents or guardians, peers and more recently, social media. In low- and middle-income countries, decision-making influences may vary due to the varied construct of adolescence and the prevalence of early marriage. In general terms, adolescent decision-making, behaviours and the ways in which problems are solved often differ from that of an adult (Blakemore & Robbins, 2012). One reason for this is that the frontal cortex – the area that controls reasoning, thinking and action – is still changing and maturing in the adolescent (Casey, Giedd, & Thomas, 2000). This may account for why adolescents are occasionally deemed to behave in impulsive or irrational ways. Indeed, adolescent parents are likely to continue to display ego-centric, unpredictable behaviours during their early parenting years until more mature, adult behaviour patterns develop (Collins & Steinberg, 2008). Moreover, adolescents often make decisions under the influence of emotion, social pressure or time constraints that interfere with a careful consideration of the options and consequences (Albert & Steinberg, 2011; Weinberger, Elvevåg, & Giedd, 2005). Midwives caring for adolescent mothers need to understand these processes when presenting information and in their interactions with pregnant and parenting adolescents to avoid misinterpretation of behaviours that may lead to unnecessary judgement and/or condescending communication.

Furthermore, when promoting contraception and healthy lifestyle options, remembering that adolescents' involvement in risky behaviours is historically attributed to their thinking of themselves as invulnerable (Quadrel, Fischhoff, & Davis, 1993) means midwives should be careful not to appear prescriptive, but to present options as choices – to facilitate shared and informed decision-making. In Western countries, adolescence is often characterised as a turbulent period of development as children gain independence in readiness for adulthood (Curtis, 2015). Whilst parents maintain a considerable influence, the roles of friends and other adults and the importance of peer-group acceptance becomes increasingly significant during adolescence (Collins & Steinberg, 2008). As a result, midwives need to ascertain where adolescents are obtaining their information from and who is likely to influence their decisions. It needs to be acknowledged that in this era of ever-increasing digital technology, mobile phone use is entrenched in the daily lives of most adolescents in high-income countries (Boyd, 2014; Mascheroni & Ólafsson, 2016); it acts as a valuable source of communication, information and often support. Whilst information is freely available online, not all information sourced in this context is considered accurate or helpful in terms of health-related decision-making (Bratu, 2018; Collier, 2018; Moorhead et al., 2013; Sommariva, Vamos, Mantzarlis, Đào, & Martinez Tyson, 2018). Notwithstanding, as adolescent mothers are using social media to inform their decision-making (Logsdon et al., 2014; Nolan, Hendricks, & Towell, 2015), midwives may, in the first instance, need to engage in respectful dialogue about reputable sources of online information and support. Nolan, Hendricks, Williamson, and Ferguson (2018) attest that midwives worldwide should consider engaging in online platforms to optimise accurate information-sharing, enhance peer support opportunities and provide links to community health and education services. Midwives' online engagement and involvement in app and/or website development is likely to become increasingly important if midwives, as primary healthcare providers, are to successfully engage with a generation of mothers who have known little other than a digitally connected existence.

Increasing levels of social support are demonstrated to improve outcomes for adolescent mothers and their children (Leahy-Warren, McCarthy, & Corcoran, 2012; McGeechan et al., 2018), improving parenting efficacy and reducing feelings of isolation, anxiety and depression (Angley, Divney, Magriples, & Kershaw, 2015; Brown, Harris, Woods, Buman, & Cox, 2012). It is, therefore, imperative that midwives consider ways to enhance supports when providing care. Some countries have successfully adopted support interventions using peer mentors to harness the benefits of peer support and peer-led education. For example, in Australia, 'Talking Realities' is a service provided for students in high school environments by adolescents who have experienced pregnancy and parenting (http://talkingrealities.karitane.com.au/). This initiative also incorporates tertiary education qualifications for participant adolescent mothers, increasing their educational prospects whilst maximising peer support opportunities. Equally, in Turkey, training Kurdish-speaking women as peer educators for communities of childbearing women, including adolescents, successfully increased women's engagement with healthcare services and their consent for health-related interventions (Coskun & Karakaya, 2013).

How can midwives optimise shared decision-making with pregnant and parenting adolescents?

- Midwives need to display a *non-judgemental, welcoming attitude* and reinforce this with body language: sustained eye contact, a friendly smile and an open stance. It is important to clearly explain your role, to describe what you will be doing and to minimise assumptions.
- Primarily, midwives should use *strengths-based approaches* that celebrate what is working well. As discussed, adolescents often have differing priorities and needs to adult women based on their stage of development. Harm minimisation should be the overarching goal whilst demonstrating an empathetic understanding of the challenges faced during adolescence.
- When sharing information, midwives need to use *age-appropriate language and visual aids* if required. Language should be free of medical jargon and materials should contain images of young mothers/fathers to create a sense of identity and acceptance, focusing on the concerns and risks of this age group.
- Ensure *consent is adequately informed* and appropriately provided (issues surrounding consent will be explored in more detail later in the chapter). Ask adolescents to explain in their own words what they have understood to ensure they have gained an accurate understanding and ensure adequate time for them to ask questions.
- Ideally, midwives should *involve influential/chosen support people* (with the adolescent's agreement), including husband/partner/mother/family/friends/peers in information-sharing sessions and care provision to enhance engagement and optimise safety and supports.
- Midwives need to *consider online extensions to midwifery-led models of care* to engage with adolescents using their preferred sources of information and support and dominant mode of communication.

Midwives are responsible for child safeguarding. What decisions may relate to this legal and professional responsibility?

Primarily, midwives should clarify that young women and men under 16 years of age have the same right to confidentiality as older people. Midwives must, however, clearly explain limits in relation to child safeguarding and any perceived risk of harm. Second, the age of consent must be considered by midwives, both in terms of sexual activity, and in gaining informed consent for medical treatment or procedures (Bird, 2011; Griffith, 2015; Jackman & McRae, 2013). The legal age for sexual consent varies significantly across the globe, ranging from 11 to 21 years of age, although is commonly legislated at 16 (World Population Review, 2018). Some countries require individuals to be married before they can legally have sex, and variations also exist between the ages of consent for males/females and within same-sex relationships. In low- or middle-income countries, child safeguarding processes may be hindered due to issues of gender inequality, the varied construct of adolescence/adulthood, a lack of protection of girls' human rights, persistent traditions in favour of early marriage and motherhood, poverty, humanitarian crises and tough economic realities. Moreover, in certain religious and cultural jurisdictions, such as those of Iranian Islamic practices, the transition to adulthood and associated ages of consent can occur as early as 9 years of age for girls and 15 years of age for boys (Parsapoor, Parsapoor, Rezaei, & Asghari, 2014). In these contexts, few legislative rulings may be enforced around age-appropriate consent (Chandra-Mouli, Camacho, & Michaud, 2013). There are, however, an increasing number of low and middle-income countries that now have laws and policies to prevent early marriages, pregnancies and motherhood (UNFPA, 2013; United Nations [UN], 2015). This is further supported by the International Confederation of Midwives [ICM] (2014), who provide guidance relating to abuse recognition and the collaborative requirements of midwives supporting vulnerable women and families. In high-income countries, the challenge for legislators, and for those making clinical practice decisions is finding the balance that ensures laws protect young people from adult sexual exploitation yet do not disempower them or criminalise the sexual experimentation with peers that is expected at their stage of development. Midwives, therefore, need an awareness of cultural and legal expectations in their relevant country of practice to guide decisions that relate to the provision of consent.

In some high-income countries, such as Australia and the UK, mandatory reporting requirements relating to cases of adolescent pregnancy may prove challenging for midwives. In the UK and Australia, pregnancies to adolescents aged 13 and under are generally reported to child safeguarding agencies (Australian Institute of Family Studies [AIFS], 2017; Family Planning Association [FPA], 2015), with individual risk assessments generally undertaken for pregnant adolescents aged 14 and over. In Australia, mandatory reporting guidelines vary significantly between individual states and territories and decisions are largely guided by legislation related to suspected abuse and/or risk of harm (Australian Institute of Family Studies [AIFS], 2019). In most high-income countries, evidence of a sexual relationship between a 14-year-old female and a 30-year-old male (as presented in the scenario with 'Sumaya') would necessitate a mandatory report being made to a child safeguarding agency. Indeed, with greater age differences between partners come greater concerns for the coercive or exploitative nature of the couple's relationship processes (Department of Education, 2017). Conversely, midwives in low- or middle-income countries may find legal and professional guidelines difficult to apply, particularly in countries where early marriage between young adolescent girls and mature-aged men is culturally accepted. Midwives, therefore, need to become familiar with locally and nationally relevant legal and professional guidelines to ensure that decisions around the safeguarding of adolescents and their infants are appropriately applied. Midwives' decisions need to be appropriately guided by the laws and expectations in their country of midwifery practice. The WHO (www.who.int/) and the UNFPA (www.unfpa.org/) provide regular updates and guidance relating to the progress being made to protect the rights of women and children across jurisdictions and in every global context.

Future decision-making implications

Midwives worldwide need to consider innovative and culturally appropriate ways to reach out to and engage pregnant and parenting adolescents. This includes understanding what influences adolescent decision-making processes, particularly around health, in any given context of midwifery practice. In high-income countries, this likely means developing supportive apps or websites to disseminate evidence-based information around pregnancy, birth and parenting in a timely and accessible format. Whilst a number of peak professional bodies have created social media policies and guidelines (Nursing and Midwifery Board of Australia [NMBA], 2014; Nursing and Midwifery Board of Ireland [NMBI], 2013; Nursing and Midwifery Council [NMC], 2017; Nursing Council of New Zealand, 2013), most focus on the potential blurring of personal and professional boundaries and minimising misconduct as opposed to providing explicit guidance relating to online care provision. As a result of this, some midwives are concerned about navigating social media use in professional practice (Nolan et al., 2018) and likely need specific training from education providers if online care platforms are to be embraced, particularly to engage and support vulnerable women. Healthcare providers likely need to consider creating purpose-built online platforms to avoid data breach scandals such as the Cambridge Analytica scandal that implicated Facebook in 2018 (Nine Digital Pty Ltd, 2018). Ultimately, it must be understood that pregnant and parenting adolescents are highly motivated to improve the quality of both their own and their children's lives (Anwar & Stanistreet, 2014; Aparicio, 2017; Clarke, 2015; Ford, 2016); thus midwives have a responsibility to engage in decisions that may contribute to any such improvements.

Conclusion

Like all pregnant women, pregnant and parenting adolescents must be assisted in making informed decisions about their care. They require the supportive nurturing of reflexive, non-judgemental, welcoming midwives; willing to embrace 'youth-friendly', innovative and culturally appropriate midwifery approaches. Midwives require knowledge of adolescent development and decision-making processes and require strong links to a multitude of agencies to provide valuable liaison between ongoing support providers and health/education services. Additionally, midwives require area-specific knowledge of legislation pertaining to child safeguarding and the provision of consent to ensure they appropriately apply legislation that ensures pregnant and parenting adolescents and their children are appropriately protected from harm. Further investment is needed to encourage midwives to embrace new and innovative models of care; to reach pregnant and parenting adolescents in 'their space'. This will undoubtedly help adolescent mothers build social capital, feel confident to make informed decisions and achieve their long-term goals.

References

Albert, D., & Steinberg, L. (2011). Judgment and decision making in adolescence. *Journal of Research on Adolescence, 21*(1), 211–224.

Allen, J., Kildea, S., & Stapleton, H. (2016). How optimal caseload midwifery can modify predictors for preterm birth in young women: Integrated findings from a mixed methods study. *Midwifery, 41*, 30–38. doi:10.1016/j.midw.2016.07.012

Althabe, F., Moore, J.L., Gibbons, L., Berrueta, M., Goudar, S.S., Chomba, E., . . . McClure, E.M. (2015, June 8). Adverse maternal and perinatal outcomes in adolescent pregnancies: The global network's maternal newborn health registry study. *Reproductive Health, 12*(2), S8. doi:10.1186/1742-4755-12-s2-s8

Angley, M., Divney, A., Magriples, U., & Kershaw, T. (2015). Social support, family functioning and parenting competence in adolescent parents. *Maternal and Child Health Journal, 19*(1), 67–73. doi:10.1007/s10995-014-1496-x

Anwar, E., & Stanistreet, D. (2014). 'It has not ruined my life; it has made my life better': A qualitative investigation of the experiences and future aspirations of young mothers from the North West of England. *Journal of Public Health, 37*(2), 269–276.

Aparicio, E.M. (2017). 'I want to be better than you': Lived experiences of intergenerational child maltreatment prevention among teenage mothers in and beyond foster care. *Child & Family Social Work, 22*(2), 607–616.

Australian Institute of Family Studies [AIFS]. (2017). *Age of consent laws – CFCA resource sheet.* Retrieved January 14, 2019, from https://aifs.gov.au/cfca/publications/age-consent-laws

Australian Institute of Family Studies [AIFS]. (2019). *Mandatory reporting of child abuse and neglect, CFCA resource sheet – September 2017.* Canberra: Australian Government. Retrieved from https://aifs.gov.au/cfca/publications/mandatory-reporting-child-abuse-and-neglect

Australian Institute of Health and Welfare [AIHW]. (2018). *Teenage mothers in Australia 2015.* Canberra: AIHW. Retrieved from www.aihw.gov.au/reports/mothers-babies/teenage-mothers-in-australia-2015/formats

Baker, E.C., & Rajasingam, D. (2012, February 1). Using trust databases to identify predictors of late booking for antenatal care within the UK. *Public Health, 126*(2), 112–116. doi:https://doi.org/10.1016/j.puhe.2011.10.007

Best, J. (2017). Typification and social problems construction. In *Images of issues* (2nd ed., pp. 3–10). New York: Routledge.

Bird, S. (2011, March). Consent to medical treatment: The mature minor. *Australian Family Physician, 40*(3), 159–160.

Blakemore, S.J., & Robbins, T.W. (2012). Decision-making in the adolescent brain. *Nature Neuroscience, 15*(9), 1184–1191. doi: 10.1038/nn.3177

Boyd, D. (2014). *It's complicated: The social lives of networked teens.* New Haven: Yale University Press.

Brand, G., Morrison, P., & Down, B. (2014, September 1). How do health professionals support pregnant and young mothers in the community? A selective review of the research literature. *Women and Birth, 27*(3), 174–178. doi:https://doi.org/10.1016/j.wombi.2014.05.004

Bratu, S. (2018). Fake news, health literacy, and misinformed patients: The fate of scientific facts in the era of digital medicine. *Analysis and Metaphysics, 17*, 122. doi:10.22381/AM1720186

Brown, J., Harris, S., Woods, E., Buman, M., & Cox, J. (2012). Longitudinal study of depressive symptoms and social support in adolescent mothers. *Maternal and Child Health Journal, 16*(4), 894–901. doi:10.1007/s10995-011-0814-9

Butcher, A., Williams, P., & Jones, F. (2016). Is the introduction of a named midwife for teenagers associated with improved outcomes? A service development project. *British Journal of Midwifery, 24*(5), 331–338.

Casey, B. J., Giedd, J. N., & Thomas, K. M. (2000, October). Structural and functional brain development and its relation to cognitive development. *Biological Psychology, 54*(1–3), 241–257.

Cense, M., & Ruard Ganzevoort, R. (2018). The storyscapes of teenage pregnancy: On morality, embodiment, and narrative agency. *Journal of Youth Studies*, 1–16.

Chandra-Mouli, V., Camacho, A. V., & Michaud, P-A. (2013). WHO guidelines on preventing early pregnancy and poor reproductive outcomes among adolescents in developing countries. *Journal of Adolescent Health, 52*(5), 517–522.

Chikalipo, M. C., Nyondo-Mipando, L., Ngalande, R. C., Muheriwa, S. R., & Kafulafula, U. K. (2018). Perceptions of pregnant adolescents on the antenatal care received at Ndirande health centre in Blantyre, Malawi. *Malawi Medical Journal: The Journal of Medical Association of Malawi, 30*(1), 25. doi:10.4314/mmj.v30i1.6

Clarke, J. (2015, October 2). It's not all doom and gloom for teenage mothers – exploring the factors that contribute to positive outcomes. *International Journal of Adolescence and Youth, 20*(4), 470–484. doi: 10.1080/02673843.2013.804424

Collier, R. (2018). Containing health myths in the age of viral misinformation. *CMAJ: Canadian Medical Association Journal = Journal de l'Association Medicale Canadienne, 190*(19), E578. doi:10.1503/cmaj.180543

Collins, W. A., & Steinberg, L. (2008). Adolescent development in interpersonal context. In W. A. Damon & R. M. Lerner (Eds.), *Child and adolescent development: An advanced course*. Hoboken, NJ: Wiley and Sons.

Coskun, A., & Karakaya, E. (2013). Supporting safe motherhood services in Diyarbakir: A community-based distribution project. *Maternal and Child Health Journal, 17*(6), 977–988. doi:10.1007/s10995-012-1102-z

Curtis, A. C. (2015). Defining adolescence. *Journal of Adolescent and Family Health, 7*(2), 2.

Dahlen, H. G. (2016). Continuity of midwifery care models improve outcomes for young women and babies. *Evidence Based Nursing, 19*(3). doi:10.1136/eb-2015-102233

Damle, L. F., Gohari, A. C., McEvoy, A. K., Desale, S. Y., & Gomez-Lobo, V. (2015). Early initiation of postpartum contraception: Does it decrease rapid repeat pregnancy in adolescents? *Journal of Pediatric and Adolescent Gynecology, 28*(1), 57–62.

Department of Education. (2017). *Child protection: Supporting pregnant and parenting young people*. Government of Western Australia. Retrieved from http://det.wa.edu.au/childprotection/detcms/inclusiveeducation/child-protection/public/resources/Guidelines.en?page=3&oid=MultiPartArticle-id-13332213

Department of Health. (2010). *Teenage pregnancy strategy: Beyond 2010*. London: Retrieved from www.education.gov.uk/consultations/downloadableDocs/4287_Teenage%20pregnancy%20strategy_aw8.pdf

Department of Health. (2015). *Getting maternity services right for pregnant teenagers and young fathers*. London: PHE Publications. Retrieved from www.rcm.org.uk/sites/default/files/Getting%20maternity%20services%20right%20for%20pregnant%20teenagers%20and%20young%20fathers%20pdf.pdf

Department of Health & Human Services, & Office of Adolescent Health. (2016). *Teen pregnancy prevention program*. Retrieved from www.hhs.gov/ash/oah/oah-initiatives/tpp_program/about/

Dubber, S., Reck, C., Müller, M., & Gawlik, S. (2015). Postpartum bonding: The role of perinatal depression, anxiety and maternal – fetal bonding during pregnancy. *Archives of Women's Mental Health, 18*(2), 187–195.

Duncan, S., Edwards, R., & Alexander, C. (2010). *Teenage parenthood: What's the problem?* London: Tufnell Press.

Ebeigbe, P. N., Ndidi, E. P., Igberase, G. O., & Oseremen, I. G. (2010). Reasons given by pregnant women for late initiation of antenatal care in the Niger Delta, Nigeria. *Ghana Medical Journal, 44*(2), 47. doi:10.4314/gmj.v44i2.68883

Every Woman Every Child. (2015). *The global strategy for women's, children's and adolescent's health (2016–2030)*. Geneva. Retrieved from www.who.int/life-course/partners/global-strategy/globalstrategy report2016-2030-lowres.pdf

Fall, C.H.D., Sachdev, H.S., Osmond, C., Restrepo-Mendez, M.C., Victora, C., Martorell, R., . . . Richter, L.M. (2015, July 1). Association between maternal age at childbirth and child and adult outcomes in the offspring: A prospective study in five low-income and middle-income countries (COHORTS collaboration). *The Lancet Global Health, 3*(7), e366–e377. doi:https://doi.org/10.1016/S2214-109X(15)00038-8

Falster, K., Hanly, M., Banks, E., Lynch, J., Chambers, G., Brownell, M., . . . Jorm, L. (2018). Maternal age and offspring developmental vulnerability at age five: A population-based cohort study of Australian children.(Research Article) (Report). *PLoS Medicine, 15*(4), e1002558. doi:10.1371/journal.pmed.1002558

Family Planning Association [FPA]. (2015). *The law on sex.* Retrieved from www.fpa.org.uk/factsheets/law-on-sex

Ford, K. (2016). *Negotiating identities: Adolescent mothers' journey to motherhood: A research study.* Bloomington, IN: Balboa Press.

Ganchimeg, T., Ota, E., Morisaki, N., Laopaiboon, M., Lumbiganon, P., Zhang, J., . . . Tunçalp, Ö. (2014). Pregnancy and childbirth outcomes among adolescent mothers: A World Health Organization multicountry study. *BJOG: An International Journal of Obstetrics & Gynaecology, 121*(Suppl. 1), 40–48.

Griffith, R. (2015). What is Gillick competence? *Human Vaccines & Immunotherapeutics, 12*(1), 244–247. doi:10.1080/21645515.2015.1091548

Harden, A., Brunton, G., Fletcher, A., & Oakley, A. (2009). Teenage pregnancy and social disadvantage: Systematic review integrating controlled trials and qualitative studies. *British Medical Journal, 339*, b4254–b465.

Harrison, M., Clarkin, C., Rohde, K., Worth, K., & Fleming, N. (2017, April 1). Treat me but don't judge me: A qualitative examination of health care experiences of pregnant and parenting youth. *Journal of Pediatric and Adolescent Gynecology, 30*(2), 209–214. doi:https://doi.org/10.1016/j.jpag.2016.10.001

Harrison, M., Clarkin, C., Worth, K., Norris, M., & Rohde, K. (2016). But we're not like the people on TV: A qualitative examination of how media messages are perceived by pregnant and parenting youth. *Maternal and Child Health Journal, 20*(3), 684–692. doi:10.1007/s10995-015-1868-x

Hollowell, J., Oakley, L., Kurinczuk, J.J., Brocklehurst, P., & Gray, R. (2011, February 11). The effectiveness of antenatal care programmes to reduce infant mortality and preterm birth in socially disadvantaged and vulnerable women in high-income countries: A systematic review. *BMC Pregnancy and Childbirth, 11*(1), 13. doi:10.1186/1471-2393-11-13

Ickovics, J.R., Earnshaw, V., Lewis, J.B., Kershaw, T.S., Magriples, U., Stasko, E., . . . Bernstein, P. (2016). Cluster randomized controlled trial of group prenatal care: Perinatal outcomes among adolescents in New York city health centers. *American Journal of Public Health, 106*(2), 359–365.

International Confederation of Midwives [ICM]. (2014). *Midwives and violence against women and children.* The Hague, Netherlands: ICM. Retrieved from www.internationalmidwives.org/assets/files/statement-files/2018/04/midwives-and-violence-against-women-and-children-eng.pdf

Ireson, D. (2015). *Antenatal clinic: Using ethnographic methods to listen to the voices of pregnant adolescents* (Unpublished PhD thesis), Edith Cowan University.

Jackman, M., & McRae, A. (2013). *1.5. 2 medical decision-making and mature minors.* Canada: Royal College. Retrieved from www.royalcollege.ca/rcsite/documents/bioethics/medical-decision-making-mature-minors-e.pdf

Jahromi, L.B., Umaña-Taylor, A.J., Updegraff, K.A., & Lara, E.E. (2012, March 1). Birth characteristics and developmental outcomes of infants of Mexican-origin adolescent mothers. *International Journal of Behavioral Development, 36*(2), 146–156. doi:10.1177/0165025411430777

Jutte, D., Roos, N., Brownell, M., Briggs, G., MacWilliam, L., & Roos, L. (2010). The ripples of adolescent motherhood: Social, educational, and medical outcomes for children of teen and prior teen mothers. *Academic Pediatrics, 10*(5), 293–301.

Kapaya, H., Mercer, E., Boffey, F., Jones, G., Mitchell, C., & Anumba, D. (2015, November 25). Deprivation and poor psychosocial support are key determinants of late antenatal presentation and poor fetal outcomes-a combined retrospective and prospective study. *BMC Pregnancy and Childbirth, 15*(1), 309. doi:10.1186/s12884-015-0753-3

Kumar, N. R., Raker, C. A., Ware, C. F., & Phipps, M. G. (2017, September 1). Characterizing social determinants of health for adolescent mothers during the prenatal and postpartum periods. *Women's Health Issues*, 27(5), 565–572. doi:https://doi.org/10.1016/j.whi.2017.03.009

Leahy-Warren, P., McCarthy, G., & Corcoran, P. (2012). First-time mothers: Social support, maternal parental self-efficacy and postnatal depression. *Journal of Clinical Nursing*, 21(3–4), 388–397. doi:10.1111/j.1365-2702.2011.03701.x

Linders, A., & Bogard, C. (2014). Teenage pregnancy as a social problem: A comparison of Sweden and the United States. In *International handbook of adolescent pregnancy* (pp. 147–157). New York: Springer.

Logsdon, M. C., Bennett, G., Crutzen, R., Martin, L., Eckert, D., Robertson, A., . . . Flamini, L. (2014). Preferred health resources and use of social media to obtain health and depression information by adolescent mothers. *Journal of Child and Adolescent Psychiatric Nursing*, 27(4), 163–168. doi:10.1111/jcap.12083

Macvarish, J. (2010, August 1). The effect of 'risk-thinking' on the contemporary construction of teenage motherhood. *Health, Risk & Society*, 12(4), 313–322. doi:10.1080/13698571003789724

Makowharemahihi, C., Lawton, B., Cram, F., Ngata, T., Brown, S., & Robson, B. (2014). Initiation of maternity care for young Maori women under 20 years of age. *The New Zealand Medical Journal (Online)*, 127(1393), 52–61.

Marino, J., Lewis, L., Bateson, D., Hickey, M., & Skinner, S. (2016). Teenage mothers. *Australian Family Physician*, 45(10), 712–717.

Martin, J. A., Hamilton, B. E., Osterman, M. J., Driscoll, A. K., & Drake, P. (2018). *Births: Final data for 2016*. Hyattsville, MD. Retrieved from www.cdc.gov/nchs/data/nvsr/nvsr67/nvsr67_01.pdf

Mascheroni, G., & Ólafsson, K. (2016). The mobile internet: Access, use, opportunities and divides among European children. *New Media & Society*, 18(8), 1657–1679. doi:10.1177/1461444814567986

McCarthy, F. P., O'Brien, U., & Kenny, L. C. (2014). The management of teenage pregnancy. *BMJ: British Medical Journal*, 349. doi:10.1136/bmj.g5887

McGeechan, G. J., Baldwin, M., Allan, K., O'Neill, G., & Newbury-Birch, D. (2018). Exploring young women's perspectives of a targeted support programme for teenage parents. *BMJ Sexual & Reproductive Health*, 44(4), 272–277.

Miklush, L., & Connelly, C. D. (2013). Maternal depression and infant development: Theory and current evidence. *MCN: The American Journal of Maternal/Child Nursing*, 38(6), 369–374.

Mombo-Ngoma, G., Mackanga, J. R., González, R., Ouedraogo, S., Kakolwa, M. A., Manego, R. Z., . . . Kabanywany, A. M. (2016). Young adolescent girls are at high risk for adverse pregnancy outcomes in Sub-Saharan Africa: An observational multicountry study. *BMJ Open*, 6(6), e011783.

Moore, A., & Reynolds, P. (2018). Constructing and managing risk: The example of teenage pregnancy. In *Childhood and Sexuality* (pp. 99–120). New York: Springer.

Moorhead, S. A., Hazlett, D. E., Harrison, L., Carroll, J. K., Irwin, A., & Hoving, C. (2013). A new dimension of health care: Systematic review of the uses, benefits, and limitations of social media for health communication. *Journal of Medical Internet Research*, 15(4).

Morinis, J., Carson, C., & Quigley, M. A. (2013, October 14). Effect of teenage motherhood on cognitive outcomes in children: A population-based cohort study. *Archives of Disease in Childhood*. doi:10.1136/archdischild-2012-302525

Morris, J. L., & Rushwan, H. (2015). Adolescent sexual and reproductive health: The global challenges. *International Journal of Gynecology & Obstetrics*, 131, S40–S42.

Muzik, M., Kirk, R., Alfafara, E., Jonika, J., & Waddell, R. (2016). Teenage mothers of black and minority ethnic origin want access to a range of mental and physical health support: A participatory research approach. *Health Expectations*, 19(2), 403–415.

Narring, F., & Yaron, M. (2014). Adolescent pregnancy in Switzerland. In A. L. Cherry & M. E. Dillon (Eds.), *International handbook of adolescent pregnancy* (pp. 599–604). New York: Springer.

National Institute for Health and Care Excellence [NICE]. (2010). *Pregnancy and complex social factors: A model for service provision for pregnant women with complex social factors*. London: NICE. Retrieved from www.nice.org.uk/guidance/cg110

Nine Digital Pty Ltd. (2018). *Facebook CEO Mark Zuckerberg admits mistakes over user data.* Retrieved from www.9news.com.au/world/2018/03/22/06/47/facebook-privacy-scandal-mark-zuckerberg-admits-mistakes

Nolan, S., Hendricks, J., & Towell, A. (2015). Social networking sites (SNS); exploring their uses and associated value for adolescent mothers in Western Australia in terms of social support provision and building social capital. *Midwifery, 31*(9), 912–919. doi:http://dx.doi.org/10.1016/j.midw.2015.05.002

Nolan, S., Hendricks, J., Williamson, M., & Ferguson, S. (2018). Social networking sites (SNS) as a tool for midwives to enhance social capital for adolescent mothers. *Midwifery, 62,* 119–127. doi:10.1016/j.midw.2018.03.022

Norman, C., Moffatt, S., & Rankin, J. (2016). Young parents' views and experiences of interactions with health professionals. *Journal of Family Planning and Reproductive Health Care, 42*(3), 179–186.

Nursing Council of New Zealand. (2013). *Guidelines: Social media and electronic communication.* Wellington. Retrieved from www.nursingcouncil.org.nz/content/download/549/2254/file/Guidelines%20Social%20Media.pdf

Nursing and Midwifery Board of Australia [NMBA]. (2014). *Social media policy.* Melbourne. Retrieved from www.nursingmidwiferyboard.gov.au/documents/default.aspx?record=WD14%2f13327&dbid=AP&chksum=PvNCit4JNxlpCjqOenrKvQ%3d%3d

Nursing and Midwifery Board of Ireland [NMBI]. (2013). *Guidance to nurses and midwives on social media and social networking.* Dublin. Retrieved from www.nmbi.ie/Standards-Guidance/More-Standards-Guidance/Social-Media-Social-Networking

Nursing and Midwifery Council [NMC]. (2017). *Guidance on using social media responsibly.* London. Retrieved from www.nmc.org.uk/globalassets/sitedocuments/nmc-publications/social-media-guidance.pdf

Nyambe, S., Lungowe, S., Musonda, P., & Michelo, C. (2016). Factors associated with late antenatal care booking: Population based observations from the 2007 Zambia demographic and health survey. *The Pan African Medical Journal, 25.* doi:10.11604/pamj.2016.25.109.6873

Office for National Statistics [ONS]. (2017). *Births by parents' characteristics in England and Wales: 2016.* London: ONS. Retrieved from www.ons.gov.uk/peoplepopulationandcommunity/birthsdeathsandmarriages/livebirths/bulletins/birthsbyparentscharacteristicsinenglandandwales/2016

Parsapoor, A., Parsapoor, M-B., Rezaei, N., & Asghari, F. (2014). Autonomy of children and adolescents in consent to treatment: Ethical, jurisprudential and legal considerations. *Iranian Journal of Pediatrics, 24*(3), 1–8.

Penman-Aguilar, A., Carter, M., Snead, M. C., & Kourtis, A. P. (2013). Socioeconomic disadvantage as a social determinant of teen childbearing in the US. *Public Health Reports, 128*(2_Suppl1), 5–22.

Price-Robertson, R. (2010). *Supporting young parents.* Australian Institute of Family Studies. Retrieved from www.aifs.gov.au/cafca/pubs/sheets/ps/ps3.pdf

Quadrel, M. J., Fischhoff, B., & Davis, W. (1993). Adolescent (in) vulnerability. *American Psychologist, 48*(2), 102.

Raphael-Leff, J. (2018). *The psychological processes of childbearing* (4th ed.). New York: Routledge.

Reibel, T., Morrison, L., Griffin, D., Chapman, L., & Woods, H. (2015). Young aboriginal women's voices on pregnancy care: Factors encouraging antenatal engagement. *Women and Birth, 28*(1), 47–53.

Robinson, A., O'Donohue, M., Drolet, J., & Di Meglio, G. (2015). Tackling teenage pregnancy together: The effect of a multidisciplinary approach on adolescent obstetrical outcomes. *Journal of Adolescent Health, 56*(2), S64–S65.

Robling, M., Bekkers, M. J., Bell, K., Butler, C. C., Cannings-John, R., Channon, S., . . . Torgerson, D. (2016). Effectiveness of a nurse-led intensive home-visitation programme for first-time teenage mothers (Building Blocks): A pragmatic randomised controlled trial. *The Lancet, 387*(10014), 146–155. doi:10.1016/S0140-6736(15)00392-X

Romagnoli, A., & Wall, G. (2012, May 1). 'I know I'm a good mom': Young, low-income mothers' experiences with risk perception, intensive parenting ideology and parenting education programmes. *Health, Risk & Society, 14*(3), 273–289. doi:10.1080/13698575.2012.662634

Rukundo, G. Z., Abaasa, C., Natukunda, P. B., Ashabahebwa, B. H., & Allain, D. (2015). Antenatal services for pregnant teenagers in Mbarara municipality, Southwestern Uganda: Health workers and community leaders' views. *BMC Pregnancy and Childbirth, 15*(351), 351. doi:10.1186/s12884-015-0772-0

Sagili, H., Pramya, N., Prabhu, K., Mascarenhas, M., & Reddi Rani, P. (2012, March). Are teenage pregnancies at high risk? A comparison study in a developing country. *Archives of Gynecology and Obstetrics, 285*(3), 573–577. doi:10.1007/s00404-011-1987-6

Secura, G. M., Madden, T., McNicholas, C., Mullersman, J., Buckel, C. M., Zhao, Q., & Peipert, J. F. (2014). Provision of no-cost, long-acting contraception and teenage pregnancy. *New England Journal of Medicine, 371*(14), 1316–1323.

Sedgh, G., Finer, L. B., Bankole, A., Eilers, M. A., & Singh, S. (2015). Adolescent pregnancy, birth, and abortion rates across countries: Levels and recent trends. *Journal of Adolescent Health, 56*(2), 223–230. doi:https://doi.org/10.1016/j.jadohealth.2014.09.007

Siegel, R. S., & Brandon, A. R. (2014). Adolescents, pregnancy, and mental health. *Journal of Pediatric and Adolescent Gynecology, 27*(3), 138–150.

Skinner, S. R., & Marino, J. L. (2016). England's teenage pregnancy strategy: A hard-won success. *The Lancet, 388*(10044), 538–540. doi:10.1016/S0140-6736(16)30589-X

SmithBattle, L., Loman, D. G., Chantamit-o-pas, C., & Schneider, J. K. (2017). An umbrella review of meta-analyses of interventions to improve maternal outcomes for teen mothers. *Journal of Adolescence, 59*(Suppl. C), 97–111. doi:https://doi.org/10.1016/j.adolescence.2017.05.022

Smyth, S., & Anderson, G. (2014). Family nurse partnership: Meeting the needs of teenage mothers. *British Journal of Midwifery, 22*(12), 870–875. doi:10.12968/bjom.2014.22.12.870

Sommariva, S., Vamos, C., Mantzarlis, A., Đào, L. U-L., & Martinez Tyson, D. (2018). Spreading the (fake) news: Exploring health messages on social media and the implications for health professionals using a case study. *American Journal of Health Education, 49*(4), 246–255. doi:10.1080/19325037.2018.1473178

Teenage Pregnancy Independent Advisory Group. (2010). *Teenage pregnancy: Past successes – future challenges.* London: TPIAG. Retrieved from www.gov.uk/government/publications/teenage-pregnancy past-successes-future-challenges

Tocce, K. M., Sheeder, J. L., & Teal, S. B. (2012). Rapid repeat pregnancy in adolescents: Do immediate postpartum contraceptive implants make a difference? *American Journal of Obstetrics & Gynecology, 206*(6), 481.e481–481.e487. doi:10.1016/j.ajog.2012.04.015

Torvie, A. J., Callegari, L. S., Schiff, M. A., & Debiec, K. E. (2015, July 1). Labor and delivery outcomes among young adolescents. *American Journal of Obstetrics and Gynecology, 213*(1), 95.e91–95.e98. doi:https://doi.org/10.1016/j.ajog.2015.04.024

UNFPA. (2013). *Adolescent pregnancy: A review of the evidence.* New York. Retrieved November 28, 2018, from www.unfpa.org/sites/default/files/pub-pdf/ADOLESCENT%20PREGNANCY_UNFPA.pdf

UNFPA. (2017). *Adolescent pregnancy.* Retrieved November 28, 2018, from www.unfpa.org/adolescent-pregnancy

United Nations [UN]. (2015). *Transforming our world: The 2030 agenda for sustainable development.* New York. Retrieved from www.un.org/ga/search/view_doc.asp?symbol=A/RES/70/1&Lang=E

Weinberger, D. R., Elvevåg, B., & Giedd, J. N. (2005). *The adolescent brain.* Washington, DC: National Campaign to Prevent Teen Pregnancy.

Wellings, K., Palmer, M. J., Geary, R. S., Gibson, L. J., Copas, A., Datta, J., … Erens, B. (2016). Changes in conceptions in women younger than 18 years and the circumstances of young mothers in England in 2000–12: An observational study. *The Lancet, 388*(10044), 586–595.

Whitworth, M., Cockerill, R., & Lamb, H. (2017, February 1). Antenatal management of teenage pregnancy. *Obstetrics, Gynaecology & Reproductive Medicine, 27*(2), 50–56. doi:https://doi.org/10.1016/j.ogrm.2016.11.005

WHO. (2018). *Adolescent pregnancy – fact sheet.* Geneva. Retrieved November 28, 2018, from www.who.int/mediacentre/factsheets/fs364/en/

Wilson, E. K., Samandari, G., Koo, H. P., & Tucker, C. (2011). Adolescent mothers' postpartum contraceptive use: A qualitative study. *Perspectives on Sexual and Reproductive Health, 43*(4), 230–237.

World Health Organization [WHO]. (2014a). *Adolescent pregnancy*. Retrieved from www.who.int/mediacentre/factsheets/fs364/en/

World Health Organization [WHO]. (2014b). *Health for the world's adolescents: A second chance in the second decade. Summary*. Geneva: World Health Organization. Retrieved March 2019, from http://apps.who.int/iris/bitstream/10665/112750/1/WHO_FWC_MCA_14.05_eng.pdf?ua=1

World Health Organization [WHO]. (2016). *Global health estimates 2015: Deaths by cause, age, sex, by country and by region, 2000–2015*. Geneva: World Health Organization. Retrieved March 2019, from https://www.who.int/healthinfo/global_burden_disease/estimates/en/index1.html

World Population Review. (2018). *Age of consent by country 2018*. US. Retrieved from http://worldpopulationreview.com/countries/countries-by-age-of-consent/

Yakubu, I., & Salisu, W.J. (2018). Determinants of adolescent pregnancy in Sub-Saharan Africa: A systematic review. *Reproductive Health, 15*(1), 15–26. doi:10.1186/s12978-018-0460-4

12

DECIDING TO TRANSFER

Tools to navigate the crossroads of expectations, values and models of care when making transfer decisions at a midwifery birth center

Jennifer Stevens

Chapter overview

Midwifery centers offer a unique space for a woman to birth, utilising the midwifery model of care. This chapter explores the dilemma of decision-making in the context of transferring a woman from a midwifery center in the community to a higher level care facility, commonly a hospital providing a medical model of care. Such a decision is packed with expectations and potential disappointments for both the woman and the midwife. The context in which the midwifery center functions and how the decision is made can have a significant impact on the experience and quality of care provided. The potential for an optimal experience for the woman and her family, as well as the midwife and collaborative medical partner if a transfer is needed, can be enhanced by the use of clear, but not rigid guidelines, and honest communication based on mutual respect and awareness of individual values. This chapter will explore the non-emergent transfer decision to demonstrate ideal decision-making tools and common pitfalls in this collaborative model.

Introduction

In recent years there is a growing demand for alternative birth settings such as midwifery centers (Declercq et al., 2013; Murray-Davis et al., 2014; Hodnett, Downe, & Walsh, 2012). Different countries have different names for these alternative birth settings, for example they are known as birth centers in the United States (US) or midwifery-led care units in the United Kingdom (UK). Regardless of their name, midwifery centers can be found around the world in high-, middle- and low-income countries. A midwifery center is defined as:

> a health care facility, which can provide sexual and reproductive health services for women and newborn care. Midwifery centers are rooted in the midwifery philosophy and model of care. They are in a home-like, shared space. Midwifery centers ensure basic emergency maternal and neonatal care for all births. They are integrated within the health care system, align the level of care to optimal outcome, are

responsive to the needs of their community, and have the woman's experience as their heart and center.

(Goodbirth.net, 2017)

Midwifery centers developed in response to the needs of midwives and women. They can be found in or alongside hospitals, and/or in a community setting (Cheyney, 2019). The common theme they all share is they are staffed by midwives using the midwifery model of care (Hermus et al., 2017). Midwives specialise in healthy women with normal pregnancies. Care provided at a midwifery birth center is specially designed for normal birth (American Association of Birth Centers, 2017). At a midwifery center there are no other healthcare providers, equipment is focused on physiological birth and, if needed, initial stabilisation of emergencies. Because of this focused scope of care, a midwifery center commonly uses risk assessment to identify women appropriate to birth there and use guidelines for transferring a woman, usually to a hospital, if she requires more interventions.

Tension between the models

Internationally, the midwifery model of care is founded on the relationship between the midwife and woman, built on trust, support, and education (Rooks, 1999; Thorstensen, 2000; ICM, 2018). This model embraces birth as a normal process focusing on non-intervention and women's self-determination, requiring the midwife to protect and trust the women (Thorstensen, 2000). The American Association of Birth Centers embrace this model of care, stating: 'While the practice of midwifery and the support of physiologic birth and newborn transition may occur in other settings, this is the exclusive model of care in a birth center' (AABC, 2017).

By working separate from the medical model, the midwifery center creates a space designed for the midwifery model of care to be fully expressed. Care at a midwifery center represents a deep commitment to the midwifery model of care, and in a way a rejection of the medical model approach to physiological birth. In other words, midwifery care is unencumbered by the normal dominant medical model present in a hospital (Walsh, 2005, 2007). The differences in philosophy of care between the midwifery and medical model result in different ways of identifying problems and how to respond. Yet the midwifery center must still function as part of the healthcare system to provide high-quality care that is safe. The professions of midwife and medicine are '*complementary* professions with *different* philosophies and overlapping but *distinct* purposes and bodies of knowledge' (Rooks, 1999, p. 370). Consequently, the center, run by midwives, commonly has a collaborating medical provider to consult with and refer to if variations in normal are identified.

A midwifery center considers the midwife, the woman and the collaborating medical provider (when involved) to be a team, each with unique knowledge and all equally valued in the decision-making process (Stevens et al., 2012). An obstetrician (gynecologist) is an expert in pathology and thus focuses on this potential occurring throughout pregnancy and birth (Rooks, 1999). The medical lens, therefore, when applying clinical reasoning has a 'reductionist focus and privileging of reason to the exclusion of emotional and contextual factors' (Jefford, Fahy, & Sundin, 2011, p. 246). This juxtaposes the midwifery model, where the primary focus is the woman, and her experience. The contextual and emotional factors are more significant. While the medical model in the hospital focuses on the potential for complications during pregnancy and birth for the midwife, Rooks (1999) states, 'The possi-bility of complications is not allowed to preempt all other values associated with the woman's experience of bearing and giving birth to a child' (Rooks, 1999, p. 370). It is these values that are at the heart of the challenge of a transfer from a midwifery center to a hospital. Jefford (2012) states, 'none of the existing theories (of decision making) place the woman at the cen-tre of decision-making' (p. 251). As a result, the tension that exists between the medical and midwifery models, values and expectations becomes heightened during a transfer decision as different models of care collide when the rejection of the mainstream is suddenly what is needed. To complicate this process further, most transfers from a midwifery center to a hos-pital are not clear-cut emergency issues, but more subjective non emergent decisions.

Transfers

Although there are midwifery centers around the world, the majority of studies on maternal outcomes in these environments have been undertaken in developed countries including the United States, UK, Sweden, Denmark, Germany, Australia, Canada and Scotland (Alli-man & Phillippi, 2016). Stapleton, Osborne, & Illuzzi (2013), in their prospective study of over 15,000 planned births at midwifery centers in the United States, found that roughly 12% of clients admitted to a midwifery center in labour were transferred to a higher level care facility. Of these women, over 80% were nulliparous. Stapleton et al. (2013) identified the majority of the intrapartum transfers from a midwifery center to hospital for non-emergent issues were primarily for prolonged labour and arrest of labour. Other less common reasons to transfer included psychological challenges, as well as physiological issues such as meconium-stained amniotic fluid, malpresentation, hypertension, abnormal bleeding and prolonged rupture of membranes. Less than 1% of the transfers from a midwifery center to hospital were for emer-gent reasons. These findings on intrapartum transfers from midwifery centers to hospitals have been replicated in the few studies done in low- and middle-income countries. For example, a study in Iran of over 22,000 midwifery center births found 2.1% of mostly nul-liparous women were transferred to the hospital during labour. Of these, the majority were transferred for poor labour progress (Moudi et al., 2013). The transfer rate in a Brazilian study of over 3,900 cases found an intrapartum transfer rate of 5.8%, with prolonged labour and cephalopelvic disproportion as the most common reasons cited. Again, most of the women transferred were nulliparous (Bonadio, 2011).

Less common, emergent causes for transfer, such as non-reassuring fetal heart rate, cord prolapse, seizure and abruption, offer clear clinical assessments and little decision-making dilemmas, especially with well-written clinical practice guidelines. But with the majority of transfers from midwifery centers to hospitals being for non-emergent issues, these decisions are filled with potential conflicts because of the somewhat subjective influence of risk assess-ment in the non-urgent setting. Additionally, variations in decision-making threshold, and the underlying philosophy and values of the different models of care between midwifery center and hospital add a political and relational tension as well. It is therefore imperative for all mid-wives to have strong clinical knowledge and understanding of risk, irrespective of geographic location around the world, when considering a transfer for non-emergent reasons. Further, each midwife needs an awareness of the politics in her healthcare system and the environ-ment's available resources at the transfer facility. Yet fundamentally and most importantly, the midwifery model of care demands midwives have knowledge of the woman, her desires, her values and a 'dignity-protective' midwife-woman relationship to optimise the experience of a transfer decision (Kuliukas et al., 2015; Berg, 2005; Thompson, 2004)

Contextual and emotional challenges for midwifery centers and decision-making

Factors impacting midwifery decision-making can be divided into three domains: the midwife, the woman and the environment (Daemers et al., 2017; Berg, 2005). Embedded within the environment influencing factors are contextual and emotional factors. These are at the root of a decision dilemma and can vary depending on the country and environment the midwifery center is in, as well as the midwife-woman relationship. For example, *contextual factors* such as culture, collaboration and the organisation of care (Daemers et al., 2017) are often dictated by the greater context of a country's global status, the political context, education and regulation of providers, as well as how well resourced the healthcare system is (Kruk et al., 2018), whilst the *emotional factors* are rooted in the relationship between midwife and woman as being 'dignity protective' (Berg, 2005). This human rights approach to midwifery places the values, priorities and expectations of the individual people, the midwife and woman, at the heart of ethical decision-making (Thompson, 2004). Relational autonomy acknowledges how situations impact the way decisions are made and how individual autonomy is honoured (Newnham & Kirkham, 2019). A midwife's responsibility in this relationship is to protect the woman's autonomy. To do this, awareness of her values and priorities and aligning decision options and processes to them can optimise the quality of the decision and experience as well as preserving one's rights and dignity.

Environment challenges

High- and middle-income countries

The income status of a country usually reflects its health resources and midwifery regulation (Kruk et al., 2018). This can impact a midwifery center, as an environment that has little resources (i.e. lacks emergency medications, ability to undertake caesarean sections or even have doctors at the local hospital) offers the midwife little incentive to transfer. Nevertheless, high and middle income countries (i.e. US, UK, EU, Japan, Brazil, and Mexico) generally have strong, stable healthcare systems although they are often highly medicalised, with interventions frequently occurring. In childbirth care this has resulted in the phenomena known as, 'too much too soon' (Miller et al., 2016). These phenomena have a tendency to lead to medically inappropriate caesarean section rates without improvement in outcomes or women's satisfaction in their care. Such an approach to childbirth is becoming a global concern, particularly in middle-income countries (Boerma et al., 2018), as evidence-informed care can slip away when the focus is on intervention. Further, midwives may feel a need to be validated by the well-established dominant system, which can result in the midwife-institution relationship having priority over the midwife-woman relationship (Newnham & Kirkham, 2019). Yet it could be suggested that midwives in these settings may lean towards protecting the woman's autonomy to choose her birthing environment and wish to experience a birth within a midwifery center irrespective of clinical need. Such an environment and midwifery philosophy could impact upon midwives' clinical reasoning and subsequent decision to transfer a woman to a medicalised environment.

Low-income countries

In low income countries the situation is more complicated. Maternal healthcare suffers from 'too little care, too late' (Miller et al., 2016). Healthcare systems in low-income countries are often poorly resourced and lack healthcare facilities, basic lifesaving medicine and skills to use them as well as medical practitioners. This is further hindered by the disparities in access and outcomes between urban and rural, and wealthy and poor demographics, even within individual communities (Lisonkova et al., 2016; Lehmann et al., 2008). Healthcare facilities are administered and governed by many different entities, from the government to public-private partnerships, private ownership and non-governmental organisations, all with varying management systems and governance (Bradley, 2015). The fragmentation of the healthcare system has serious impacts on the basics of healthcare. This may be compounded by governments that may not be politically committed to healthcare quality. This can result in minimal or no standard processes for quality systems or the oversight needed to enforce them. For example, one study found 35% of healthcare facilities in such countries lacked basic soap and water (WHO & UNICEF, 2015). The impact of these factors adds further complexities to midwives' clinical reasoning and decision to transfer.

There are a couple of other pertinent influencing factors impacting upon midwives decision-making that need to be taken into consideration in low income countries. The first is that in many countries midwives have no mechanisms to be licensed as an autonomous healthcare provider as defined by the International Confederation of Midwives (ICM, 2018). Additionally, they lack accreditation and regulation of their education (Thompson et al., 2011) and/or practice. As a result of these disparities, there is a wide range of quality in basic education and little enforced (if any) maintenance of skills or professional development once practicing. If a healthcare provider does not have access to basic level midwifery education, then the impact on how one develops as an autonomous provider with critical thinking (Carter, Creedy, & Sidebotham, 2018) and clinical reasoning skills and makes subsequent decisions becomes problematic. Clinical knowledge can vary in low-resourced environments where education and thus clinical competence may be weaker, or when working with unlicensed or unregulated providers (Schwerdtle, Morphet, & Hall, 2017).

The second influencing factor affecting midwives' decision-making is gender inequities. There is growing evidence of the impact of gender inequities on the quality of care experienced by women, especially poor women (Kinney, Boldosser-Boesch, & McCallon, 2016; Hartmann et al., 2016; Hartigan, 2001). Gender inequalities will and do impact upon midwives' autonomy, clinical reasoning and decision-making. For example, if a midwife who is a female practices in a country where the patriarchal systems is alive, then her ability to be an autonomous practitioner and decision-maker is severely limited and challenged. These gender barriers seem to be not just related to economic and professional issues but social and political issues as well (Filby et al., 2016).

Because of the greater inequities present and the lack of available healthcare for women locally, development of midwifery centers has occurred in some countries. For example in Brazil, the highly medicalised environment and high caesarean rates promoted groups of midwives and the government to work together to open a birth center to 'counter-hegemony established in providing care during pregnancy and physiological birth' – clearly a political act for an alternative care model (Pereira & Moura, 2009, p. 868). For women in remote areas, midwifery centers offer local care and thus increase access in women's communities. One such development of midwifery centers is in Nepal, which were supported and expanded by the government and UNICEF (UNICEF, 2013, pp. 36–40). Goodbirth Network, a global network of midwifery centers in low- and middle-income countries, reports that in Haiti in recent years, birth centers have opened throughout the country, even in hard-to-reach rural mountains, by NGOs looking to bring care to where the women live. This pattern is repeated in many low- and middle-income countries such as Mexico, Uganda, the Philippines and Bangladesh. This global movement towards development of midwifery centers is because they have been recognised as meeting the need to increase access to care for women, provide personalised care for those in minority or marginalised groups and be a viable financial option for women's healthcare (Moudi et al., 2013; Mahato et al., 2017). Despite these steps forward in childbirth provision, if mechanisms to license a healthcare provider as a midwife or regulation of their education and/or practice do not exist, the outcomes for childbearing women and their babies will not improve.

The ideal – enabled and integrated

'The politics and power relationship of birth are most often visible when someone resists them' (Newnham & Kirkham, 2019, p. 3). A midwifery center is usually resisting the dominant medical philosophy of birth as pathological and the healthcare system that propagates it. Whether a country is high, middle or low income, a midwifery center and the teams' decision-making function optimally when the center is well integrated in an enabling healthcare system, not in opposition to it. When developed as part of such a healthcare system, it works in an environment that enables its success. Such an enabling environment is one where there is space, permission and even support to resist the medicalised birth system. The woman feels confident and empowered to state what she needs and wants, yet humble enough to know birth is not entirely in her control and sometimes compromises need to be made. The midwife is well educated, feels comfortable providing birth out of the dominant system, yet feels valued and supported as part of that system. The healthcare team has a collaborative relationship that is based on trust, curiosity and an aligned philosophy and approach to care practices and goals. This encourages a free flow of communication so no one is surprised by a change of events or plans when the clinical situation changes. Logistics are easily accessible, resources (such as ambulance, medications and care at a transfer facility) are available, and there are clear clinical practice guidelines that support physiological birth. In an environment, such enabled midwives can work autonomously and to the full scope of their practice (ICM, 2018), decisions are impacted solely by the midwife and woman, their communication, the clinical situation and the decision threshold. Yet the midwife acknowledges the expertise of medical colleagues and seeks guidance and assistance if warranted and together as a tripartite relationship (woman, midwife, doctor), decisions are made that meet the woman's needs and enable her to remain empowered during her birthing journey.

Weakly integrated or enabled

In countries where midwifery centers develop outside of the healthcare system, many barriers to quality care are present, although a complete lack of integration or working in parallel to the dominant healthcare is most common in low- and middle-income countries (Cole & Avery 2017). At the extreme, midwives and midwifery centers often have no legal status, no standards and no rights or regulations. This lack of integration reinforces a lack of access to care and removes options for women. Further barriers to effective collaboration such as hierarchy and competitive models, as well as the restriction of independent autonomous midwifery practice, risk safety for the women who desire this model (Corry, Williams, & Stapleton, 1997). Compounding this may be a healthcare system that has considerably fewer resources. If such barriers, based on perceived alternatives rather than what is medically necessary, are allowed to exist these environments can often become adversarial. Ultimately this impacts on midwives' decision-making, especially around the decision threshold, timing and final decision to transfer. Nevertheless, irrespective of geographical location around the world, making a decision to transfer a woman from the community midwifery-model of care to an obstetric model within a hospital setting is complex, multifactorial and has implications for both the woman, her baby and the midwife. Some of the influencing factors a midwife needs to consider are:

- The skills and knowledge required to identify the necessity for transfer
- The time frame to make that decision especially in regards to the environment
- How to negotiate this with the woman within a midwife-woman partnership based on care ethics (Newnham & Kirkham, 2019).

Women

All women approach birth with plans, expectations and fears which are grounded within their personal lives and their culture. For various reasons, a woman choosing to birth at a midwifery center has stepped outside of the dominant medical healthcare system and thus has unique expectations, values, preferences and priorities. In some environments, especially high-resourced environments such as the US, UK or EU, women choose midwifery centers to increase their chance for a non-medicalised birth (Sperlich, Gabriel, & Seng, 2017; Coxon, 2015). It reflects and supports their belief and commitment to physiological birth (Wood, 2016). To help increase their chances of being successful in their plan to achieve this, women at midwifery centers often have increased engagement and accountability in their care (Wood et al., 2016). Yet in middle- and low-income countries, giving birth at a midwifery center is less a matter of choice, as much as midwifery centers in these environments are often developed to increase access to care (Schrag, 2017). It is well documented that if given the choice, women in these countries will avoid hospital birth because of the distance, poor treatment and higher cost (Bohren, 2014). This adds another dimension to the complexity of midwifery decision-making, if a woman is at a midwifery birth center and the midwife needs to transfer her to a hospital for medical reasons. Such a decision can result in significant resistance from the woman, especially as the referral hospital is often a distance away and thus requiring transportation, which costs more money.

Regardless of where around the world a midwife practices, in midwifery centers where the need to transfer a woman is inevitable at some point, they must be aware of these additional expectations as well as the woman's focus on the outcome instead of the process. Further is there is a lack of affirming communication, as it can create a sense of failure for the woman who has 'failed' to achieve her planned physiological birth (Berg, 2005). It is imperative all midwives, therefore, explore with a woman the underlying values for her expectations, priorities and preferences prenatally and educate them about the process. Allowing grief to be part of that discussion (Lylerly, 2017) can mitigate some of the potential conflict. The strength of the relationship between midwife and woman and the ability to trust in each other while making shared decisions can impact how successful they will both feel (Berg, 2005). Ideally the relationship should provide a structure of equality between midwife and woman. The inherent challenge in this healthcare relationship is the tension that exists with the power imbalance of knowledge and authority between the midwife and woman (Newnham & Kirkham, 2019). The woman will always have less knowledge regarding her care than the midwife, and the midwife has the absolute authority to remove her care, or decide to transfer, at any time. This tension between expressing equality in a relationship with power inequity requires awareness and humility, especially on the part of the midwife.

Midwives

The midwifery center is the ideal place for the full expression of the midwifery model of being 'with woman'. Developing one or working in one can be a political act of advocating for women (Walsh, 2005). Midwives at midwifery centers in lower income countries often work in systems they are actively trying to change (Pereira & Moura, 2009; da Silva et al., 2013). Midwives may view providing care in a midwifery center as advocating for women in opposition to the medical model (Keating & Fleming, 2007; Walsh, 2007). In other words, they deeply desire to provide women compassionate, high-quality care they believe is lacking in the medical model (Lakko, 2016). Yet the midwife needs to balance her commitment and relationship with the mother, as well as her sociocultural-political perceptions of available options (e.g. medicalised model within a hospital) to the reality of the unfolding clinical situation. If not the situation becomes ripe for conflict between the developing clinical need for a transfer and the current transfer environment, especially if the midwife believes she is trying to protect the woman from the medical model and all that may entail. As a result, her clinical reasoning and judgement will impact her decision threshold as she feels ultimate accountability for experiences/circumstances she cannot control especially if the transfer of 'information, authority and responsibility for patient care' (Cole & Avery, 2017, pp. 92–95) results in sending a woman into a system where the midwifery center is poorly integrated and there isn't a strong, mutually respectful collaborative environment. This may cause a loss (real or perceived) of autonomy, agency and control for the midwife. The responsibility for decisions made is present in all healthcare decisions, but there is an increased sense of awareness of it as a midwife in a midwifery center because of working outside the dominant model. It can potentially become a heavy burden laden with expectations, emotions, values, preferences and priorities for midwives, thus it may be tempting to avoid and/or delay the decision to transfer.

Making decisions

There is limited research available regarding midwives decision-making around transfers. One study found midwives and obstetricians make similar risk assessments but have different decision thresholds (Cheyne et al., 2012). They found three elements that are useful as a framework for the decision-making process. These can be applied to the midwife, the referral provider and the woman:

1 A judgement or *assessment*. This is influenced by professional knowledge, education and the individual's assessment of level of risk.
2 *The decision*. To make an informed decision, clear alternative choices need to be identified and presented as options.

3   The individual's *decision threshold*. This is the moment the decision to transfer is made. It is 'the link between the assessment and the decision'. An individual's assessment threshold is influenced by the individual's philosophy, approach to care, past experiences and biases.

A lack of alignment between the assessment, the decision options and the decision threshold will cause tension and be a source of disagreement between the members of the healthcare team and result in a poor experience for all.

Assessment

Generally, the clinical assessment itself should not be a source for disagreement. Although the assigned level of risk may be influenced by an individual's philosophy or bias, the assessment is based on clinical knowledge. One research study found that the midwife and obstetrical providers have high correlation in assessments of clinical factors determining risk (Cheyne et al., 2012). A thorough understanding of research, evidence-informed care and experience is necessary to know not every birth follows the same path. There is significant 'gray space' around what is clearly normal and what is clearly not normal and potentially unsafe. The threshold to make a decision can be reached at different times and for different reasons for those involved. When the risk, values, priorities, clinical assessment and options come together in a way that the care team decides the woman needs to be moved from the midwifery center to the hospital, this is when the impact of environment, emotions and different models of care have their greatest influence. An enabled environment minimises the potential clashes and allows a decision to be based on the identified values and clinical assessment. Being aware of factors that impact a decision threshold can aid in keeping the decision process transparent and as objective as possible. These factors include the persons' attitude toward physiological birth, woman-centred care, collaboration and shared decision-making and the individual's experience, intuition, personal circumstances and history (Daemers et al., 2017). Care should also be taken to know the members of the healthcare team, their knowledge, risk assessment, practice style and beliefs in physiological birth. While the midwifery model of care and the medical model have different priories and can have very different approaches, the midwife should make all efforts to understand her own capabilities, practice style and knowledge. Knowing who you are and how you are different, and what is valuable about those differences and how you handle variations is important and can strengthen the quality of care. When presented with a variation, many midwives create the habit of identifying the most common and worse case cause of the variation. Then they look and constantly assess for more information or data (this is discussed in Chapter 1) that would cause the variation to lean more one way or the other to confirm a decision to transfer or stay, constantly communicating with the woman. Making decisions based on probability alone removes the context and meaning from the factors and it removes the woman and her unique experience from the decision-making process (Lyerly et al., 2007).

Decision-making – values and options

A clinical decision is based on the clinical presentation and the available options. Our values offer direction and a framework to our life and decisions we make (Thompson, 2004). Based on their philosophies and values, the woman, midwife and collaborating partner have a unique understanding of what those options are. The collaborating partner specialises in complications and interventions, all of which are lifesaving when used appropriately. The woman knows her body and how it reacts, although if a primigravida this knowledge may be limited. The midwife should have a deep understanding of the woman's desires and values to help her clarify what she needs and a bank of midwifery care options for her to use in non-emergent situations. When considering options, discussions should always include a sound, evidence-informed basis including risks and benefits of doing something and of doing nothing at all. There is a tendency to prioritise an incremental risk over a woman's experience, and value action above all else, rather than considering no intervention as a choice as well (Lyerly et al., 2007).

When variations are identified, a midwife's management can be independent or collaborative. Ultimately, however, the final decision-maker is the woman. Whilst the midwifery philosophy embraces this totally, it is important to address the challenges for midwives that surrounding this. As a midwife becomes more aware of the possible need to transfer, they may want the woman to make the decision. If the woman chooses, then the midwife doesn't have to be accountable for taking away what was desired. By presenting all the negative information and our opinion about lack of progress, we can discourage the woman so they choose to transfer. A decision needs options. By presenting all the information and all the choices and possible impacts of those choices, an empowered choice can be made together. Yet some midwives fear influencing a woman or letting her down. Alternatively, some midwives may want to please the collaborating partner or the medical system by 'prioritizing the midwife-institution relationship over the midwife-woman relationship' (Newnham & Kirkham, 2019). This is an example of abdicating the midwifery model (Jefford & Jomeen, 2015 see Chapter 6) and can potentially lower the decision threshold of the midwife to transfer. Yet some midwives may believe that by making a decision to recommend a transfer or not makes them vulnerable to being wrong. A midwife should not be afraid to say they feel a transfer is necessary. Perhaps they will be proven wrong and it undermines the need for alternatives such as a woman's choice and the midwifery model of care. Or perhaps not. Skilled communication, self-knowledge and confidence with a touch of humility are required to present options for managing a case that is a variation in physiological birth. In an honest relationship, such discussions and shared decision-making will only strengthen it, and the midwife and woman will know they at least tried all they reasonable could.

Conclusion

All midwives who work in community-based midwifery centers have the opportunity and privilege to work freely, express the midwifery model of care how they interpret it and have deep, satisfying relationships with the women the serve. With this right, midwives around the globe have the responsibility and accountability to make quality decisions. These decisions need to take into account not just the clinical situation but also the woman's values and the midwifery center's greater environment. By utilising evidence-informed care discussion, collaboration and decision-making, midwives can provide sensitive, safe, respectful care that is satisfying for all involved, even if a decision to transfer is made.

References

AABC 2017, 'Definition of a "birth center" clarified', 11 May 2017, American Association of Birth Centers. Perkiomenville, PA. Available from: www.birthcenters.org/news/344953/Definition-of-Birth-Center-Clarified.htm. [23 January 2019].

Alliman, J, & Phillippi, JC., 2016, 'Maternal outcomes in birth centers: An integrative review of the literature', *Journal of Midwifery & Women's Health*, pp. 1–31.

Berg, M 2005, 'A midwifery model of care for childbearing women at high risk: Genuine caring in caring for the genuine', *Journal of Perinatal Education*, vol. 14, no. 1, pp. 9–21.

Boerma, T, Ronsmans, C, Melesse, DY, Barros, AJD, Barros, FC, Juan, L, Moller, AB, Say, L, Hosseinpoor, AR, Yi, M, Neto, DLR, & Temmerman, M 2018, 'Global epidemiology of use of and disparities in caesarean sections', *Lancet*, vol. 392, pp. 1341–1348.

Bohren, M, Hunter, E, Munthe-Kaas, HM, Souza, JP, Vogel, JP, & Gulmerzoglu, AM 2014, 'Facilitators and barriers to facility-based delivery in low- and middle-income countries: A qualitative evidence synthesis', *Reproductive Health*, vol. 11, no. 71.

Bonadio, IC, Schneck, CA, Pires, LG, Osava, RH, da Silva, FMB, de Oliveira, SMJV, & Riesco, MLG 2011, 'Transferring mothers from a free-standing birth center to a reference hospital, *Revista da Escola de Enfermagem da U S P*, vol. 45, no. 6, pp. 1301–1307.

Bradley, EH, Taylor, LA, & Cuellar, CJ 2015, 'Management matters: A leverage point for health systems strengthening in global health', *International Journal of Health Policy and Management*, vol. 4, pp. 411–15.

Carter, AG, Creedy, DK, & Sidebotham, M 2018, 'Critical thinking in midwifery practice: A conceptual model', *Nurse Education in Practice*, vol. 33, pp. 114–120.

Cheyne, H, Dalgleish, L, Tucker, J, Kane, F, Shetty, A, McLeod, S, & Niven, C 2012, 'Risk assessment and decision making about in-labour transfer from rural maternity care: A social judgement and signal detection analysis', *BMC Medical Informatics and Decision Making*, vol. 12, no. 122.

Cheyney, M, Bovbjerg, ML, Leeman, L, & Vedam, S 2019, 'Community versus out-of-hospital birth: What's in a name?' *Journal of Midwifery & Women's Health*, vol. 64, no. 1.

Cole, L & Avery, MD (eds) 2017, *Freestanding birth centers, innovation, evidence, optimal outcomes*, Springer Publishing Company, New York.

Corry, M, Williams, D, & Stapleton, SR 1997, 'Models of collaborative practice: Preparing for maternity care in the 21st century', *Women's Health Issues*, vol. 7, no. 5, pp. 279–284.

Coxon, K, Sandall, J, & Fulop, NJ 2015, 'How do birth experiences influence planned place of birth in future pregnancies? Findings from a longitudinal, narrative study', *Birth*, vol. 42, pp. 141–148.

Daemers, D, van Limbeek, EBM, Wijnen, HAA, Nieuwenhuijlze, M, & de Vries, RG 2017, 'Factors influencing the clinical decision-making of midwives: A qualitative study', *BMC Pregnancy and Childbirth*, vol. 17, no. 345.

da Silva, FMB, da Paixão, TCR, de Oliveira, SMJV, Leite, JS, Riesco, MLG, & Osava, RH 2013, 'Care in a birth center according to the recommendations of the World Health Organization', *Revista da Escola de Enfermagem da U S P*, vol. 47, no. 5, pp. 1031–1038.

Declercq, ER, Sakala, C, Corry, MP, Applebaum, S, & Herrlich, A 2013, 'Listening to mothers III: New mothers speak out', *Childbirth Connection*, New York. Available from: http://transform.childbirth connection.org/reports/listeningtomothers/. [5 January 2019].

Filby, A, McConville, F, & Portela, A 2016, 'What presents quality midwifery care? A systematic mapping of barriers in low and middle income countries from the providers' perspective', *PLoS One*, vol. 11, no. 5.

Goodbirth Network 2017, *About goodbirth network, what is a midwifery center*. Mexico. Available from: https://goodbirth.net/about/. [21 January 2019].

Hartigan, P 2001, 'The important of gender in defining and improving care: Some conceptual issues', *Health Policy and Planning*, vol. 16 (Suppl.1), pp. 7–12.

Hartmann, M, Khosla, R, Krishnan, S, George, A, Gruskin, S, & Amin, A 2016, 'How are gender equity and human rights interventions included in sexual and reproductive health programming and policies: A systemative review of existing research foci and gaps', *PLoS One*, vol. 11, no. 12.

Hermus, MAA, Boesveld, IC, Hitzert, M, Franx, A, de Graaf, JP, Steegers, EAP, Weigers, TA, & van der Pal-deBruin, KM 2017, 'Defining and describing birth centres in the Netherlands – a component study of the Dutch birth centre study', *BMC Pregnancy and Childbirth*, vol. 17, no. 210.

Hodnett, ED, Downe, S, & Walsh, D 2012, 'Alternative versus conventional institutional settings for birth (review)', *Cochrane Database of Systematic Reviews*, no. 8, Issue. CD000012.

ICM, 2018. 'ICM definitions', International Confederation of Midwives. The Hague. Available from: www.internationalmidwives.org/our-work/policy-and-practice/icm-definitions.html. [5 February 2019].

Jefford, E 2012. *Optimal midwifery decision-making during 2nd stage labour: The integration of clinical reasoning into practice.* PhD Research, Southern Cross University. NSW, Australia.

Jefford, E, & Jomeen, J 2015. ' "Midwifery abdication": A finding from an interpretive study', *International Journal of Childbirth*, vol. 5, no. 3, pp. 116–125.

Jefford, E., Fahy, K. & Sundin, D 2011. Decision-making theories and their usefulness to the midwifery profession both in terms of midwifery practice and the education of midwives. *International Journal of Nursing Practice*, vol. 17, pp. 246–253.

Keating, A, & Fleming, VEM 2007, 'Midwives' experiences of facilitating normal birth in an obstetric-led unit: A feminist perspective', *Midwifery*, vol. 25, pp. 518–527.

Kinney, MV, Boldosser-Boesch, A, & McCallon, B 2016, 'Quality, equity, and dignity for women and babies', *Lancet Online*, September 15. http://dx.doi.org/10.1016/S0140-6736(16)31525-2

Kruk, ME, Gage, AG, Arsenault, C, Jordan, K, Leslie, HH, Roder-DeWan, S, Adeyi, O, Barker, P, Daelmans, B, Doubova, SV, English, M, Elorrio, EG, Guanais, F, Gureje, O, Hirschhorn, LR, Jiang, L, Kelley, E, Lemango, ET, Liljestrand, J, Malata, A, Marchant, T, Matsoso, MP, Meara, JG, Mohanan, M, Ndiaye, Y, Norheim, OF, Reddy, KS, Rowe, AK, Salomon, JA, Thapa, G, Twum-Danso, NAY, & Pate M 2018, 'High-quality health systems in the sustainable development goals era: Time for a revolution', *The Lancet Global Health Commission*, vol. 6, pp. e1196–e1252.

Kuliukas, LJ, Lewis, L, Hauck, YL, & Duggan, R 2015, 'Midwives' experiences of transfer in labour from a Western Australian birth centre to a tertiary maternity hospital', *Women Birth*, vol. 29, no. 1, pp. 18–23.

Lakko, H 2016, 'Los derechos humanos en los movimientos sociales: el caso de las parteras autónomas en México', *Revista Mexicana de Ciencias Políticas y Sociales*, UNAM, May–August, no. 227, pp. 167–195.

Lehmann, U, Dieleman, M, & Martineau, T 2008 'Staffing remote rural areas in middle- and low-income countries: A literature review of attraction and retention', *BMC Health Services Research*, vol. 8, no. 19.

Lisonkova, S, Haslam, M, Dahlgren, L, Chen, I, Synnes, AR, & Lim, K 2016, 'Maternal morbidity and perinate outcome amount women in rural versus urban areas, *Canadian Medical Association Journal*, doi:10.1503/cmaj.151382.

Lylerly, AD 2017, 'Of pain and childbirth', *Narrative Inquiry in Bioethics*, vol. 2017, no. 2, pp. 221–224.

Lyerly, AD, Mitchell, LK, Armstrong, EM, Harris, LH, Kukla, R, Kuppermann, M, & Little, MO 2007, 'Risks, values and decision making surrounding pregnancy', *Obstetrics & Gynecology*, vol. 109, no. 4, pp. 979–984.

Mahato, PK, van Veijlinger, E, Simkhada, P, Sheppard, P, Sheppard, ZA, & Silwal, RC 2017, 'Factors related to choice of place of birth in a district in Nepal', *Sexual & Reproductive Healthcare*, vol. 13, pp. 91–96.

Miller, S, Abalos, E, Chamillard, M, Ciapponi, A, Colaci, D, Comandé, D, Diaz, V, Geller, S, Hanson, C, Langer, A, Manuelli, V, Millar, K, Morhason-Bello, I, Castro, CP, Pileggi, VN, Robinson, N, Skaer, M, Souza, JP, Vogel, JP, & Althabe F 2016, 'Beyond too little, too late and too much, too soon: A pathway towards evidence-based, respectful maternity care worldwide', *Lancet*, vol. 388, pp. 2176–2192.

Moudi, Z, Tabatabaie, MG, Tabatabaei, SM, & Vedadhir, A 2013, 'Safe delivery posts: An intervention to provide equitable childbirth care services to vulnerable groups in Zahedan, Iran', *Midwifery*, pp. 6–11.

Murry-Davis, B, McDonald, H, Rietsma, A, Coubrough, M, & Hutton, E 2014, 'Deciding on home or hospital birth: Results of the Ontario choice of birthplace survey', *Midwifery*, vol. 30, pp. 869–876.

Newnham, E, & Kirkham, M 2019, 'Beyond autonomy: Care ethics for midwifery and the humanizing of birth', *Nursing Ethics*, pp. 1–11.

Pereira, ALF, & Moura, MAV 2009, 'Hegemony and counter-hegemony in the process of implementing the Casa de Parto birth center in Rio de Janeiro', *Revista da Escola de Enfermagem da U S P*, vol. 43, no. 4, pp. 868–874.

Rooks, J 1999, 'The midwifery model of care', *Journal of Nurse-Midwifery*, vol. 44, no. 4, pp. 370–374.

Schrag, K 2017, 'Birth centers in the global area', in L Cole & MD Avery (eds), *Freestanding birth centers, innovation, evidence, optimal outcomes*, pp. 337–354, Springer Publishing Company, New York.

Schwerdtle, P, Morphet, J, & Hall, H 2017, 'A scoping review of mentorship of health personnel to improve the quality of health care in low and middle-income countries', *Global Health*, October 13, no. 1, p. 77.

Sperlich, M, Gabriel, C, & Seng, J 2017, 'Where do you feel safest? Demographic factors and place of birth', *Journal of Midwifery & Women's Health*, vol. 63, no. 1.

Stapleton, SR, Osborne, C, & Illuzzi, J 2013, 'Outcomes of care in birth centers: Demonstration of a durable model', *Journal of Midwifery &Women's Health*, vol. 58, no. 1, pp. 3–14.

Stevens, J, Witmer, T, Grant, R, & Cammarano, D 2012, 'Description of a successful collaborative birth center practice among midwives and an obstetrician', *Obstetrics and Gynecology Clinics of North America*, vol. 39, pp. 347–357.

Thompson, JB 2004, 'A human rights framework for midwifery care', *Journal of Midwifery & Women's Health*, vol. 49, pp. 175–181.

Thompson, JB, Fullerton, JT, Sawyer, AJ, & International Confederation of Midwives 2011, 'The international confederation of midwives: Global standards for midwifery education (2010) with companion guidelines', *Midwifery*, vol. 27, no. 4, pp. 409–416.

Thorstensen, KA 2000, 'Trusting women: Essential to midwifery', *Journal of Midwifery & Women's Health*, vol. 44, no. 5, pp. 405–407.

UNICEF, 2013, 'Nepal: Establishing and sustaining birthing centres closer to communities', in *Innovative approaches to maternal and newborn health: Compendium of case studies*, pp. 36–40, United Nations Children's Fund (UNICEF), New York.

Walsh, D 2005, 'Subverting the assembly-line: Childbirth in a free-standing birth centre', *Social Science & Medicine*, vol. 62, pp. 1330–1340.

Walsh, D 2007, 'A birth centre's encounters with discourses of childbirth: How resistance led to innovation', *Sociology of Health & Illness*, vol. 29, pp. 216–232.

WHO & UNICEF 2015, 'Water, sanitation and hygiene in health care facilities: Status in low and middle income countries and way forward', WHO. Geneva. Available from: http://apps.who.int/iris/bitstream/10665/154588/1/9789241508476_eng.pdf. [21 January 2019].

Wood, R, Mignone, J, Robinson, K, & Roger, K 2016, 'Choosing an out-of-hospital birth centre: Exploring women's decision-making experiences', *Midwifery*, vol. 39, pp. 12–19.

13

DECISION-MAKING AROUND PAIN AND ITS MANAGEMENT DURING LABOUR AND BIRTH

Sigfríður Inga Karlsdóttir, Elizabeth Newnham, Hildur Kristjánsdóttir and Ruth Sanders

Chapter overview

In this chapter, we take a critical approach to the way that childbirth pain and its management has been viewed. We examine the influence of various paradigms on the way that pain-management decisions are made, including the way that information is shared with women. Rather than listing the pros and cons of various pharmacological analgesic methods, as can be found in many midwifery texts, we present emerging research that sheds light on how women themselves view labour pain, the impact of the midwife on women's experiences, and how belief systems and environments can influence decision-making. By discussing pain management decision-making in this way, we aim to encourage reflection on midwifery practice and maternity services more broadly. The primary midwifery theories we draw on in this chapter are the 'working with pain' approach (Leap et al., 2010a), the 'woman's paradigm of pain' (Karlsdottir et al., 2014), the 'circle of trust' (Newnham et al., 2018) and identifying labour pain as 'functional discomfort' (Sanders, 2015a). These theories are underpinned by a 'salutogenic' approach to labour pain. This approach identifies the positive physiological effects of pain in an uncomplicated labour, therefore throughout this chapter we work with the idea of supporting women through pain rather than avoiding or relieving it, no matter the setting or system of care, although some settings are better equipped to support physiological birth. However, we are not advocating that women should be denied analgesia if they choose it. We are simply looking underneath some of the everyday assumptions that midwives, doctors and women themselves may have about approaching pain in labour.

Introduction

Engaging with the key tenet of the book, that of midwifery decision-making, we encourage a critical and reflexive approach to labour pain, based on the premise that woman are able to cope with the physiological pain of normal labour and birth, that labour pain can be seen as 'salutogenic' (that it can contribute to the well-being of women and their babies) and the importance of all midwives irrespective of model of care or geographical location around the world to support women to achieve this. First, we introduce the concept of decision-making in midwifery practice, with reference to Elwyn and colleagues' (2017) three-talk model. Following that, provide an overview of the positive pain approach with a basis in salutogenic theory. We then outline the theories introduced in relation to midwifery philosophy and practice when considering decision-making for the management of labour pain.

Decision-making for midwifery practice

Users of the healthcare system, such as pregnant women and women in childbirth, are encouraged to be active decision-makers in their care especially when it comes to making informed choices to accept or decline treatment or intervention, and this is often clearly set out in international ethical codes (International Confederation of Midwives, 2014a) and national healthcare laws. For example, in Icelandic law, if pregnant women are to be able to make an informed decision about whether or not to have an epidural, they must get accurate and unbiased information (health education) that promotes a comprehensive understanding of the intervention involved and its purpose, benefits and possible complications (Lög um réttindi sjúklinga 74/1997. E: Icelandic patient law). There are similar legal precedents and ethical codes of conduct guiding healthcare decisions in most countries around the world. Informed consent is grounded in the ethical principle of respect for autonomy. Midwives with their emphasis on holistic care, autonomy and empowerment can provide women with the support needed to make informed decisions consistent with their values and preferences (Benyamini et al., 2017), however it is useful to explore how decision-making occurs within such partnerships of care.

One model for decision-making is presented by Elwyn et al. (2012, 2017), who suggest a three-talk model for shared decision-making and highlight that the decision-making process should be based on what matters most to women. The model and its strengths and limitations are discussed in Chapter 1. This is an empowering model whereby women are encouraged to make informed decisions about their care as an ongoing conversation with healthcare providers. An ongoing discursive process is also recommended by Edwards (2004), who challenges the idea that 'informed consent' is static and suggests that consent should be seen as an ongoing process. The three-talk model is easily adaptable for antenatal care and as preparation for childbirth. However, use of this model is more difficult in fragmented models of care or if discussions about pain management are not initiated until the woman is in labour. In order to experience the positive benefits of shared decision-making (Nieuwenhuijze et al., 2014), women require support and facilitation from midwives sharing their beliefs and a common philosophy of labour pain. A risk-oriented hospital environment, the attitude of the attending midwife towards pain, the amount of support the woman receives, and medicalised birth practices not only affect a woman's ability to cope with labour pain, but they can also influence the information that she receives and therefore the decisions that she is able to make (Benyamini et al., 2017; Leap et al., 2010b; Newnham et al., 2018).

Childbirth pain as salutogenic

Salutogenesis is a theory of health that focuses on maximising the strength and well-being of each individual rather than focusing on risk and disease. In the childbirth literature, salutogenesis has been in the spotlight in recent years, with various authors expressing how this approach can be used to improve healthcare systems including maternity care (Ferguson et al., 2015). Although the Ferguson et al. (2015) study was conducted within a high-income country, the impact of salutogenesis on healthcare systems can be applied to any maternity care location around the world. A salutogenic approach focuses on personal resources and the direction towards health, instead of looking at individuals as only either healthy or sick (Antonovsky, 1979). A key concept of the theory is a 'sense of coherence', which consists of three components: meaningfulness, manageability and comprehensibility. A person's sense of coherence is a predictor of health and has been shown to influence the outcome of childbirth (Ferguson et al., 2015). However, the theory of salutogenesis entails more than a sense of coherence; it is a broad theory which focuses on resources, competencies, abilities and assets of the individual, the group and society.

There is an assumption in the medical literature about pain relief that women do not want to, nor should have to cope with the pain of labour (Newnham et al., 2017). These ideas, documented here through western medical ideology, also have purchase in low- and middle-income countries (see, for example, Ogboli-Nwasor and Adaji, 2014; Panjabi et al., 2018) where medicalised birth practices are increasing (Miller et al., 2016). However, more recent research has shown that most women expect to feel some pain in labour, and some welcome it as a positive experience (Karlsdottir et al., 2014; Newnham et al., 2018; Van der Gucht and Lewis, 2015). There is a scientific basis to this, because labour pain increases the hormonal feedback loop, stimulating the release of oxytocin and endorphins, which contribute to feelings of well-being, relaxation, ecstasy and bonding and breastfeeding behaviours (Buckley, 2015). According to Downe and McCourt (2008), salutogenic theory is useful in the identification and acknowledgement of the benefits of physiological birth to maternal and fetal/neonatal health and well-being. Furthermore, women's experience of childbirth pain has been identified as a salutogenic birth outcome, together with normal vaginal birth (Smith et al., 2014).

Working with pain

The 'working with pain' approach (Leap, 1997) incorporates the belief that labour pain is salutogenic, contributing to the promotion of physiological labour and birth, which then positively influences other aspects of women's lives (Leap et al., 2010a). The crucial element of this approach is enabling good support in labour, which has been shown to be central to the quality of women's experiences of childbirth and reduce obstetric intervention (Leap and Hunter, 2016; Bohren et al., 2017).

If childbirth pain can be a positive and salutogenic experience for women, then all midwives need to know how to support this pain. This can be difficult if the midwife has not examined her/his own attitudes towards or fear about pain. It is recognised in the most recent intrapartum NICE guideline (UK) (2014) that 'healthcare professionals should think about how their own values and beliefs inform their attitude to coping with pain in labour and ensure their care supports the woman's choice' (p. 3). Regardless of the geographical situation or the model of care midwives practice within, midwives' decisions surrounding pain are interwoven with their individual perceptions of risk, vulnerability and how autonomously they are able to practice. Midwives must acknowledge how women prepare for the pain of childbirth during pregnancy and support them in this, for example by giving them encouragement in their body's ability to birth, normalising birth pain and providing evidence-informed information about coping mechanisms and pain management (Karlsdottir et al., 2014; Leap et al., 2010a). These options are highly dependent on culture, location and financial resources, and rather than basing advice and decisions on a pharmacological outlook, midwives need a diverse range of tools and alternatives including mobility, comfort measures and trustful communication to reflect women's aspirations for negotiating pain. Through creating a flexible sphere of midwifery support, autonomy of decision-making becomes possible on both sides of the care relationship.

This means avoiding the discussion of pain management as a 'pain relief menu'. If midwives are to challenge ideologies about relieving pain, they must feel enabled to promote the biophysical event of birth. However, this only becomes realistic and realisable if applied to the wider context of midwife-mother care provision. If midwives experience what Walsh (2012) describe as 'professional unease', they may default to a seemingly humanistic approach of offering pharmacological relief which can undermine both women's endogenous ability and midwives' facilitation capabilities (Sanders, 2015b). Usually beginning with physiological coping strategies, the other items on the 'menu' are offered on an increasing scale, commonly mobility, water, heat, nitrous oxide and oxygen, pethidine and then epidural offered as the final, most effective (but perhaps most interventionist) option. This 'menu' approach can undermine a woman's confidence by its implicit assumption that she may be unable to cope, that she has unrealistic expectations of labour or just has to make the right 'choice' for pain relief (Leap et al., in press). However, the working with pain approach also acknowledges the need for all midwives to be cognisant of 'abnormal' pain, which can accompany a labour complication or lack of support, and may result in a requirement for analgesia.

Women's paradigm of pain in labour

Pain relief is an important option, particularly in difficult labours, but it comes with side effects that can affect birth and the immediate postnatal period. While pain relief should remain an option, it should not be viewed as necessary or even as the most important issue for women as they approach birth. As pharmacological analgesia was being introduced into the birthing environment, it displaced older traditions that we now know decrease analgesic requirements in labour, such as use of upright positions, massage or warm water, and the presence of supportive female companions, including midwives (Bohren et al., 2017; Cluett and Burns, 2009; Lawrence et al., 2013).

The medical paradigm has been mainly proactive in its support of pharmaceutical analgesia in the birth space and has viewed labour pain as being of primary concern for women (Newnham et al., 2018). However, when women have been asked, it is clear that these older practices described earlier are actually more important for women and that pain is not necessarily perceived as solely negative but has positive connotations (Lundgren and Dahlberg, 1998). Karlsdottir et al. (2014) have identified the need to describe labour pain from the perspective of the childbearing woman, as prior theories have been either medical or midwifery-oriented.

A study conducted in Iceland has shown that most pregnant women, early in pregnancy, have a positive attitude towards managing the pain of labour without medication (77% compared to 35% who wanted to use medication for pain management) (Karlsdottir et al., 2015). When asked about the experience of pain after they had given birth, the majority of these women experienced childbirth pain as positive. The women's attitudes to their impending birth and their sense of security affected their experience of pain in childbirth; in fact, these factors were predictors for positive experiences of pain and the same applied for women's overall satisfaction with care during labour. According to an Icelandic study, shared decision-making around pain management in childbirth was one of the issues that contributed to women's satisfaction with care during labour, including their experience of pain in childbirth (Karlsdottir et al., 2018).

Furthermore, according to an Icelandic study the quality of the midwife's presence and professionalism was of great importance to women; they identified this as being conducive to the managing of their pain. It was crucial for them to have a midwife who they felt connected with, and someone who made them feel in charge of managing the pain (Karlsdottir et al., 2014). Midwifery presence, birth environment, fear and self-efficacy have significant impact on the uptake of intrapartum analgesia and this needs to be considered when planning maternity care services (Sanders, 2015a).

This 'women's paradigm' of pain shows how women often describe labour pain as transformative – linked to the meaningfulness of birth and the transition to motherhood and of inducing feelings of power, capability and positive self-image (Lundgren and Dahlberg, 1998; Leap et al., 2010b; Karlsdottir et al., 2014). Midwives are in the privileged position of being able to positively support this transformative process, which, if it achieves these things, provides a salutogenic start to motherhood.

More recent research has supported this idea of a positive pain paradigm. A review of qualitative literature on women's capacity to cope with the pain of labour found that the two most important influences were individualised and continuous support, and acceptance of pain during birth (Van der Gucht and Lewis, 2015). Other research has identified the importance of how pain is perceived: when pain is understood as productive and purposeful, women are more likely to feel they can cope, but if it is seen as threatening, they are more likely to feel they need help from external sources. The social environment (including beliefs and behaviours of midwives and support people) thus shapes experiences of pain by influencing how pain is interpreted (Whitburn et al., 2017). A literature review on the nature of labour pain itself identified three aspects that mark it out from other kinds of pain. Labour pain is intense and emotional (including positive descriptors), unique (not like other kinds of pain) and meaningful (shaped by cultural and personal beliefs and context). It is influenced not only by a woman's cognitive predisposition and social support but also by the environment and culture in which she gives birth (Whitburn et al., In press). It is vital then that clinical reasoning and decision-making around 'pain management' includes the attitude of attending midwives towards pain, the presence or absence of support people and the availability (or lack) of physiological support, such as access to water, and environmental factors such as space to walk, space for privacy, and preferably architectural and design features that support the hormones of birth physiology (Foureur, 2008; Hammond et al., 2013; Harte et al., 2016).

The circle of trust

The midwife–woman relationship lies at the heart of woman-centred midwifery care, with trust central to this relationship (Hunter et al., 2008; Kirkham, 2000). Women rely on information, guidance and support from their midwife, especially during labour and birth, even if the midwife is not previously known to them. This relationship during labour not only enables women to cope better with labour pain (Halldorsdottir and Karlsdottir, 1996; Van der Gucht and Lewis, 2015) but also supports them to follow their bodies' cues in the knowledge that all is well (Halldorsdottir and Karlsdottir, 1996; Maher, 2010; Leap et al., 2010a) and reduce fear of birth (Fisher et al., 2006). Conversely, women who are not supported well in labour often report higher pharmacological pain relief requirements (Hodnett, 2002; Newnham et al., 2018; Van der Gucht and Lewis, 2015). Women can approach labour with negative or positive expectations of pain (Lally et al., 2008), however drivers for analgesia requirements may in fact be more related to fear, loss of control or lack of support rather than actual levels of pain experienced (Newnham et al., 2018). A recent meta-ethnography exploring women's psychological experiences of physiological childbirth found that two main elements affected their experience of pain: women trusting their bodies and managing to work with the pain (Olza et al., 2018). These are reflected in the 'circle of trust' model. Again, these issues are relevant to women across the globe. For example, many women in low- to middle-income countries are not able to utilise a birth companion of their choice, despite wanting to (Miller et al., 2016).

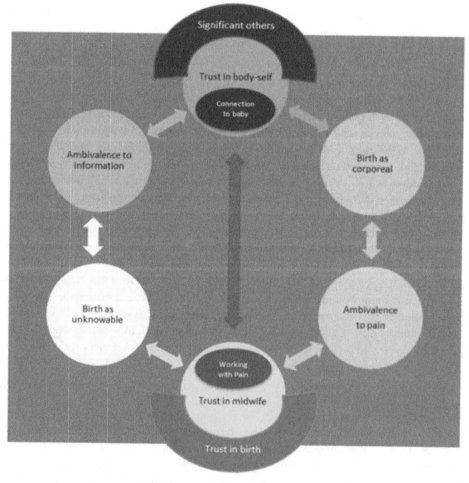

FIGURE 13.1 The circle of trust

Source: Newnham et al. (2018, p. 196)

The circle of trust is a conceptual model of this trusting relationship during labour which was developed from findings of a hospital within a high-income country ethnography looking at epidural analgesia use (Newnham et al., 2018). It shows a circular process of women trusting themselves to do the work of birthing, influenced or surrounded by their significant others, and needing to trust their midwife to support this process. The second concept in this model is that women view birth as a corporeal (or physiological) event, believing that their bodies will 'do' birth as have millions of women before them. The third is the anticipation of labour pain. Women expect to feel some pain during birth and although this is not always seen as positive, neither is it wholly negative. Rather, the women approached pain with an ambivalence that could range from fear to excitement. There is a symbiotic relationship between the woman and the midwife as represented by the central arrow. The woman looks to the midwife to support her and the midwife needs to communicate her trust in the woman's body and the process of birth. Although developed from research in a high-income country labour ward, there are reflections in the international literature, for example women's belief in the 'normality' of birth (Bohren et al., 2017; Downe et al., 2018) and similarities in how women cope with labour pain that exist across cultural and socioeconomic contexts (Van der Gucht and Lewis, 2015). This reinforces the idea that to facilitate reflective clinical reasoning skills and effective decision-making with women around pain management, midwives and other care providers need to work with their own fears around birth and pain and have knowledge of the positive aspects of labour pain, as suggested by the working with pain approach (Leap et al., 2010a).

Moving up from the lowermost circle, 'trust in the midwife' is necessary for women because birth is 'unknowable', even for those women who have given birth before. Women trust the midwife to guide them through this uncharted territory and they expect this guidance to support their own belief in their bodies to birth. 'Ambivalence to information' illustrates the discrepancy between the overload of information that pregnant women get from any number of sources including family and their community, which carry some weight in women's decision-making (Bohren et al., 2014; Downe et al., 2018), and their actual need for tailored, timely and individualised information. This brings it back to the trust that women have in their bodies and the connection to their babies, which for some women is strengthened by feeling the pain of labour. Although this research took place in a high-income country, the uncovered assumptions within practice regarding women's approaches to pain management can be applied to various models of care located anywhere around the world, as globally, women report an understanding of birth as a normal, physiological function, an acceptance of the role of labour pain, and the desire for support and respectful care during labour (Downe et al., 2018; Miller, 2016; Van der Gucht and Lewis, 2015).

Need for critical thinking

Because our understanding of labour pain is complex and influenced by historic and social events and beliefs, midwives need to stay reflexive and committed to critical thinking about labour pain and pain-management. (Critical thinking and reflection are discussed further in Chapters 7 and 8.)

While respect for autonomy means that information should be non-directive, midwives and other healthcare professionals can unwittingly reinforce institutional norms, practitioner preference or risk-orientated protocols when presenting 'information' (Newnham et al., 2017;

Kirkham, 2004). More alarmingly, women in the maternity system have been subject to bullying and coercion when making decisions outside of recommended guidelines (Jenkinson et al., 2017).

As a profession, midwives are philosophically bound to support the physiological process of birth (International Confederation of Midwives, 2014b), however midwives can be challenged to provide optimal birth environments within the parameters of a medicalised birth culture and practices which increase demand for analgesia. Browne et al. (2014) argue that what constitutes core midwifery philosophy – midwives' belief in normality and trust in the process of physiological birth – is becoming increasingly challenging. Thus, midwives risk becoming further separated from normality, boxed into the space of pathology, with women only accessing advice if there is a potential problem. It is vital that all midwives are aware of these subtler influences on pain-management decision-making and reflexive in the practice of supporting and managing pain in labour.

Discussing labour pain with women

We have identified how the pain relief menu should be avoided if midwives are to use a working with pain approach, however this leaves a question as to how midwives should manage discussions and subsequent decisions of labour pain with women in their care. Guidance surrounding how pain management should be presented to women is scarce, focusing primarily on pharmacological strategies and placing the benefit and drawbacks of each strategy at the forefront of discussions. Although midwives are prompted to consider their own belief systems and ideologies and how these may influence women's own expectations and experiences of labour pain (National Institute for Health and Care Excellence, 2014; Nursing and Midwifery Council, 2018 Leap and Hunter, 2016), currently no policy or guidance exists about how midwives should facilitate discussions about pain.

Furthermore, women report experiencing a 'professional lack' (Sanders and Crozier, 2018) arising from their perceptions of limited contact time with midwives and concern regarding coping strategies and potential suffering (Simkin and Anchetta, 2017; Simkin and Bolding, 2004), expressing worry that they do not have the capacity to negotiate labour without recourse to pain management (Leap et al., 2010a). Women can also be influenced by broader societal beliefs of pain as pathological. If midwives are able to change this pathological focus when discussing labour, it is possible to shift women's pain expectations from the fear of pathology to the understanding of physiological experience. Women may feel uncertain about their role within the experience of labour (Rachmawati, 2012), distrusting their own ability to birth. Because pain can be associated with damage and suffering (Simkin and Anchetta, 2017), bringing the purposeful nature of labour pain to the fore and exploring this experience as one of 'functional discomfort' (Sanders, 2015a) changes a painful process which is passively received into an experience of active and potentially empowering participation.

The intransigence of the current ideology likening labour pain to powers outside the woman's body are in opposition to midwives' encouragement for women to work with their bodies in labour. The persistent avoidance of physiological terminology and use of environmental imagery such as 'waves', situate contractions as external forces of nature, potentially confirming women's fear that labour sensations will become overwhelming, and further disconnecting women from their bodies and birthing abilities. Emphasising labour pain as 'functional discomfort' arising from women's physiological process could alleviate reliance on pharmacology whilst increasing women's own sense of agency. Antonovsky (1993) theorises health as a fluctuating point on a trajectory between ease and dis-ease, with the facility to comprehend the whole journey formulating a sense of coherence. This can be likened to women's journey through the rhythm of labour, with functional discomfort creating a sense of coherence, forming a new articulation of the experience of pain without bringing pathology into the birthing environment.

Conclusion

In a maternity climate where professionals are attempting to balance interventions between 'too much too soon' and 'too little too late' (Miller et al., 2016), women's decision-making processes surrounding pain management formulate an important part of the global discussion. Communication often focuses around the emphasis of relieving pain rather than a working with pain outlook, and care providers' perceptions of what women want in terms of pain management may be radically different from what women require. The transformative potential of labour pain must be championed by midwives, considering women's individual needs as each labour progresses, explored from an approach of trusting and shared decision-making. If this is to be achieved, then midwives must have a wide range of supportive strategies at their disposal, reflexive to the needs of women but also aware of the potential challenges of working within the medical paradigm and its increasing sequalae of intervention.

References

Antonovsky, A., 1979. *Health, stress and coping.* Jossey-Bass, San Francisco.

Antonovsky, A., 1993. The structure and properties of the sense of coherence scale. *Social Science and Medicine* 36, 725–733.

Benyamini, Y., Molcho, M. L., Dan, U., Gozlan, M., & Preis, H., 2017. Women's attitudes towards the medicalization of childbirth and their associations with planned and actual mode of birth. *Women and Birth* 30, 424–430. https://doi:10.1016/j.wombi.2017.03.007

Bohren, M. A., Hofmeyr, G., Sakala, C., Fukuzawa, R. K., & Cuthbert, A., 2017. Continuous support for women during childbirth. *Cochrane Database of Systematic Reviews*, Issue 7, Art. No. CD003766. doi:10.1002/14651858.CD003766.pub6

Bohren, M. A., Hunter, E. C., Munthe-Kaas, H. M., Souza, J. P., Vogel, J. P., & Gülmezoglu, A. M., 2014. Facilitators and barriers to facility-based delivery in low- and middle-income countries: A qualitative evidence synthesis. *Reproductive Health* 11, 71. https://doi.org/10.1186/1742-4755-11-71

Browne, J., O'Brien, M., Taylor, J., Bowman, R., & Davis, D., 2014. 'You've got it within you': The political act of keeping a wellness focus in the antenatal time. *Midwifery* 30, 420–426.

Buckley, S. J., 2015. Hormonal Physiology of Childbearing: Evidence and implications for women, babies, and maternity care. Washington, DC: Childbirth Connection Programs, National Partnership for Women and Families.

Cluett, E.R., & Burns, E., 2009. Immersion in water in labour and birth. *Cochrane Database of Systematic Reviews*, Issue 2, Art. No. CD000111.

Downe, S., Finlayson, K., Oladapo, O. T., Bonet M., & Gülmezoglu A. M., 2018. What matters to women during childbirth: A systematic qualitative review. *PLoS ONE* 13(4): e0194906. https://doi.org/10.1371/journal.pone.0194906

Darvish, B., Gupta, A., Alahuhta, S., Dahl, V., Helbo-Hansen, S., Thorsteinsson, A., …Dahlgren, G., 2011. Management of accidental dural puncture and post-dural puncture headache after labour: A Nordic survey. *Acta Anaesthesiologica Scandinavica* 55, 46–53. https://doi:10.1111/j.1399-6576.2010.02335.x

Downe, S., & McCourt, C., 2008. From being to becoming: Reconstructing childbirth knowledges. In S. Downe (ed.), *Normal childbirth evidence and debate* (2nd ed., pp. 3–27). Churchill Livingstone, Edinburgh.

Edwards, N.P., 2004. Why can't women just say no? And does it really matter? In M. Kirkham (ed.) *Informed choice in maternity care* (pp. 1–30). Palgrave Macmillan, Basingstoke, Hampshire.

Elwyn, G., Durand, M.A., Song, J., Aarts, J., Barr, P.J., Berger, Z., . . . Van der Weijden, T., 2017. A three-talk model for shared decision making: Multistage consultation process. *British Medical Journal* 359, 4891. https://doi:10.1136/bmj.j4891www.bmj.com/content/bmj/359/bmj.j4891.full.pdf

Elwyn, G., Frosch, D., Thomson, R., Joseph-Williams, N., Lloyd, A., Kinnersley, P., . . . Barry, M., 2012. Shared decision making: A model for clinical practice. *Journal of General Internal Medicine* 27, 1361–1367.

Ferguson, S., Davis, D., Browne, J., & Taylor, J., 2015. Sense of coherence and childbearing choices: A cross sectional survey. *Midwifery* 31, 1081–1086.

Fisher, C., Hauck, Y., & Fenwick, J., 2006. How social context impacts on women's fears of childbirth: A western Australian example. *Social Science and Medicine* 3, 64–75.

Foureur, M., 2008. Creating birth space to enable undisturbed birth. In K. Fahy, M. Foureur, & C. Hastie (eds.), *Birth territory and midwifery guardianship: Theory for practice, education and research* (pp. 57–77). Elsevier, Sydney.

Halldorsdottir, S., & Karlsdottir, S.I., 1996. Journeying through labour and delivery: Perceptions of women who have given birth. *Midwifery* 12, 48–61.

Hammond, A., Foureur, M., Homer, C., & Davis, D., 2013. Space, place and the midwife: Exploring the relationship between the birth environment, neurobiology and midwifery practice. *Women and Birth* 26, 277–281.

Harte, J.D., Sheehan, A., Stewart, S.C., & Foureur, M., 2016. Childbirth supporters' experiences in a built hospital birth environment: Exploring inhibiting and facilitating factors in negotiating the supporter role. *HERD: Health Environments Research and Design Journal* 9, 135–161.

Hodnett, E., 2002. Pain and women's satisfaction with the experience of childbirth: A systematic review. *American Journal of Obstetrics and Gynecology* 186(5, Supplement 1), S160–S172.

Hunter, B., Berg, M., Lundgren. I., Ólafsdóttir, Ó.Á., & Kirkham, M., 2008. Relationships: The hidden threads in the tapestry of maternity care. *Midwifery* 24, 132–137.

International Confederation of Midwives, 2014a. International code of ethics for midwives. www. internationalmidwives.org/assets/files/general-files/2019/01/cd2008_001-eng-code-of-ethics-for-midwives.pdf

International Confederation of Midwives, 2014b. Philosophy and model of care. www.internationalmidwives.org/assets/files/definitions-files/2018/06/eng-philosophy-and-model-of-midwifery-care.pdf

Jenkinson, B., Kruske, S., & Kildea, S., 2017. The experiences of women, midwives and obstetricians when women decline recommended maternity care: A feminist thematic analysis. *Midwifery* 52, 1–10.

Karlsdottir, S.I., Halldorsdottir, S., & Lundgren, I., 2014. The third paradigm in labour pain preparation and management: The childbearing woman's paradigm. *Scandinavian Journal of Caring Sciences* 28, 315–327.

Karlsdottir, S.I., Sveinsdottir, H., Kristjansdottir, H., Aspelund, T., & Olafsdottir, O.A., 2018. Predictors of women's positive childbirth pain experience: Findings from an Icelandic national study. *Women and Birth* 31, e178–e184.

Karlsdottir, S.I., Sveinsdottir, H., Olafsdottir, O.A., & Kristjansdottir, H., 2015. Pregnant women's expectations about pain intensity during childbirth and their attitudes towards pain management: Findings from an Icelandic national study. *Sexual and Reproductive Healthcare* 6, 211–218. https://doi.org/10.1016/j.srhc.2015.05.006

Kirkham, M. (ed.), 2000. *The midwife-mother relationship* (2nd ed). Palgrave Macmillan, London.

Kirkham, M., 2004. Choice and bureaucracy. In M. Kirkham (ed.), *Informed choice in maternity care* (pp. 265–290). Palgrave MacMillan, Houndmills, Basingstoke.

Lally, E., Murtagh, M., Macphail, S., & Thomson, R., 2008. More in hope than expectation: A systematic review of women's expectations and experience of pain relief in labour. *BMC Medicine* 6, 1–10.

Lawrence, A., Lewis, L., Hofmeyr, G.J., & Styles, C., 2013. Maternal positions and mobility during first stage labour. *Cochrane Database of Systematic Reviews*, Issue 10, Art. No. CD003934. https://doi:10.1002/14651858.CD003934.pub4

Leap, N., 1997. Being with women in pain – Do midwives need to re-think their role? *British Journal of Midwifery* 5, 263.

Leap, N., Dodwell, M., & Newburn, M., 2010a. Working with pain in labour: An overview of evidence. *New Digest* 49, 22–26.

Leap, N., & Hunter, B., 2016. *Supporting women for labour and birth: A thoughtful guide.* Routledge, London.

Leap, N., Newnham, E., & Karlsdottir, S.I., In press. Approaches to pain in labour: Implications for midwifery practice. In S. Downe & S. Byrom (eds.), *Squaring the circle: Researching normal childbirth in a technological world.* Churchill Livingstone, Elsevier, Edinburgh.

Leap, N., Sandall, J., Buckland, S., & Huber, U., 2010b. Journey to confidence: Women's experiences of pain in labour and relational continuity of care. *Journal of Midwifery and Women's Health* 55, 234–242.

Lundgren, I., & Dahlberg, K., 1998. Women's experience of pain during childbirth. *Midwifery* 14, 105–110.

Lög um réttindi sjúklinga nr. 74/1997. (Icelandic patient law). www.althingi.is/lagas/nuna/1997074.html

Maher, J., 2010. Beyond control? Resituating childbirth pain in subjectivity. *Outskirts Online Journal*, 22.

Miller, S., Abalos, E., Chamillard, M., Ciapponi, A., Colaci, D., Comandé, D., . . . Althabe, F., 2016. Beyond too little, too late and too much, too soon: A pathway towards evidence-based, respectful maternity care worldwide. *Lancet* 388, 2176–2192.

National Institute for Health and Care Excellence [NICE] Intrapartum care: Care of healthy women and their babies during childbirth, 2014. Clinical Guideline 190, Methods, evidence and recommendations. National Institute for Health and Care Excellence.

Newnham, E., McKellar, L., & Pincombe, J., 2017. 'It's your body, but . . .' Mixed messages in childbirth education: Findings from a hospital ethnography. *Midwifery* 55, 53–59.

Newnham, E., McKellar, L., & Pincombe, J., 2018. *Towards the humanisation of birth: A study of epidural analgesia and hospital birth culture.* Palgrave Macmillan, Cham.

Nieuwenhuijze, M., Korstjens, I., de Jonge, A., de Vries, R., & Lagro-Janssen, A., 2014. On speaking terms: A Delphi study on shared decision-making in maternity care. *BMC Pregnancy Childbirth* 223, 1–11.

Nursing and Midwifery Council, 2018. The Code: Professional standards of practice and behaviour for nurses, midwives and nursing associates. Nursing and Midwifery council, London.

Ogboli-Nwasor, E.O., & Adaji, S.E., 2014. Between pain and pleasure: Pregnant women's knowledge and preferences for pain relief in labor, a pilot study from Zaria, Northern Nigeria. *Saudi Journal of Anesthesia* 8, S20–S24.

Olza, I., Leahy-Warren, P., Benyamini, Y., Kazmierczak, M., Karlsdottir, S.I., . . . Nieuwenhuijze, M., 2018. Women's psychological experiences of physiological childbirth: A meta-synthesis. *BMJ Open* 8, e020347. https://doi:10.1136/bmjopen-2017-020347

Panjabi, G.M., Prajapati, K.N., & Pandya, P.D., 2018. Awareness, attitude and knowledge of antenatal women towards labour analgesia in a medical college hospital in India. *National Journal of Integrated Research in Medicine* 9, 20–24.

Rachmawati, I.N., 2012. Maternal reflection on labour pain management and influencing factors. *British Journal of Midwifery* 20(4), 263–270.

Sanders, R., 2015a. Functional discomfort and a shift in midwifery paradigm. *Women and Birth* 28, e87–e91.

Sanders, R., 2015b. Midwifery facilitation: Exploring the functionality of labor discomfort. *Birth Issues in Perinatal Care* 42, 202–205.

Sanders, R., & Crozier, K., 2018. How do informal information sources influence women's decision-making for birth? A meta-synthesis of qualitative studies. *BMC Pregnancy and Childbirth* 18, 21. https://doi:10.1186/s12884-017-1648-2

Simkin, P., & Anchetta, R., 2017. Normal labor and labor dystocia: General considerations. In P. Simkin, L. Hanson, & R. Anchetta (eds.), *The labor progress handbook early interventions to prevent and treat dystocia* (4th ed., pp. 9–42). John Wiley & Sons, New Jersey.

Simkin, P., & Bolding, A., 2004. Update on non-pharmacological approaches to relieve labour pain and prevent suffering. *Journal of Midwifery and Women's Health* 49, 489–504.

Smith, V., Daly, D., Lundgren, I., Eri, T., Benstoem, C., & Devane, D., 2014. Salutogenically focused outcomes in systematic reviews of intrapartum interventions: A systematic review of systematic reviews. *Midwifery* 30, e151–e156. doi:10.1016/j.midw.2013.11.002

Van der Gucht, N., & Lewis, K., 2015. Women's experiences of coping with pain during childbirth: A critical review of qualitative research. *Midwifery* 31, 349–358.

Walsh, D., 2012. *Evidence and skills for normal labour and birth. A guide for midwives* (2nd ed.). Routledge, Oxford.

Whitburn, L. Y., Jones, L. E., Davey, M., & McDonald, S., In press. The nature of labour pain: An updated review of the literature, *Women and Birth.* https://doi.org/10.1016/j.wombi.2018.03.004

Whitburn, L. Y., Jones, L. E., Davey, M., & Small, R., 2017. The meaning of labour pain: How the social environment and other contextual factors shape women's experiences. *BMC Pregnancy and Childbirth* 17, 157. https://doi.org/10.1186/s12884-017-1343-3

14

MIDWIVES' DECISION-MAKING FOR FETAL HEART MONITORING

Robyn Maude

Chapter overview

Monitoring maternal and fetal well-being during labour and birth is fundamental to midwifery practice and an extension of the monitoring of well-being that takes place during the antenatal period. Decision-making for intrapartum fetal heart rate monitoring is made in partnership with the woman and informed by evidence. A midwifery model of care, underpinned by continuity of care(r), empowers women's informed choice and decision-making. The choice of fetal monitoring modality may influence the outcomes of care for both the woman and baby. For this reason, this chapter will explore a number of considerations that will inform decision-making. Further this chapter will consider the application of ethical principles and provide understanding of maternal and fetal physiology while critically appraising the current evidence and fetal heart monitoring guidelines. The need for midwives to be cognisant of how place of birth choice influences outcomes, and to apply the principles of cultural awareness, will also be discussed. A decision-making framework for intelligent structured intermittent auscultation (ISIA) will be used to demonstrate critical thinking and informed decision-making for fetal heart monitoring.

Introduction

Fetal heart rate monitoring is an important component of intrapartum care in all birth settings. Fetal well-being is determined by listening to the fetal heart rate during labour to determine how it responds to maternal uterine contractions and taking into account other aspects that might have an influence. There are two main fetal heart rate monitoring modalities: intermittent auscultation (IA) using a Pinard stethoscope or a handheld Doppler device, and continuous electronic fetal monitoring using the cardiotocograph (CTG) machine. There is international consensus that IA is recommended for fetal heart rate monitoring in healthy women with uncomplicated pregnancies (also known as low risk) during labour and birth (FIGO, 2015; ICM, 2017b; WHO, 2018). Though there is no evidence for improved outcomes for routine use of CTG on admission to a maternity unit or in complicated labours (high risk), some professional bodies' guidelines recommend that this is the optimal approach to use in these situations especially where more than one such risk factor is present such as advanced maternal age, high BMI, and gestational hypertension (RANZCOG, 2014)

Midwives around the world are well positioned to support informed choice and decision-making for women during their pregnancy, labour and birth, and after birth. The philosophy of midwifery is holistic by nature, dynamic in its approach and takes place in partnership with women (ICM, 2014a). Partnership supports shared decision-making as evidenced by the ICM's Philosophy and Model of Midwifery Care (2014a) statement. The partnership relationship between a woman and a midwife acknowledges individual and shared responsibilities, open communication, shared information and negotiated choices and decisions (ICM, 2014a). Midwife-led continuity of care enhances the partnership (ICM, 2014a).

A midwife-led continuity of care model is where the midwife is the lead professional from early pregnancy through labour and birth and including the early days of parenting (ICM, 2017a). A systematic review found women who received midwife-led continuity of care were more likely to be cared for in labour by midwives they already knew, less likely to experience interventions, had increased chance of spontaneous vaginal birth and increased satisfaction with their care (Sandall, Soltani, Gates, Shennan, & Devane, 2016). Where continuity of care is not possible, a midwifery philosophy of understanding, promoting, protecting and facilitating normal physiological birth will guide informed choices and decision-making (ICM, 2014a).

Underpinning midwives' decision-making for fetal heart rate monitoring during labour and birth is an assumption of pregnancy and birth as a normal physiological event for the majority of women. This perspective of normal physiology is within the international scope of practice of a midwife and reinforced by the standards for practice and clinical competencies (ICM, 2014b, 2017a, 2019). Some countries have also expanded on the ICM (2017c) statement on heritage and culture by developing their own cultural competencies; example of this are the regulatory (www.midwiferycouncil.health.nz) and professional (www.midwife.org.nz) bodies of New Zealand. Whilst it is acknowledged that for some women there are significant challenges impacting on the health and well-being of themselves and their babies, interventions in the normal physiological processes of birth must be used appropriately. 'The unthinking application of technology is counterproductive' (Gibb & Arulkumaran, 2008). In the foreword of the third edition of their fetal monitoring in practice handbook the authors state: '[e]xcessive technology should not be applied to those [women] who are manifestly at low risk. It may confer no benefit, can generate both non-medical and medical anxiety, and through subtle effects may cause significant harm' (Gibb & Arulkumaran, 2008, p. vii).

As midwives, we must have clear understanding of the fetal heart rate monitoring modalities available for the assessment of fetal well-being during labour, apply these appropriately and according to evidence-informed guidelines. Importantly, we must also take into account the wishes of the well-informed woman and the status of her current health and well-being. Midwives should take responsibility for educating themselves in how to interpret what we see and hear during fetal heart rate monitoring. Midwives should know the appropriate actions to take when there are concerns, and find and refine methods of communicating this to women and our colleagues – this includes using an agreed standard language, asking for a second opinion or a 'fresh eyes' approach to validate our clinical reasoning, and importantly documenting our decision-making in a way that provides evidence of this clinical reasoning. It is acknowledged that midwives practising in remote, rural and village settings in a low-income country may not have access to education, colleagues or indeed opportunities for transferring women to another health centre when concerns arise. The use of decision-making pathways, written for the birth context, which are practical, uncomplicated and easy to follow may support midwives who are impacted by workforce shortages and lack of resources or geographical issues (Housseine et al., 2018).

Fetal heart monitoring and the evidence

During labour there are two main fetal heart rate monitoring modalities: intermittent auscultation (IA) using a Pinard stethoscope or a handheld Doppler device, and continuous electronic fetal monitoring using the cardiotocograph (CTG) machine. More recently, a form of continuous monitoring using a Doppler device (Moyo) for the purpose of detecting abnormal fetal heart rate has been trialled in Tanzania (Mdoe et al., 2018; Kamala et al., 2019).

Professional midwifery and obstetric organisations from Australasia, UK, the US and Canada, and key stakeholders such as the World Health Organization (WHO), International Confederation of Midwives (ICM) and the International Federation of Gynecology and Obstetrics (FIGO) (Lewis, Downe, Panel & FIFMEC, 2015) recommend IA of the fetal heart rate over continuous CTG for healthy women with uncomplicated pregnancies during labour (American College of Nurse-Midwives [ACNM], 2007; American College of Obstetricians & Gynecologists [ACOG], 2005; National Institute for Health and Clinical Excellence [NICE], 2017, New Zealand College of Midwives [NZCOM], 2005; Royal Australian and New Zealand College of Obstetricians and Gynaecologists [RANZCOG], 2014; Liston, Sawchuck, & Young, 2007).

Studies comparing intermittent auscultation with CTG monitoring found an increase in the incidence of assisted vaginal births (forceps and ventouse) and caesarean section without evidence of benefit for mothers and babies (cerebral palsy, mortality, admission to neonatal units) (Alfirevic, Devane, Gyte, & Cuthbert, 2017). Most of the studies in this review were from high-income countries with one being from a middle- to lower-income country and one from a lower-income country. A recent study from the United States has also concluded that the universal application of continuous CTG in pregnancies that are low risk and at term is not supported (Heelan-Fancher et al., 2019). In contrast, the recent studies from Tanzania comparing the continuous Doppler device during labour versus IA found that the Doppler device detected abnormal fetal heart rates more frequently, facilitating higher rates of intrapartum resuscitation, however there were higher than acceptable delays in expediting delivery in both groups (Mdoe et al., 2018; Kamala et al., 2019). Whilst use of the continuous Doppler device positively affected women's birth experience (Lafontan et al., 2018), rates of caesarean section were significantly higher in the continuous Doppler device group, with adverse perinatal outcomes similar between the groups (Mdoe et al., 2018; Kamala et al., 2019).

It has long been established that the 'admission CTG' for low-risk women is associated with an increase in the caesarean section rate by approximately 20% (Devane et al., 2017; Alfirevic et al., 2017). Despite this knowledge, there continues to be widespread use of the 'admission CTG' in many maternity environments around the world. Midwives must take some responsibility for this, as we are the ones who are applying the CTG machine. We must know what the evidence says about 'admission CTG' and be prepared to debate this with our colleagues. Facilitating informed decision-making supports us to share this research evidence with women to enable them to make an informed choice without compromising the normality of labour.

Informed choice and decision-making

Empowering women to engage in informed choices about their pregnancy, labour and birth care and early parenthood is fundamental to the midwifery model of care (ICM, 2017c). The right to informed choice, decision-making and consent are enshrined in many patient rights charters from around the world (Flood & May, 2012), as well as in statements on midwives' philosophy, scope of practice, competencies for entry to the register of midwives, the code of ethics and the standards for practice (ICM, 2014b, 2019). The context for informed choice and consent in the woman-midwife partnership model, irrespective of geographical location or model of care provision, is the provision of accurate and unbiased information including an explanation of the condition, options available for the treatment and/or management of the condition, an assessment of the risks, potential side effects, benefits and costs of those treatment/management options. The woman also has the right to refuse the advice and services and withdraw from services (HDC, 1996).

Applying ethical principles to decision-making for fetal heart monitoring

Despite a lack of evidence, the choice of fetal monitoring modality for women with complicated pregnancies is usually limited. For this reason, midwives draw upon the current fetal heart rate monitoring international guidelines such as those of the National Institute for Health and Clinical Excellence (NICE) (2014 update 2017) or the Royal Australian and New Zealand College of Obstetricians and Gynaecologists (RANZCOG) (2014), which recommend continuous CTG where there is a high likelihood that the foetus may become hypoxic during labour. For low-risk women the choices are greater, and it is in this situation that midwives face a moral conundrum around fetal heart rate monitoring, particularly in the hospital setting (Wood, 2003). The model of care, place of birth and decision-making frameworks influence choices around fetal heart monitoring for this group of low-risk women and ultimately may influence the outcomes of the labour and birth for the woman and the baby.

Although ethics is discussed in Chapter 4, this chapter draws upon the Lagana-Duderstadt Deontological Ethical Model (1995), described by Woods (2003). This model is based on the application of the ethical principles of *autonomy* (self-determination), *beneficence* (to do good), *non-maleficence* (to prevent harm), *justice* (fair and equal treatment), *respect, informed consent* and *veracity* (duty to tell the truth) to decision-making for fetal heart rate monitoring for low-risk women. The dilemma is whether it is ethical for intrapartum care providers to offer low-risk labouring women a fetal heart monitoring modality that can increase risk to them without benefitting the baby. Using a four step approach – identifying the ethical dilemma; describing possible solutions; evaluating the solutions in light of the ethical principles and choosing a solution – Wood (2003) concluded that there is no ethical support for the use of continuous electronic fetal monitoring for low-risk women. This conclusion is further supported by Sartwelle, Johnston, and Arda (2017), who claim the three principles of autonomy, beneficence and non-maleficence are violated every day by the ongoing application of electronic fetal heart monitoring, especially for low-risk women, and have knowingly been violated for 50 years.

The application of the ethical principles to the decision-making processes around intrapartum fetal heart monitoring results in an understanding that the use of intermittent auscultation of the fetal heart in labour for low-risk women is supported by the midwives' scope of practice, the midwifery model of care (partnership, continuity of care, informed choice/consent) (Maude, 2012), research and ethics (Wood, 2003). Therefore, the knowledge that IA as a fetal heart monitoring modality for low-risk women is well supported should be reassuring for practising midwives around the globe.

Using a decision-making framework for intermittent auscultation of the fetal heart

To support midwives in their decision-making around fetal heart rate monitoring for low-risk women, a robust framework for the conduct of IA and an education session, overtly informed by an understanding of fetal physiology and research evidence, was developed and evaluated in practice (Maude, 2012; Maude, Foureur, & Skinner, 2014, 2016). Although this decision-making framework was designed and evaluated within a high-income country, there is no reason readers could not apply it to their own location and midwifery practice, irrespective of where this is around the world. The IA decision-making framework is called Intelligent Structured Intermittent Auscultation (ISIA). The ISIA framework guides women and maternity care providers in their decision-making regarding monitoring choice, clinical practice, interpretation and action on the use of IA of the fetal heart during labour for low-risk women. It is presented with two parts: 'Admission Assessment or First Contact in Labour' and 'Ongoing IA in Active Labour'. The Admission Assessment or First Contact in Labour component (Figure 14.1) is used by the midwife when a woman is first admitted to an institutional birth setting or when first seen during early labour, which may be in her home. The second component, Ongoing IA in Active Labour (Figure 14.2), is used when the findings of the assessment phase indicate the woman is suitable for ISIA as the ongoing FHR monitoring modality.

Labour is one part of the whole childbearing continuum from conception to the postnatal period (Gibb & Arulkumaran, 2008) and risk factors may develop at any stage throughout pregnancy. A thorough assessment by the midwife on admission to the birth suite or at the first contact at home will help midwives to determine whether there are risk factors, either previously present or recently developed, that signal potential for fetal compromise during labour. An absence of risk factors, accompanied by findings from the physical assessment, means the woman is suitable to receive IA in labour.

As part of routine antenatal care, the midwife introduces the concept of monitoring fetal well-being by listening to the fetal heart and will discuss the methods in which this can occur, thereby empowering the woman to make choices. Limited health literacy in some medium- and low-income countries may impact women's autonomy and decision-making on fetal heart monitoring (Lafontan et al., 2018). Some women in this study did not understand the purpose of the new intrapartum monitoring device and said they would have preferred to receive this information antenatally rather than in labour (Lafontan et al., 2018). Where intrapartum care is provided by a midwife not known to the woman antenatally, the ISIA framework can be used to triage labouring women into appropriate levels of fetal heart rate monitoring (Housseine et al., 2018).

There are two key decision points during labour where the midwife and woman discuss and decide on a method of fetal heart rate monitoring. The first decision point is at the time of the admission to the birth room or at the first contact at home. At this time, the midwife

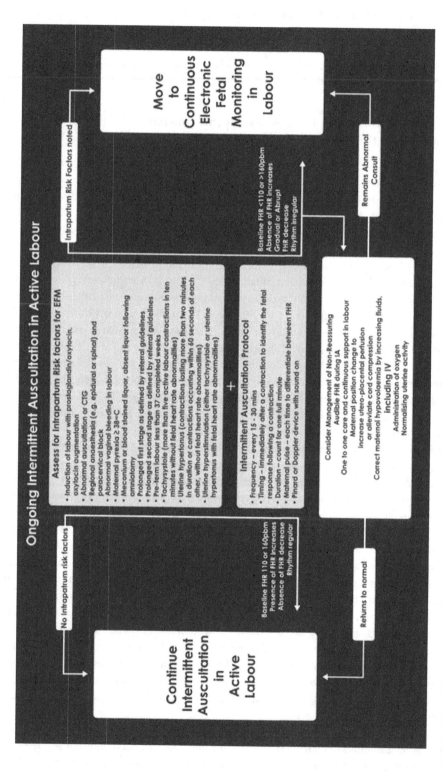

Ongoing Intermittent Auscultation in Active Labour

Intrapartum Risk Factors noted

Move to Continuous Electronic Fetal Monitoring in Labour

No Intrapartum risk factors

Assess for Intrapartum Risk Factors for EFM

- Induction of labour with prostaglandin/oxytocin, oxytocin augmentation
- Abnormal auscultation or CTG
- Regional anaesthesia (e.g. epidural or spinal) and paracervical block
- Abnormal vaginal bleeding in labour
- Maternal pyrexia ≥ 38°C
- Meconium or blood stained liquor, absent liquor following amniotomy
- Prolonged first stage as defined by referral guidelines
- Prolonged second stage as defined by referral guidelines
- Pre-term labour less than 37 completed weeks
- Tachysystole (more than five active labour contractions in ten minutes without fetal heart rate abnormalities)
- Uterine hypertonus (contractions lasting more than two minutes in duration or contractions occurring within 60 seconds of each other, without fetal heart rate abnormalities)
- Uterine hyperstimulation (either tachysystole or uterine hypertonus with fetal heart rate abnormalities)

+

Intermittent Auscultation Protocol

- Frequency – every 15 - 30 mins
- Timing – Immediately after a contraction to identify the fetal response following a contraction
- Duration – count for one full minute
- Maternal pulse – each time to differentiate between FHR
- Pinard or Doppler device with sound on

Baseline FHR 110 or 160bpm
Presence of FHR increases
Absence of FHR decrease
Rhythm regular

Continue Intermittent Auscultation in Active Labour

Returns to normal

Consider Management of Non-Reassuring Audible FHR during IA
One to one care and continuous support in labour
Maternal position change to increase utero-placental perfusion or alleviate cord compression
Correct maternal hypovolaemia by increasing fluids, including IV
Administration of oxygen
Normalising uterine activity

Baseline FHR <110 or >160pbm
Absence of FHR increases
Gradual or Abrupt
FHR decrease
Rhythm irregular

Remains Abnormal
Consult

FIGURE 14.1 ISIA decision-making framework: Admission Assessment or First Contact in Labour

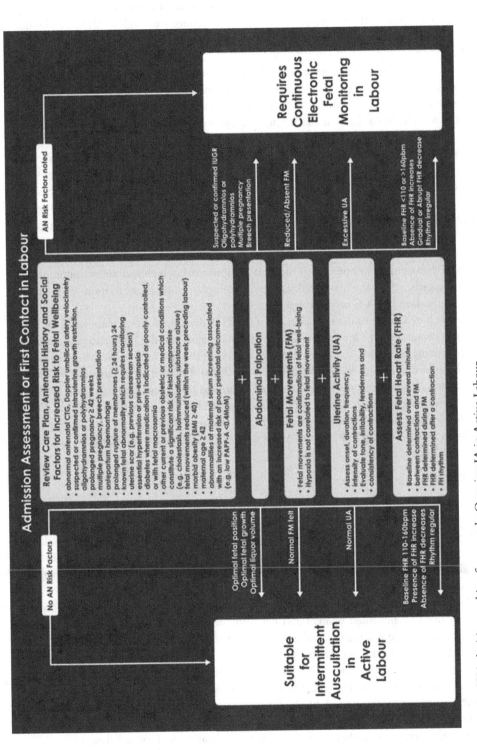

FIGURE 14.2 ISIA decision-making framework: Ongoing IA in Active Labour

Sources: Maude (2012) and Maude et al. (2014, 2016)

and the woman share information about how she is coping, what supports are needed moving forward, and review of the maternity care plan, as well as information gleaned from a physical assessment of the woman and her unborn baby (NZCOM, 2008; Rattray, Flowers, Miles, & Clarke, 2010).

The second decision point occurs after the initial assessment has been completed and the risk status determined with a discussion and decision-making around ongoing fetal heart rate monitoring (Rattray et al., 2010). The collective findings from the assessment are discussed with the woman and a decision about ongoing fetal heart rate monitoring modality can be made and documented on the care plan or in the woman's notes. In the absence of any risk factors and when all other parameters are normal, it is appropriate to offer and recommend IA for ongoing FHR monitoring during labour, and a statement to this effect is entered in the woman's medical record. The second component of the ISIA framework describes the protocol for IA during active labour and the management options when the FHR findings on auscultation are abnormal. There are two main components in the central block for ongoing FHR monitoring using ISIA (Figure 14.2). They are a continuous assessment of risk factors that might develop during labour, and how IA is performed and interpreted. A third section describes management options when the FHR is abnormal, which include communication with colleagues, referral and potential transfer of birth place and change to more frequent IA or the application of CTG monitoring.

Research evaluating of the introduction of the ISIA decision-making framework for fetal heart rate monitoring for low-risk women in New Zealand found a 12% relative increase in the appropriate use of IA, and a significant reduction in the risk of low-risk women receiving an admission CTG ($p = 0.016$) (Maude et al., 2014). Following the introduction of the intervention, medical records review revealed improved documentation of clinical findings from assessments, communication with colleagues, conduct of an appropriate level of fetal well-being monitoring with continued high rates of normal birth and few babies requiring admission to the neonatal unit or with Apgar scores of < 7 at 5 minutes (Maude et al., 2014).

Conclusion

Monitoring fetal well-being during labour and birth is a central component of midwifery care, irrespective of geographical location or model of care provision. The aim of fetal monitoring during labour is to monitor the health of the foetus, to identify those that could be at risk of neonatal and long-term injury, to reassure labouring women and midwives that all is well in most cases, and to intervene in a timely manner where deviations from normal are observed.

Decision-making for fetal monitoring modality during labour and birth is negotiated between the well-informed woman and her midwife who is competent in critiquing the research and communicating the findings in an unbiased manner. Informed choice and consent underpinned by the application of ethical principles to the decision-making process empower both the woman and the midwife. A midwifery model of care (partnership, continuity of care, informed choice/consent), ethics and research, all strengthen decision-making for fetal heart rate monitoring. A model for fetal heart monitoring such as the ISIA framework supports midwives and women in any birth setting, and across high-, medium- and low-resource countries, in their decision-making for monitoring fetal well-being.

References

American College of Nurse-Midwives (ACNM). (2007). Intermittent auscultation for intrapartum fetal heart rate surveillance. *Journal of Midwifery & Women's Health*, 52(3):314–319.

American College of Obstetricians & Gynecologists (ACOG). (2005). Intrapartum fetal heart rate monitoring. Practice Bulletin. Number 62. *Obstetrics & Gynecology*, 105(5 Pt 1):1161–1169.

Alfirevic, Z., Devane, D., Gyte, G.M.L., & Cuthbert, A. (2017). Continuous cardiotocography (CTG) as a form of electronic fetal monitoring (EFM) for fetal assessment during labour. *Cochrane Database of Systematic Reviews*, 2017(2):CD006066. doi:10.1002/14651858.CD006066.pub3. Retrieved 23 February 2019 from www.cochranelibrary.com/cdsr/doi/10.1002/14651858.CD006066.pub3/epdf/full

Devane, D., Lalor, J. G., Daly, S., McGuire, W., Cuthbert, A., & Smith, V. (2017). Cardiotocography versus intermittent auscultation of fetal heart on admission to labour ward for assessment of fetal wellbeing. *Cochrane Database of Systematic Reviews*, 2017(1):CD005122. doi:10.1002/14651858.CD005122.pub5. Retrieved 3 February 2019 from www.cochranelibrary.com/cdsr/doi/10.1002/14651858.CD005122.pub5/epdf/full

Flood, C.M., & May, K. (2012). A patient charter of rights: How to avoid a toothless tiger and achieve system improvement. *CMAJ*. doi:10.1503/cmaj111050

Gibb, D., & Arulkumaran, S. (2008). *Fetal monitoring in practice* (3rd ed.). Oxford: Elsevier Ltd.

The HDC Code of Health and Disability Services Consumers' Rights Regulation. (1996). Retrieved 9 February 2019 from www.hdc.org.nz/your-rights/the-code-and-your-rights/

Heelan-Fancher, L., Shi, L., Zhang, Y., Cai, Y., Nawai, A., & Leveille, S. (2019). Impact of continuous electronic fetal monitoring on birth outcomes in low-risk pregnancies. *Birth*, 1–7. doi:10.1111/birt.12422

Housseine, N., Punt, M., Browne, J., van't Hooft, J., Maaløe, N., Meguid, T., Theron, G., Franx, A., Grobbee, D., Visser, G., & Rijken, M. (2018). Delphi consensus statement on intrapartum fetal monitoring in low-resource settings. *International Journal of Gynecology & Obstetrics*, 1–9. doi:10.1002/ijgo.12724

International Confederation of Midwives (ICM). Use of intermittent auscultation for assessment of foetal wellbeing during labour. 2017d. Retrieved from www.internationalmidwives.org/assets/files/statementfiles/2018/04/eng-use_intermittend_auscultation.pdf

International Confederation of Midwives (ICM). (2014a). Philosophy and model of midwifery care (CD2005_001 V2014). The Hague, Netherlands.

International Confederation of Midwives (ICM). (2014b). International code of ethics for midwives (CD2008_001 V2014 ENG). The Hague, Netherlands.

International Confederation of Midwives (ICM). (2017a). International definition of the midwife (CD2005_001 V2017 ENG). The Hague, Netherlands.

International Confederation of Midwives (ICM). (2017b). Bill of rights for women and midwives (CD2011_002 V2017 ENG). The Hague, Netherlands.

International Confederation of Midwives (ICM). (2017c). Heritage and culture in childbearing (PS2011_009 V2017 ENG). The Hague, Netherlands.

International Confederation of Midwives (ICM). (2019). Essential competencies for midwifery practice. The Hague, Netherlands.

Kamala, B., Kidanto, H., Dalen, I., Ngarina, M., Abeid, M., Perlman, J., & Erdsal, H. (2019). Effectiveness of a novel continuous Doppler (Moyo) versus intermittent Doppler in intrapartum detection of abnormal foetal heart rate: A randomized controlled study in Tanzania. *International Journal of Environmental Research and Public Health*, 16:315. doi:10.3390/ijerph16030315

Lafontan, S., Sundby, J., Erdsal, H., Abeid, M., Kidanto, H., & Mbekenga, C. (2018). 'I was relieved to know that my baby was safe': Women's attitudes and perceptions on using a new electronic fetal heart rate monitor during labour in Tanzania. *International Journal of Environmental Research and Public Health*, 15:302. doi:10.3390/ijerph15020302

Lewis, D., Downe, S., Panel & FIFMEC. (2015). FIGO consensus guidelines on intrapartum fetal monitoring: Intermittent auscultation. *International Journal of Gynaecology & Obstetrics*, 131(1):9–12.

Liston, R., Sawchuck, D., & Young, D. (2007). Fetal health surveillance: Antepartum & intrapartum consensus guideline. *Journal of Obstetrics and Gynaecology Canada*, 29(9, Supp. 4):S3–S56.

Maude, R. (2012). Intelligent Structured Intermittent Auscultation (ISIA): A mixed methods evaluation of an informed decision-making framework for fetal heart monitoring. Unpublished PhD Thesis. Victoria University of Wellington, New Zealand. Retrieved March 2019 from http://hdl.handle.net/10063/2481

Maude, R., Foureur, M., & Skinner, J. (2014). Intelligent Structured Intermittent Auscultation (ISIA): Evaluation of a decision-making framework for fetal monitoring of low-risk women. *BMC Pregnancy and Childbirth*, 14:184. doi:10.1186/1471-2393-14-184. Retrieved March 2019 from www.biomedcentral.com/1471-2393/14/184

Maude, R., Foureur, M., & Skinner, J. (2016). Putting intelligent structured intermittent auscultation (ISIA) into practice. *Women and Birth*, 29:285–292. doi:10.1016/j.wombi.2015.12.001. Published on-line 19 December 2015. http://dx.doi.org/10.1016/j.wombi.2015.12.0013

Mdoe, P., Erdsal, H., Mduma, E., Moshiro, R., Dalen, I., Perlman, J., & Kidanto, H. (2018). Randomized controlled trial of continuous Doppler versus intermittent fetoscope fetal heart rate monitoring in a low resource setting. *International Journal of Gynecology and Obstetrics*, 143:344–350. doi:10:1002/ijgo.12648

National Institute for Health and Clinical Excellence (NICE). (2014). Intrapartum care for healthy women and babies. Clinical guideline [CG190]. Updated 2017. National Collaborating Centre for Women's and Children's Health. London: RCOG Press; 2007. Retrieved 3 February 2019 from www.nice.org.uk/guidance/cg190

New Zealand College of Midwives (NZCOM). (2005). Foetal monitoring in labour, NZCOM Consensus Statement. Christchurch: NZCOM.

New Zealand College of Midwives (NZCOM). (2008). *Midwives handbook for practice*. Christchurch: NZCOM.

Rattray, J. Flowers, K., Miles, S., & Clarke, J. (2010). Foetal monitoring: A woman-centred decision-making pathway. *Women & Birth*, doi:10.1016/j.wombi.2010.08.003

Royal Australian and New Zealand College of Obstetricians and Gynaecologists (RANZCOG). (2014). *Intrapartum fetal surveillance. Clinical guidelines* (2nd ed.). Melbourne: RANZCOG.

Sandall, J., Soltani, H., Gates, S., Shennan, A., & Devane, D. (2016). Midwife-led continuity models versus other models of care for childbearing women. *Cochrane Database of Systematic Reviews*, 2016(4):CD004667. doi:10.1002/14651858.CD004667.pub5. Retrieved January 2019 from www.cochranelibrary.com/cdsr/doi/10.1002/14651858.CD004667.pub5/media/CDSR/CD004667/CD004667_abstract.pdf

Sartwelle, T., Johnston, J., & Arda, B. (2017). The ethics of teaching physicians electronic fetal monitoring: And now for the rest of the story. *Surgery Journal*, 3(1):e42–e47. doi:http://dx.doi.org/

Wood, S. (2003). Should women be given a choice about fetal assessment in labour? *MCN*, 28(5):292–299.

World Health Organization. 2018. *Intrapartum care for a positive childbirth experience*. Geneva: World Health Organization. Retrieved March 2019 from www.who.int/reproductivehealth/publications/intrapartum-care-guidelines/en/

15

THIRD STAGE OF LABOUR AND OPTIMAL CORD CLAMPING

Implications for midwives' decision-making

Amanda Burleigh and Elaine Jefford

Chapter overview

Management of the third stage of childbirth involves care practices regarding cutting of the umbilical cord and expulsion of the placenta and membranes. Yet, there is a growing amount of evidence to show routine intervention of immediate/early cord clamping practices in the third stage of childbirth are known to impact upon a range of important maternal and infant health outcomes, such as early onset infant anaemia. Several international organisations across the world are recommending delayed cord clamping (hereinafter known as optimal cord clamping) for all babies (NICE 2014; RCOG 2015; WHO 2014, ACOG 2017, ACNM 2014), This chapter provides the history of optimal cord clamping and focuses on the midwife's role and the decision-making within this practice.

Introduction

To be able to inform and support midwives and student midwives within the international context in safe clinical decision-making during the third stage of labour, it is essential that midwives understand the historical medical risk-averse implementation of what has become a routine midwifery practice: cutting and clamping of the umbilical cord. Further, all midwives must understand of the physiology of transition of all aspects of third stage of labour and the short- and long-term impacts for both the mother and baby of prematurely interrupting placental blood flow.

History

Immediate cord clamping is an intervention. By clamping and cutting the cord, it prematurely intervenes in fetal to neonatal physiology (Ashish et al., 2016, 2017; McDonald et al., 2013). Immediate or premature cord clamping became routine practice with the advent of the use of oxytocic drugs, which were introduced in the late 1960s. By the late 1980s, oxytocic drugs were routinely used in many countries around the world after a UK study showed a significant reduction in postpartum haemorrhage (PPH) when immediate or premature cord clamping was practiced (Prendiville et al., 1988). This finding was and continues to be significant, especially in middle- and low-income countries where appropriate health professionals and resources are not always readily available. Nevertheless, the effect of early cord clamping on the baby was not really considered despite documentation, at that time, showing an awareness that baby lost approximately 30% of their intended blood volume (Bennett & Brown, 1993). The resulting implications of neonatal and baby/childhood anaemia remain prevalent across the world today (Ashish et al., 2016, 2017; McDonald et al., 2013). Other potential implications of early cord clamping and cutting specifically in preterm babies or babies that are compromised, include

- Cardiovascular function, which may impede stabilisation
- Increases the incidence of intraventricular haemorrhage
- Late onset sepsis
- Increased need for blood transfusion
- Necrotising enterocolitis (Mercer & Erickson-Owens, 2012, 2014; Rabe et al., 2004)
- Decreased myelin (Mercer, 2018).

Physiology

Natural physiology allows a baby to receive a placental transfusion of approximately 30% of their blood volume following birth (Royal College of Obstetricians and Gynaecologists, 2017). At birth, delayed umbilical cord clamping for one minute permits approximately 80 ml of placental blood to transfer to the baby. If delayed for three minutes, placental transfusion is approximately 100ml (Royal College of Obstetricians and Gynaecologists, 2017). This physiological transfusion aids the transition of the infant from intrauterine to extrauterine life and transfers iron-rich, oxygenated blood, resulting in higher ferritin levels and iron stores (McDonald et al., 2013, Hutton & ES, 2007), and prevents hypovolaemia while supporting optimal perfusion of all organs. It has been shown delayed umbilical cord clamping between one and three minutes can have enormous benefits for term and preterm neonates including increased haemoglobin levels at birth, improved iron stores for the first six to eight months of life, better cardiopulmonary adaption and improved brain oxygenation, specifically in preterm neonates (World Health Organization, 2014). In 2016, American midwife Judith Mercer showed that in delaying clamping and cutting the cord for five minutes, term infants have the benefits of delayed cord clamping as described with no increase in hyperbilirubanaemia or polycythaemia (Mercer et al., 2016). Further, if umbilical cord clamping is delayed for at least three minutes, anaemia at 8 and 12 months of age is significantly reduced than when clamped and cut prior to three minutes (Ashish et al., 2017).

Midwifery decision-making and optimal cord clamping: points to consider

Midwifery practice and consequently a midwife's clinical reasoning and decision-making is supposed to be based on evidence. Yet the inconsistencies in the literature, midwifery practices, international policies and procedures around the optimal time to clamp and cut the cord places her in a difficult decision-making terrain. Other influencing factors the midwife needs to consider when making a decision are if a baby is believed to be compromised or not (ACOG, 2017Wyllie et al., 2015, WHO 2012), if the woman is undergoing an active management of labour process (National Institute of Clinical Excellence, 2014), if the baby is at the introitus or is enjoying skin-to-skin contact (American College of Nurse Midwives, 2014) or if the parents (after informed choice) wish to harvest stem cells. Consideration about the geographical location of the birthing environment, resources such as medical assistance, medications, equipment and skills of the midwife all compound the complexity of midwives' clinical reasoning and decision-making processes and optimal cord clamping.

In March 2015, the World Health Organization (WHO) Regional Office for the Western Pacific launched the 'First Embrace' campaign for 'Early Essential Newborn Care' to help support health professionals including midwives in their decision-making from third stage of labour through to the first 24 hours postnatal period. Through a series of modules, health professionals are provided simple, cost-effective, lifesaving practices and tools (WHO, 2018). Some of the key areas of practice covered are:

1 Dry immediately and thoroughly
2 Immediate skin to skin
3 Delayed cord clamping (until stops pulsating)
4 Early breastfeeding.

'First Embrace' has been introduced into 17 countries at more than 3,360 health facilities with 30,251 health facility staff coached in the 'Early Essential Newborn Care' program (WHO, 2018). Though this program was introduced primarily to support low- and middle-income countries, implementation in high-income countries is occurring. The program and the steps within it, however, do not negate the professional accountability of a midwife. The midwife must employ her professional judgement, utilise her clinical reasoning and decision-making skills and assess each clinical scenario on its own merit.

Protocols and guidelines

Encompassed within the scope of practice is a midwife's compliance obligations with midwifery regulation, as well as professional and legal governance, relevant to the country within which she is employed (please refer to Chapters 2 and 3). In relation to optimal cord clamping, the dilemma for all midwives is how one upholds her professional accountability while following institutional protocols and guidelines, which may not reflect the latest evidence. This stance is supported by a midwife's accountability to standards of practice whereby she does no harm (International Confederation of Midwives, 2018). Something all midwives must consider when making decision is the growing evidence that practicing non-optimal cord clamping, which has been proven to have negative impact upon mother and/or baby (Ashish et al., 2016, 2017; Hall & O'Neil, 2016; Laws et al., 2010). In other words, if a midwife does not practice optimal cord clamping (depending on factors noted earlier), then inadvertently harm to mother and/or baby may ensue.

Oxytocic drug administration

Midwifery decision-making around active and physiological third stage management of labour and the timing of administration of an oxytocic drug has been a contentious issue for many years. The arguments seem to centre on a combination of risk management, informed consent, policies and guidelines and safe autonomous practice as well as what the woman wants.

Over the past few decades early umbilical cord clamping has been linked to post-partum haemorrhage (PPH) (World Health Organization, 2012). Prevention of PPH is paramount as it can be life-threatening, and therefore some key organisations recommend early cord clamping as a preventative measure (Royal Australian and New Zealand College of Obstetricians and Gynaecologists, 2017, American College of Obstetricians and Gynaecologist, 2017). These recommendations come despite research such as Andersson et al. (2011, 2012), who found delayed (optimal) cord clamping offers no significant risk for PPH.

More recent research (Satrageno et al., 2018) using a RCT methodology, examining post-partum maternal administration of oxytocin and volume of placental transfusion, showed placental transfusion volume was unaffected by oxytocin administration timing. Women and their unborn babies within the study ($n = 144$ babies) were randomised in two groups: the first group of women received oxytocin (10 IU) IV within 15 seconds of birth of the baby and the second group of women received oxytocin (10 IU) IV after clamping the cord at three minutes. Completed results on 124 babies showed no difference in the primary outcome: infants in group A ($n = 70$) gained 86 g (SD 48), 95% CI 74–97 and in group B ($n = 74$) 87 g (SD 50), 95% CI 75–98, $p = 0.92$. Haematocrit was 57% (SD 5) in group A and 56.8% (SD 6) in group B. No differences were found in any secondary outcomes including jaundice, poly-cythaemia and maternal PPH. No clinically relevant adverse events in mothers or infants were recorded. In other words, physiological third stage of labour can be seen as the logical ending to a normal physiological labour (Soltani, 2008), with no ill effect. This is corroborated in the Dixon et al. (2013) study, which concluded use of physiological care during the third stage of labour should be considered and supported for healthy women who have had a spontaneous labour and birth regardless of birth place setting. This study was conducted in a high-income country, and it is the midwife's professional responsibility when making decisions about third stage of labour that caution needs to be noted if trying to implement this practice in certain situations and models of care – for example, if women are not located within easy distance of appropriate resources and skilled health professionals or available resources are limited (World Health Organization, 2012).

Cord blood gases

Historically blood gases were taken in order to assess the condition of the baby after a complicated birth or when the baby was born compromised (Sykes et al., 1982). Today, however, in a risk-averse culture, where maternity staff are at greater risk of litigation, the practice of obtaining cord blood gases is increasingly common. Hence, such a libellous culture can hinder the implementation of optimal cord clamping practices. Practice may be further hampered by the fact that optimal cord clamping does alter acid-base parameters and lactate values compared to immediate cord clamping, which may have implications in relation to making the decisions if and when intervention is required. Variations, however, depend mainly on time, prior pH and lactate. Therefore the timing of samples should be taken into consideration by midwives and medical practitioners (Valero et al., 2012). Nevertheless, the midwife must take into consideration the latest evidence and inform the mother that if indicated, umbilical artery gas analysis can be safely taken with optimal cord clamping – in other words, without the cord being clamped (Xodo et al., 2018).

Cord milking

A relatively new area of practice and evidence that needs to be taken into consideration when mid-wives undertake clinical reasoning and make decisions around third stage of labour is that of cord milking. Cord milking is the practice of gently grasping the uncut umbilical cord and squeezing the cord from the placenta several times toward the infant (Katheria et al., 2015). In 2016, Agarwal, found that term-born Indian infants who had optimal cord clamping at 60–90 seconds or cord milking showed no significant differences in ferritin and haemoglobin levels and growth parameters at 12 months of age (Agarwal et al., 2016). In obstetrical emergency situations such as caesarean section, surgical delivery or resuscitation, placental transfusion via efficient milking of the umbilical cord provides immediate placenta transfusion when resuscitation is required (Katheria et al., 2017). A systematic review found that umbilical cord milking has also been associated with some benefits and no adverse effects in the immediate postnatal period in preterm infants (gestational age < 33 weeks) (Al-wassia et al., 2015). Adding an additional ten randomised control trials to Al-wassia et al.'s (2015) systematic review, comparing umbilical cord milking to delayed cord clamping, Katheria (2018) found the benefits of cord milking consistent with optimal cord clamping.

Resuscitation of the newborn

An initiative used for teaching newborn resuscitation in low-resource settings, 'Helping Babies Breathe' (Singhal, 2012), advocates optimal cord clamping during the 'golden minute'. If a baby, however, is compromised, the first actions, while the cord is still intact, should be that of drying and stimulating the baby (30 seconds) and five rescue breaths of air using a bag and mask (30 seconds). This practice is supported by the European Resuscitation Council (Wyllie et al., 2015), however they note that should a neonate require resuscitation, this remains the immediate priority. Wyllie et al. (2015) also advocate that babies in developed countries that are 'limp' or apnoeic at birth receive optimal cord clamping. This is especially important as hypovolaemia from immediate cord clamping may decrease the effectiveness of resuscitation impacting short- and long-term outcomes. A reason for this is that access to the approximated 30% blood volume transfer occurring via optimal cord clamping may be essential for recovery and helping perfusion of the heart and brain (Mercer & Erickson-Owens, 2012) In such cases, the midwife must use her professional judgement to ensure optimal well-being of the baby.

A potential aid to help overcome the dilemma/conflict of intact cord resuscitation and immediate/early clamping comes in the form of a 'Mobile Resuscitation Unit'. The Bedside Assessment, Stabilisation and Initial Cardiorespiratory Support (BASICS) trolley, developed by a group of clinicians in 2010, is a small portable resuscitation trolley with oxygen, suction and a heated mattress. It was designed specifically to facilitate newborn resuscitation at the bedside with an intact cord and is currently used in units and trials around the world (Weeks et al., 2015). Parental (Sawyer, 2015) and clinician (Yoxall, 2015) response to bedside resuscitation has been positive to date.

Informed choice/consent

Midwives and women work in partnership (Miller & Bear, 2019). Within this partnership, mutual respect and trust is established. A woman needs to trust that a midwife will provide any information or advice from a stance of the best available evidence. This applies to all midwives around the world and in all models of care (International Confederation of Midwives, 2018). It is from this stance that a woman can then be empowered to actively participate in and ultimately make the final informed decision about her care. Informed consent is a philosophical and legal doctrine that has come to serve as the cornerstone of ethically sound clinical care in Western society. This doctrine requires that individuals truly understand and freely and knowledgeably make choices regarding their treatment (Roberts, 2015). If a midwife gatekeeps and makes the decision to withhold information, including the latest available evidence around optimal cord clamping, then the woman cannot make an informed decision. In other words, as a midwife one needs to ask, is a woman informed that in cutting the umbilical cord before it has fully finished its function, the baby may lose up to 30% of their intended blood volume? (Farrar, 2011). Are the longer-term implications of early cord clamping discussed? Whilst as midwives we do not wish to frighten women into accepting one care practice or another, it is important to consider the implications our individual attitudes, values and biases can have on the midwifery practice we give and our decision-making (see Chapters 23 and 24).

Ethical considerations

Another point for a midwife to consider is that of ethics. Although this topic is discussed in Chapter 4, to help the reader understand this concept in relation to optimal cord clamping, we draw on a quote made by Aristotle in 300 BC and Darwin (1797):

> Frequently the child appears to be born dead, when it is feeble and when, before the tying of the cord, a flux of blood occurs into the cord and adjacent parts and at once the baby, who had previously been as if drained of blood, comes to life again.
>
> *(Cresswell, 1862)*

> Another thing very injurious to the child is the tying and cutting of the navel string too soon, which should always be left till the child has not only repeatedly breathed but till all pulsation in the cord ceases. As otherwise the child is much weaker than it ought to be, a part of the blood being left in the placenta which ought to have been in the child.
>
> *(Darwin, 1797)*

Although the Hippocratic Oath ('*Primum non nocere*' or 'first do no harm') is predominately linked with medicine, it is adopted within midwifery. When providing information to women about optimal cord clamping, all midwives must engage in providing up-to-date evidence. It also the midwife's professional responsibility to translate that into practice. Repeated evidence is showing early clamping and cutting of the cord has the possibility to be detrimental to a baby both in the short and long term. If all midwives around the world employ best cord practice, then they shall be practicing safe ethical care. It could be argued that if a midwife fails to practice optimal cord clamping, that midwife will be working outside the International Confederation of Midwives Code of Ethics (2018), as noted earlier.

Learning activity

Now you have read about some of the points to consider around midwifery decision-making and third stage of labour, reflect on your practice within your current location using the following activity.

BOX 15.1   REFLECT ON YOUR PRACTICE – LINKED ACTIVITY 1

1   What is the policy that encompasses third stage of labour practices?
2   Does it include optimal cord clamping?
3   Does it marry with best evidence?
4   Do I enact this policy in my practice? If not, why not?
5   How will I approach this subject within my next midwife-woman relationship?

Conclusion

Midwifery practice within the third stage of labour is complex, diverse and contentious. There is a growing amount of evidence to show routine intervention of immediate/early cord clamping practices in the third stage of childbirth are known to impact upon a range of important maternal and infant health outcomes. Yet umbilical cord clamping is steeped in historical and traditional practices as well anti-libellous and risk-averse practices. All these elements have major implications for all midwives and their decision-making.

References

Agarwal, S., Jaiswal, V., Singh, D., Jaiswal, P., Garg, A., & Upadhyay, A. 2016. Randomised control trial showed that delayed cord clamping and milking resulted in no significant differences in iron stores and physical growth parameters at one year of age. *Acta Paediatrica*, 105, e526–e530.

Al-Wassia, H., & Shah, P. S. 2015. Efficacy and safety of umbilical cord milking at birth: A systematic review and meta-analysis. *JAMA Pediatrics*, 169(1), 18–25. doi:10.1001/jamapediatrics.2014.1906

American College of Nurse Midwives. 2014. Delayed umbilical cord clamping. Position Statement. Silver Spring, MD: ACNM. Available at: www.midwife.org/ACNM/files/ACNMLibraryData/UPLOADFILENAME/000000000290/Delayed-Umbilical-Cord-Clamping-May-2014.pdf. Retrieved September 1, 2016.

American College of Obstetricians and Gynaecologists. 2017. Delayed umbilical cord clamping after birth. Committee Opinion No. 684. *Obstetrics & Gynecology*, 129, e5–e10.

Andersson, O., Hellström-Westas, L., Andersson, D., & Domellöf, M. 2011. Effect of delayed versus early umbilical cord clamping on neonatal outcomes and iron status at 4 months: A randomised controlled trial. *British Medical Journal*, 343(1), d7157–d7157. http://dx.doi.org/10.1136/bmj.d7157

Andersson, O., Hellström-Westas, L., Andersson, D., Clausen, J., & Domellöf, M. 2012. Effects of delayed compared with early umbilical cord clamping on maternal postpartum hemorrhage and cord blood gas sampling: A randomized trial. *Acta Obstetricia Et Gynecologica Scandinavica*, 92(5), 567–574. http://dx.doi.org/10.1111/j.1600-0412.2012.01530.x

Ashish, K., Mälqvist, M., Rana, N., Ranneberg, L. J., & Andersson, O. 2016. Effect of timing of umbilical cord clamping on anaemia at 8 and 12 months and later neurodevelopment in late pre-term and term infants; a facility-based, randomized-controlled trial in Nepal. *BMC Pediatrics*, 16.

Ashish, K., Rana, N., & Mälqvist, M. 2017. Effects of delayed umbilical cord clamping vs early clamping on anemia in infants at 8 and 12 months: A randomized clinical trial. *JAMA Pediatrics*, 171, 264–270.

Bennett, R., & Brown, L. (eds.) 1993. *Myles Textbook for Midwives*. Edinburgh: Churchill Livingstone.

Cresswell, R. 1862. *Aristotle History of Animals*. Tr. London: Henry G Bohn.

Darwin, E., & Caldwell, C. 1797. *Zoonomia; or, The Laws of Organic Life* (A new edition; with an introductory address, and a short appendix.). Philadelphia: Printed by T. Dobson, at the stone house no. 41, South Second Street.

Dixon, L., Tracy, S., Guillard, K., Fletcher, L., Hendry, C., & Pairman, S. 2013. Outcomes of physiological and active third stage labour care amongst women in New Zealand. *Midwifery*, 29, 67–74.

Farrar, D., et al. 2011. Measuring placental transfusion for term births: Weighing babies with cord intact. *British Journal of Obstetrics and Gynaecology*, 118, 70–75.

Hall, J., & O'Neil, L. 2016. Northern Territory Midwives' Collection. Mothers and Babies 2014. Darwin: Department of Health.

Hutton, E. K., & Hassan, E. S. 2007. Late vs early clamping of the umbilical cord in full-term neonates: Systematic review and meta-analysis of controlled trials. *Journal of the American Medical Association*, 297, 1241–1252.

International Confederation of Midwives. 2018. International code of ethics for midwives. The Hague: International Confederation of Midwives.

Katheria, A., Brown, M., Rich, W., & Arnell, K. 2017. Providing a placental transfusion in newborns Who need resuscitation. *Frontier in Pediatrics*, 5.

Katheria, A. C. 2018. Umbilical cord milking: A review. *Frontiers in Pediatrics*, 6, 335. doi:0.3389/fped.2018.00335

Katheria, A. C., Truong, G., Cousins, L., Oshiro, B., & Finer, N. 2015. Umbilical cord milking versus delayed cord clamping in preterm infants. *Pediatrics*, 136(1), doi:10.1542/peds.2015-0368

Laws, P. J., Li, Z., & Sullivan, E. A. 2010. Australia's mothers and babies 2008. Perinatal statistics series no. 24. Catalogue No. PER 50. Canberra: AIHW.

McDonald, S. J., Middletone, P., Dowswell, T., & Morris, P. 2013. Effect of timing of umbilical cord clamping of term infants on maternal and neonatal outcomes. *Evidence-Based Child Health: A Cochrane Review Journal*.

Mercer, J. S., & Erickson-Owens, D. A. 2012. Rethinking placental transfusion and cord clamping issues. *Journal of Perinatal & Neonatal Nursing*, 26, 202–217.

Mercer, J. S., & Erickson-Owens, D. A. 2014. Is it time to rethink cord management when resuscitation is needed? *Journal of Midwifery & Womens Health*, 59, 635–644.

Mercer, J. S., Erickson-Owens, D. A., Collins, J., Barcelos, M., Parker, A., & Padbury, J. 2016. Effects of delayed cord clamping on residual placental blood volume, hemoglobin and bilirubin levels in term infants: A randomized controlled trial. *Journal of Perinatology*, 37(3), 260–264.

Mercer, J. S., Erickson-Owens, D. A., Deoni, S., Dean, D., Collins, J., Parker, A., Wang, M., Joelson, S., Mercer, E., & Padbury, J. 2018. Effects of delayed cord clamping on 4-month ferritin levels, brain myelin content, and neurodevelopment: A randomized controlled trial. *Journal of Pediatrics*, 203, 266–272.e2.

Miller, S., & Bear, R. 2019. Midwifery partnership. In S. Pairman, S. Tracy, H. Dahlen, & L. Dixon (eds.), *Midwifery: Preparation for Practice* (4th ed.). Chatswood, NSW: Elsevier.

National Institute of Clinical Excellence. 2014. Intrapartum care: Care of healthy women and their babies during childbirth | Guidance and guidelines. London: National Institute of Clinical Excellence.

Prendiville, W., Elboumed, D., & Chalmers, I. 1988. The effects of routine oxytocic administration in the management of the third stage of labour: An overview of the evidence from controlled trials. *British Journal of Obstetrics and Gynaecology*, 95, 3–16.

Rabe, H., Reynolds, G., & Diaz-Rossello, J. 2004. Early versus delayed umbilical cord clamping in preterm infants. *Cochrane Database of Systematic Reviews*, Oct 18(4): CD003248.

Roberts, L. W. 2015. *International Encyclopedia of the Social & Behavioral Sciences* (2nd ed.). Florida: Elsevier, pp. 320–325.

Royal College of Obstetricians and Gynaecologists. 2015. Scientific impact paper no. 14: Clamping of the umbilical cord and placental transfusion. *Obstetrics & Gynecology*, 17, 216–216. DOI:10.1111/tog.12205

Royal College of Obstetricians and Gynaecologists. 2017. *Delayed Umbilical Cord Clamping After Birth. Obstetrics and Gynecologists*. London: Wolters Kluwer Health, Inc.

Satrageno, D., Vain, N., Gordillo, J., Fernandez, A., Carroli, G., Romero, N., & Prudentt, L. 2018. Postpartum maternal administration of oxytocin and volume of placental transfusion, an RCT. *American Journal of Obstetrics & Gynecology*, 218, S26.

Sawyer, A., Ayers, S., Bertullies, S., et al. 2015. Providing immediate neonatal care and resuscitation at birth beside the mother: Parents' views, a qualitative study. *BMJ Open*, 5, e008495. doi:10.1136/bmjopen-2015-008495

Singhal, N., Lockyer, J., Fidler, H., Keenan, W., Little, G., Bucher, S., Qadir, M., & Niermeyer, S. (2012). Helping Babies Breathe: Global neonatal resuscitation program development and formative educational evaluation. *Resuscitation*, 83(1), 90–96.

Soltani, H (2008). Global implications of evidence 'biased' practice: Management of the third stage of labour. *Midwifery*, 24(2): 138–142.

Sykes, G., Johnson, P., Ashworth, F., et al. 1982. Do Apgar scores indicate asphyxia. *Lancet*, 319, 494–496.

Valero, J., Desantes, D., & Perales-Puchalt, A. 2012. Effect of delayed umbilical cord clamping on blood gas analysis. *European Journal of Obstetrics and Gynecology and Reproductive Biology*, 162, 21–23.

Weeks, A., Watt, P., Yoxall, C., Gallagher, A., Burleigh, A., Bewley, S., Heuchan, A., & Duley, L. 2015. Innovation in immediate neonatal care: Development of the Bedside Assessment, Stabilisation and Initial Cardiorespiratory Support (BASICS) trolley. *British Medical Journal Innovations*, 1, 53–58.

World Health Organization. 2012. *The evolving threat of antimicrobial resistance: Options for action.* Geneva: World Health Organization.

World Health Organization. 2014. Optimal timing of cord clamping for the prevention of iron deficiency anaemia in infants. *Who.int.* Retrieved 11 March 2015, from www.who.int/elena/titles/cord_clamping/en/

World Health Organization. 2018. Second biennial progress report: 2016–2017 (Action Plan for Health Newborn Infants in the Western Pacific Region: 2014–2020). Manila. World Health Organization Regional Office for the Western Pacific. 2018. Licence: CC BY-NC-SA 3.0 IGO. Cataloguing-in-Publication (CIP) data. 1. Infant, Newborn. 2. Infant care. 3. Research report. I. World Health Organization Regional Office for the Western Pacific. (NLM Classification: WS420).

Wyllie, J., Bruinenberg, J., Roehr, C., Rüdiger, M., Trevisanuto, D., & Urlesberger, B. 2015. European Resuscitation Council Guidelines for Resuscitation. *Resuscitation*, 95, 249–263.

Xodo, S., Xodo, L., & Berghella, V. 2018. Timing of cord clamping for blood gas analysis is of paramount importance. *Acta Obstetricia et Gynecologica Scandinavica*, 97, 1533–1534.

Yoxall, C. W., Ayers, S., Sawyer, A., et al. 2015. Providing neonatal care and resuscitation at birth besides the mother: Clinicians' views, a qualitative study. *BMJ Open*, 5, e008494. doi:10.1136/bmjopen-2015-008494

16

CHOICES AFTER TRAUMATIC BIRTH

Mari Greenfield

Chapter overview

This chapter provides the reader with an understanding of how previous traumatic birth, irrespective of location around the globe or model of care, may affect women's choices about future pregnancies and births, and in turn how this may impact midwifery decision-making. It gives an overview of current knowledge about prevalence and causation of traumatic births and the long-term consequences. A case study is used throughout the chapter to illustrate how a previous traumatic birth can affect women's relationships with midwives and other care providers, and the implications this has for midwifery decision-making.

Introduction

Up to 30% of women in the UK experience childbirth as a traumatic event, with many consequently going on to experience some form of anxiety, depression or post-traumatic stress disorder (PTSD) following childbirth (Slade, 2006; Ayers, 2014). Similar figures have been reported in other countries with similar healthcare systems, including 24% in Australia (Toohill, Fenwick, Gamble, and Creedy, 2014) and 34% in the United States (Soet, Brack, and DiIorio, 2003). The issue of traumatic birth is not, however, limited only to high-income countries. For example, 54.5% of women in one study in Iran had a traumatic birth experience, with 20% of the women reporting symptoms indicative of PTSD (Modarres, Afrasiabi, Rahnama, and Montazer, 2012). Rates of traumatic birth have not been measured in Nigeria, but the prevalence of PTSD after childbirth in Nigerian women is slightly higher than the rates amongst women in high-income countries (Adewuya, Ologun, and Ibigbami, 2006).

When childbirth presents as a traumatic experience, it can impose a profound effect on the lives of mothers, fathers (Nicholls and Ayers, 2007) and children (Parfitt and Ayers, 2009; Emmanuel, Creedy, John, Gamble, and Brown, 2008) and can present a challenge to future reproductive decisions (Fenech and Thomson, 2014; Thomson and Downe, 2013). Working with multiparous women who have previously experienced a traumatic birth(s) may bring specific challenges to midwifery decision-making. Pregnant women who have previously experienced a traumatic birth are more likely to make less common choices about perinatal care, which has implications for midwifery practice. This group of women may also have difficulties in establishing trusting relationships with midwives, which may impact the care that midwives are able to offer as well as shared decision-making.

BOX 16.1   INTRODUCING LUNA

Throughout this chapter, Luna (pseudonym) will be used as the case study of a woman who could be located in any country where medicalisation of childbirth occurs, as an example of how a previous traumatic birth can affect a subsequent pregnancy and midwifery decision-making. Luna had given birth twice before, but her first baby died during labour. Her first birth had begun at home with an Independent (private/home birth) Midwife, but Luna had asked to transfer into hospital during labour, as despite normal Doppler readings she felt something was wrong with her baby. In her second pregnancy Luna had been hospitalised with suspected pre-eclampsia, and her labour had been induced.

What is a traumatic birth?

The potential for mothers to experience significant psychological distress related to childbirth in the absence of severe physical trauma and operative births has been recognised only as recently as 2008 (Ayers, Joseph, Mckenzie-McHarg, Slade and Wijma). Research shows that there are many factors which contribute to a woman experiencing childbirth as traumatic. Some of the main contributory factors are summarised in Table 16.1 (table adapted from Greenfield, Jomeen, and Glover, 2016).

TABLE 16.1 Factors which may contribute to a traumatic birth

Factors which may contribute to a traumatic birth
Existing psychological condition
Previous sexual abuse
Previous traumatic experience
Physical harm to mother or baby
Warned of potential harm to mother or baby
Death of baby
Operative birth
Medical intervention
Haemorrhage
Lack of care
Care which is perceived as uncaring, unsupportive or inhumane
Experiencing high levels of pain during labour, and not being able to obtain analgesia
Having choice removed by the actions of a person (rather than events)
Not holding baby immediately after birth

We can think about these contributory factors as falling within three main groups:

1 Predisposing characteristics about the woman
2 The physical events of the birth
3 The care received.

In relation to these three groupings of contributory factors, midwives' decision-making will have no impact on the characteristics of the woman yet may sometimes affect the physical events of the birth, and will always affect the care received. Care which is perceived as uncaring, unsupportive or inhumane can result in a traumatic birth, even in the absence of other factors (Cigoli, Gilli, and Saita, 2006; Robinson, 2002). Equally, good care can be a protective factor in a birth that might otherwise have been perceived as traumatic (De Schepper et al., 2016; Ford and Ayers, 2009). Looking at the terms in Table 16.1, we can see that good care must be perceived by the woman as caring, supportive and humane, but good care has other characteristics too. Feeling in control of decisions that are made and able to exercise choice can be a protective factor against women experiencing birth as a traumatic event (Furuta, Sandall, Cooper, and Bick, 2016). Around the globe, good midwifery care must therefore also support women's choices and their sense of control. Regardless of the model of care provided, any care which does not promote this may be a contributing risk factor for a woman experiencing what she perceives as a traumatic birth.

Let's look again at Luna and see why she perceived her birth as traumatic.

BOX 16.2 LUNA'S EXPERIENCE OF TRAUMATIC BIRTH

Luna had very sadly lost her first baby during labour due to events beyond anyone's control. Her second baby was born with no medical complications to the baby, yet due to a medical condition (pre-eclampsia) her labour became medicalised, and was induced, which Luna hadn't wanted. She said:

> In actual fact, I, this sounds really bizarre and I think to most people this is quite a strange thing to hear, is that I would rather go through another [first baby] . . . my trauma, comes from [second baby]'s birth, unfortunately . . . I feel like I was incredibly bullied with [second baby]. There's no way I'm going through that again. . . . Even if we get the same outcome as [first baby].

> *(Luna, 1)*

Luna's experience shows us how important midwifery care is in preventing a traumatic birth, even when medical intervention is necessary. The midwifery care she received in her first birth may have protected her from experiencing trauma, and the care she received in her second birth was experienced by her as bullying. Beck states that 'birth trauma [is] in the eye of the beholder' – that is, the woman who has given birth (2004b, p. 28). This in itself presents a challenge to midwives; without asking, a midwife may not know whether a woman's previous birth(s) was traumatic.

In this chapter, we will use the following definition of a traumatic birth, which respects that the woman is the only person who can define whether her birth was traumatic:

> The emergence of a baby from the body of its mother, in a way which may or may not have caused physical injury. The mother finds either the events, injury or the care she received deeply distressing or disturbing. The distress is of an enduring nature.
>
> *(Greenfield, Jomeen, and Glover, 2016, p. 257)*

How a previous traumatic birth affects pregnant women's choices

Experiencing a traumatic birth has long-term negative consequences for women around the globe. These negative consequences include longer-term mental health problems (Forssen, 2012; Beck, 2004a), compromised maternal-infant relationships (Nicholls and Ayers, 2007), poorer quality marital relationships (Ayers, Eagle, and Waring, 2006) concomitant depression in partners (Nicholls and Ayers, 2007), distress on the anniversary of the birth or when faced with encountering people, places or phenomena which remind the mother of the birth (Beck, 2006), challenges to future reproductive decisions (Fenech and Thomson, 2014) and mistrust of healthcare professionals (Greenfield, 2017). The last three of those consequences have implications for midwifery decision-making, if a woman becomes pregnant again.

We know that women whose first birth was traumatic are less likely to become pregnant again than women whose first births were not traumatic (Porter, Bhattacharya, and van Teijlingen, 2006; Gottvall and Waldenstrom, 2002), or to wait a longer time before becoming pregnant again (Sydsjö et al., 2013). When these women do become pregnant again, Thomson and Downe (2013) describe their pregnancies as 'a journey of adversity and despair' (p. 766). Women may spend a great deal of their pregnancies 'riding the turbulent wave of panic' as they worry about experiencing a repeat of their previous birth experience (Beck and Watson, 2010, p. 241). Frequently, the biggest fear women report is loss of control and having their choices removed by midwives and obstetricians (Greenfield, 2017; Beck and Watson, 2010). In reaction to these emotions, women are also likely to gather lot of information ranging from research literature, to the local 'wise women' and their cultural practices, and strategise carefully throughout pregnancy to avoid a repeated experience. This may lead them to make choices which are outside the dominant paradigm for births within their local maternity systems (Thomson and Downe, 2013; Greenfield, 2017). Some women may even choose to use independent maternity services (Greenfield, 2017) or to 'freebirth' (to plan to give birth without any healthcare professional in attendance) (Edwards and Kirkham, 2012; Feeley and Thomson, 2016). Women's primary consideration throughout pregnancy may be their choices for birth, which may lead women to accept or decline tests, scans and other care during pregnancy based on whether the results could affect birth choices, rather than whether the test, scan or other care is indicated (Greenfield, 2017; Beck and Watson, 2010). If we reflect back to Chapter 5 on risk, we can see that in this case, the risks that are of most concern to the woman (a repeated traumatic birth) may be different to the multitude of risks that the midwives are considering. This situation may be challenging to midwives irrespective of location around the globe, as they may be unable to understand why the woman is making specific decisions, especially if the midwife is unaware that the woman has previously experienced a traumatic birth.

BOX 16.3 LUNA'S CHOICES FOR THIS BIRTH

Luna planned to have her third baby at home. She made plans throughout her pregnancy to accept and decline meetings and tests based on whether she felt they would
affect the choices she was able to make for birth.

Here she talks about how a meeting with a doctor made her feel:

> she started talking about negotiating, and . . . as soon as the words left her mouth,
> I thought there is absolutely no way I am negotiating with you. Because this is
> exactly what happened with [second baby], and what you just do is break me down.

Luna was happy to accept some medical tests: 'I . . . have agreed to erm thyroid testing
every 10 weeks. . . . That's not something that will exclude me from a home birth'.

Challenges to midwives

Some midwives practice in countries where a midwife knows the woman, her immediate
and extended family and may well have been part of the woman's previous birthing story. In
other countries, midwives may be unaware of which multiparous women have experienced
a traumatic birth, because maternal perceptions of birth are not recorded in a woman's notes.
This presents a challenge to these midwives in terms of offering appropriate care, as women
who have had a previous traumatic birth may make less common choices about their care
during pregnancy and birth, which at first glance a midwife may not understand. When
women make choices that are outside of local guidelines or policies, midwives may have to
find the delicate balance of supporting a woman's absolute legal right to make decisions about
herself and her baby whilst also working within the midwife's legal framework and employment contract.

However, the biggest challenge to midwives in working with pregnant women who have
previously experienced a traumatic birth is that of trust and mistrust.

Midwifery decision-making with women who
have had a previous traumatic birth

It is a common finding in the literature that women who have previously experienced a
traumatic birth may experience a lack of trust in those around them during a subsequent
pregnancy (Greenfield, 2017; Beck, 2004a). Most women enter their first pregnancies assuming that trusting midwives and obstetricians is an appropriate behaviour. The traumatic
birth serves as what Holmes (1981) describes as a 'strain-test' (p. 280) for the trust invested
in the relationship. In 'strain-test' situations, one individual is highly outcome dependent
on another person, but the actions that would promote the individual's own interests differ
from those that would benefit the other. For example, in the case of traumatic birth such as
Luna's, the birth itself provides the 'strain-test', but it is the actions, inactions or even simply
words of the trusted midwives and obstetricians during that crisis that results in the women
experiencing a loss of trust, as those actions or words demonstrated that the priorities of

the professionals differed from the priorities of the women. The women then lose trust in not only the specific individuals caring for them, but come to the conclusion that trusting either healthcare professionals as an entire group, or specific sub-groups such as midwives or obstetricians, is unsafe.

When women have had a traumatic birth, their faith in the provider's competences are necessarily damaged. Without a trusting relationship between woman and midwife, the midwife's ability to provide a caring role is limited (Gould, 2004). The midwife caring for a woman who has experienced a traumatic birth and has lost trust in midwives faces a difficult job, as the midwife must give this acknowledgement of the past, and at the same time, attempt to build trust with a woman who may present as highly suspicious of midwives. Only once these two tasks are achieved can the midwife efficiently offer healthcare.

Simpson (2007) identifies 'trust-diagnostic situations' (p. 265) that occur in interpersonal relationships, in which the first individual notices whether the second individual 'make[s] decisions that go against their own personal self-interest and support the best interests of the [first] individual or relationship' (p. 265).

In the context of women who have previously experienced a traumatic birth, a 'trust-diagnostic' situation could be characterised as one in which there is potential conflict between the interests of the woman and the midwife, or in any situation in which the midwife must act or speak in a way that shows whose interests they are following. Women who have previously experienced a traumatic birth may be hyper-vigilant to midwives' decision-making, and alert to whether recommendations for birth are presented as something the woman can choose or as something she must comply with. When women feel concerned that their choices have been removed, they may take steps to avoid further encounters with the specific midwife or obstetrician. In other cases, especially in countries where there are limited options to have a different midwife care for them, women may choose to avoid contact with all professionals who might potentially remove their choices. A woman's relationship of trust with a midwife may therefore be impacted both positively and negatively by the woman's interactions with other maternity professionals.

BOX 16.4 LUNA'S EXPERIENCE OF MIDWIFERY DECISION-MAKING DURING PREGNANCY

Luna had made the informed decision to decline a HbA1C test. However when she met the midwife, she had already written on the form that the test was to be done. Luna explained to the midwife that she had

> already declined and said no I don't want it [blood test], but [the midwife] in the clinic said I know you're not keen, but, can we do it anyway? . . . I did feel pressured. . . . I did feel pushed into that.
>
> *(Luna)*

This led to Luna experiencing a deterioration of trust, not just in the individual midwife but 'the lot of them' (Luna).

Midwifery decision-making to promote trust

Gould (2004) says effective midwifery care cannot be delivered in the absence of a trusting relationship. If women have lost trust as a result of a previous traumatic birth, midwives must find ways to promote a trusting relationship before they can deliver effective midwifery care. For these women, rebuilding trusting relationship with midwives (irrespective of the model of care) can only begin with an understanding that trust was previously given and was betrayed, or even abused in order to coerce women (Greenfield, 2017; Beck and Watson, 2010; Thomson and Downe, 2010; Gould, 2004).

All pregnant women need access to good quality information about pregnancy and birth, available in a variety of formats (McCants and Greiner, 2016). Pregnant women who have previously experienced a traumatic birth may need information in relation to both their current pregnancy and their previous pregnancy and birth(s). This group of women are also likely to have gathered information from other sources (Greenfield, 2017; Thomson and Downe, 2010; Beck and Watson, 2010) and may benefit from the opportunity to discuss what they have found with a midwife. Some women may benefit from the opportunity to review their previous maternity notes with a midwife, and to ask questions about what happened. This should be offered with caution, as debriefing for women who have experienced a traumatic birth is controversial because of the links to PTSD. Evidence for psychological debriefing following other types of traumatic events shows it can lead to increased PTSD under some circumstances (Rose, Bisson, Churchill, and Wessely, 2002). A case has been made targeted debriefings for women who have experienced a traumatic birth (Sheen and Slade, 2015). However, this research investigated whether such meetings reduced symptoms of PTSD or depression, not whether it was useful in a subsequent pregnancy. What we do know is that some pregnant women have found such meetings helpful (Greenfield, 2017; Thomson and Downe, 2010, 2016).

In most circumstances it is standard midwifery practice to discuss plans for birth at the end of a pregnancy, when all the events of the pregnancy are known. For women who have experienced a traumatic birth, making plans early in the pregnancy (to avoid a repeat traumatic experience) may be a high priority. We saw earlier in the chapter that care which removes choice and control can be a risk factor for a traumatic birth, and women who have experienced this previously may use birth plans as a form of contract with care providers to explicitly avoid any potential loss of choice and control in this birth (Greenfield, 2018). Midwives can support these women during pregnancy by reassuring them that they will be supported in their right to make choices. This could involve engaging in such discussions about plans for birth earlier in pregnancy, if the woman appears to need this. It is possible that securing midwives' support at as early a stage of pregnancy as possible would remove uncertainty, and help women to feel less anxious earlier on. In turn this might facilitate the development of trusting relationships, simply because there is a greater amount of low-anxiety time available in which to do so.

BOX 16.5   BUILDING TRUSTING RELATIONSHIPS WITH LUNA

Luna struggled to find midwives with whom she could build a trusting relationship. Knowing her history, and seeing how she was initially struggling to make relationships with midwives, a senior midwife assigned a specific midwife to have all appointments with Luna. This helped to start the process of rebuilding trust. At the midpoint of pregnancy, this midwife was unavailable for an appointment, but Luna was not informed. Luna arrived at the appointment to discover that she was instead going to be seen by a midwife who had been involved in her care when her first baby died. During the appointment this midwife 'asked me lots of questions that I didn't wanna answer about [first baby]' (Luna).

After this experience, Luna cancelled her subsequent three appointments and didn't see a midwife for 10 weeks.

When Luna did take up her offered appointments again, she was keen to agree a birth plan as soon as possible: 'I want it there in writing, to . . . give faith, to confirm . . . and then we can go into this fearless' (Luna).

Conclusions

Working with pregnant women who have previously experienced a traumatic birth brings specific challenges to midwives around the globe. Midwives may be unaware that the woman experienced the birth as a traumatic event; women may make choices about their current pregnancy based on their previous experience; and/or women may be mistrustful of midwives. The freedom that midwives have to respond to women presenting with these features will depend on the model of care and location around the globe, as well as the local and national context in which the midwife is working. In many countries, midwives are regulated as autonomous practitioners, but this is by no means universally true. Even within high-income countries such as the UK, midwives working for some employers may have the care they can offer curtailed by their employer's policies and/or insurance.

By prioritising the development of a trusting relationship, offering acknowledgement of previous trauma, providing a space for women to ask questions and receive information, and reinforcing that women's choices will be respected, midwives can support pregnant women who have previously experienced a traumatic birth. These tasks cannot be delivered as add-ons to a standard antenatal care package or separated from the administrative tasks and routine tests that the midwife offers. Rather, to be effective, the midwife must reflexively consider all their decision-making through the eyes of this group of women.

References

Adewuya, A., Ologun, Y. and Ibigbami, O. (2006). Post-traumatic stress disorder after childbirth in Nigerian women: Prevalence and risk factors. *BJOG: An International Journal of Obstetrics and Gynaecology*, 113, pp. 284–288.

Ayers, S. (2014). Fear of childbirth, postnatal post-traumatic stress disorder and midwifery care. *Midwifery*, 30(2), pp. 145–148.

Ayers, S., Eagle, A. and Waring, H. (2006). The effects of childbirth-related post-traumatic stress disorder on women and their relationships: A qualitative study. *Psychology, Health and Medicine*, 11(4), pp. 389–398.

Ayers, S., Joseph, S., Mckenzie-McHarg, K., Slade, P. and Wijma, K. (2008). Post-traumatic stress disorder following childbirth: Current issues and recommendations for future research. *Journal of Psychosomatic Obstetrics and Gynecology*, 29(4), pp. 240–250.

Beck, C.T. (2004a). Post-traumatic stress disorder due to childbirth: The aftermath. *Nursing Research*, 53(4), pp. 216–224.

Beck, C.T. (2004b). Birth trauma: In the eye of the beholder. *Nursing Research*, 53(1), pp. 28–35.

Beck, C.T. (2006). The anniversary of birth trauma: Failure to rescue. *Nursing Research*, 55(6), pp. 381–390.

Beck, C.T. and Watson, S. (2010). Subsequent childbirth after a previous traumatic birth. *Nursing Research*, 59(4), pp. 241–249.

Cigoli, V., Gilli, G. and Saita, E. (2006). Relational factors in psychopathological responses to childbirth. *Journal of Psychosomatic Obstetrics and Gynecology*, 27(2), pp. 91–97.

De Schepper, S., Vercauteren, T., Tersago, J., Jacquemyn, Y., Raes, F. and Franck, E. (2016). Post-traumatic stress disorder after childbirth and the influence of maternity team care during labour and birth: A cohort study. *Midwifery*, 32, pp. 87–92.

Edwards, N. and Kirkham, M. (2012). Why women might not use NHS maternity services. *Essentially MIDIRS*, 3(9), pp. 17–21.

Emmanuel, E., Creedy, D., John, W.S., Gamble, J. and Brown, C. (2008). Maternal role development following childbirth among Australian women. *Journal of Advanced Nursing*, 64(1), pp. 18–26.

Feeley, C. and Thomson, G. (2016). Tensions and conflicts in 'choice': Womens' experiences of free-birthing in the UK. *Midwifery*, 41, pp. 16–21.

Fenech, G. and Thomson, G. (2014). Tormented by ghosts from their past': A meta-synthesis to explore the psychosocial implications of a traumatic birth on maternal well-being. *Midwifery*, 30(2), pp. 185–193.

Ford, E. and Ayers, S. (2009). Stressful events and support during birth: The effect on anxiety, mood and perceived control. *Journal of Anxiety Disorders*, 23(2), pp. 260–268.

Forssen, A.S.K. (2012). Lifelong significance of disempowering experiences in prenatal and maternity care: Interviews with elderly Swedish women. *Qualitative Health Research*, 22(11), pp. 1535–1546.

Furuta, M., Sandall, J., Cooper, D. and Bick, D. (2016). Predictors of birth-related post-traumatic stress symptoms: Secondary analysis of a cohort study. *Archives of Women's Mental Health*, 19(6), pp. 987–999.

Gottvall, K. and Waldenström, U. (2002). Does a traumatic birth experience have an impact on future reproduction? *BJOG: An International Journal of Obstetrics and Gynaecology*, 109(3), pp. 254–260.

Gould, D. (2004). Birthwrite. trust me, I am a midwife. *British Journal of Midwifery*, 12(1), p. 44.

Greenfield, M. (2018). Choices made by women in pregnancy, birth and the early postnatal period, after a previous traumatic birth. PhD thesis, University of Hull, Hull.

Greenfield, M., Jomeen, J. and Glover, L. (2016). What is traumatic birth? A concept analysis and literature review. *British Journal of Midwifery*, 24(4), pp. 254–267.

Holmes, J.G. (1981). The exchange process in close relationships: Microbehavior and macromotives. In Lerner, M.J. and Lerner, S.C. (Eds.), *The justice motive in social behaviour*, New York: Plenum Press, pp. 261–284.

Modarres, M., Afrasiabi, S., Rahnama, P. and Montazer, A. (2012). Prevalence and risk factors of childbirth-related post-traumatic stress symptoms. *BMC Pregnancy and Childbirth*, 12(1), pp. 88–93.

McCants, B.M. and Greiner, J.R. (2016). Prebirth education and childbirth decision making. *International Journal of Childbirth Education*, 31(1), pp. 24–27.

Nicholls, K. and Ayers, S. (2007). Childbirth-related post-traumatic stress disorder in couples: A qualitative study. *British Journal of Health Psychology*, 12, pp. 491–509.

Parfitt, Y.M. and Ayers, S. (2009). The effect of post-natal symptoms of post-traumatic stress and depression on the couple's relationship and parent–baby bond. *Journal of Reproductive and Infant Psychology*, 27(2), pp.127–142.

Porter, M., Bhattacharya, S. and van Teijlingen, E. (2006) Unfulfilled expectations: How circumstances impinge on women's reproductive choices, *Social Science and Medicine*, 62(7), pp. 1757–1767.

Robinson, J. (2002). Jean Robinson's research round-up. Effects of PTSD on birth. *Association for Improvements in Maternity Services Journal*, 14(3), p. 17.

Rose, S.C., Bisson, J., Churchill, R. and Wessely, S. (2002). Psychological debriefing for preventing post traumatic stress disorder (PTSD). *Cochrane Database of Systematic Reviews*, 2, p. CD000560.

Sheen, K. and Slade, P. (2015). The efficacy of 'debriefing' after childbirth: Is there a case for targeted intervention? *Journal of Reproductive and Infant Psychology*, 33(3), pp. 308–320.

Simpson, J. (2007). Psychological foundations of trust. *Current Directions in Psychological Science*, 16, pp. 264–268.

Slade, P. (2006). Towards a conceptual framework for understanding post-traumatic stress symptoms following childbirth and implications for further research. *Journal of Psychosomatic Obstetrics and Gynecology*, 27(2), pp. 99–105.

Soet, J.E., Brack, G.A. and Dilorio, C. (2003). Prevalence and predictors of women's experience of psychological trauma during childbirth. *Birth: Issues in Perinatal Care*, 30(1), pp.36–46.

Sydsjö, G., Angerbjörn, L., Palmquist, S., Bladh, M., Sydsjö, A. and Josefsson, A. (2013). Secondary fear of childbirth prolongs the time to subsequent delivery. *Acta Obstetricia et Gynecologica Scandinavica*. 92(2), pp. 210–214.

Thomson, G. and Downe, S. (2010). Changing the future to change the past: Women's experiences of a positive birth following a traumatic birth experience. *Journal of Reproductive and Infant Psychology*, 28(1), pp. 102–112.

Thomson, G. and Downe, S. (2013). A hero's tale of childbirth. *Midwifery*, 29(7), pp. 765–771.

Thomson, G. and Downe, S. (2016). Emotions and support needs following a distressing birth: Scoping study with pregnant multigravida women in north-west England. *Midwifery*, 40, pp. 32–39.

Toohill, J., Fenwick, J., Gamble, J. and Creedy, D. (2014). Prevalence of childbirth fear in an Australian sample of pregnant women. *BMC Pregnancy and Childbirth*, 14, pp. 275–285.

17

STILLBIRTH AND MIDWIVES' DECISION-MAKING

What are the challenges?

Jane Warland and Claire Foord

Overview

This chapter is divided into two sections. The first outlines strategies midwives can use to raise awareness of stillbirth with women during pregnancy. The focus of this section is on how to empower women to get to know, protect and advocate for their unborn baby. The other main challenge is providing sensitive, evidence-informed midwifery care once a stillbirth has occurred. The second section of this chapter will therefore discuss the importance of building a strong relationship between the midwife and the bereaved family from the time of diagnosis, through labour and following the birth. The focus will be on communication, privacy and shared decision-making.

Introduction

The incidence of stillbirth after 28 weeks in most high-income countries ranges from 2.0 to 6.0 per thousand births (Flenady et al., 2016). However, the full extent of the burden of stillbirth is generally underestimated because of the differences in the definition of stillbirth, which ranges from 20 weeks in some countries to 28 weeks in others. These differences make it difficult to make international comparisons, however it is estimated that after 28 weeks in low- and middle-income nations (LMICs), stillbirth rates can range up to 22 per thousand births (McClure et al., 2015) This means that most midwives, irrespective of location around the globe or model of care, will provide care to a bereaved family at some stage in their career. However, many midwives say they feel ill-prepared to provide this care and often wonder what is best way forward (Warland, 2018).

There are two main challenges with respect to stillbirth and midwifery care. First, that midwives are frequently reluctant to discuss the possibility of stillbirth occurring during pregnancy (Warland & Glover, 2015). This is in spite of the fact that it is well recognised that consumer awareness of a health issue is one strategy in a raft of measures which may well reduce cases. For example, as a result of the international sudden infant death syndrome (SIDS) risk reduction awareness campaigns, the rate of SIDS in high-income countries has been reduced by as much as 83% (Hauck & Tanabe, 2008). The outstanding success of the SIDS public education campaigns demonstrates that increasing public awareness alongside an education campaign about protective behaviours can result in dramatic reduction in prevalence (Skadberg, Morild, & Markestad, 1998).

However, while the strategies we offer in this chapter can be applied in any setting, significant barriers can prevent the provision of quality midwifery care in LMICs. Filby and colleagues published an analytical framework from the midwifery care provider perspective which shows how such barriers interrelate, overlap and reinforce each other, and that they can arise from societal views including gender inequality. They suggest that in order to improve quality care, these kinds of barriers need to be addressed from the midwifery provider perspective (Filby, McConville, & Portela, 2016).

Nevertheless, wherever the woman resides, working with her to educate her about risk factors for stillbirth and encouraging her to be more aware of context-specific ways to protect her pregnancy and unborn baby in order to minimise her risk is an important aspect of stillbirth prevention. Maternal awareness of risks for stillbirth is dependent on someone making them aware. This responsibility naturally rests with maternity care providers such as midwives and obstetricians, but stillbirth is generally considered a taboo subject in many societies and also of concern by those providing antenatal care (Warland, 2013).

The challenge of including stillbirth prevention in routine antenatal care

There are four main challenges that we have identified with respect to including a discussion about ways of reducing the risk of stillbirth during antenatal care provision, namely, breaking silence, ongoing discussion, changing habits and imparting knowledge.

The challenge of breaking silence

In the case of stillbirth, silence is not golden, and ignorance is not bliss. Though both authors work within Australia, what we present below is applicable to all maternity care providers including midwives, irrespective of your location or the model of care within which you practice. We have extensive experience in delivering education about stillbirth awareness and prevention to maternity care providers, including midwives. We have observed that many midwives seem to want to treat the pregnant woman as if she is somehow vulnerable and needful of protection. This tendency to treat them in this way may stem from Victorian times when pregnant women often announced their pregnancy by fainting and the due time was called 'confinement' because she was literally confined to her bedroom. A Victorian pregnant woman's family protected her and nurtured her in a way that some cultures still do today. While there is nothing wrong with this, in essence, it does mean that alongside it, many countries (including maternity care providers who work in those settings) have still retained the idea that the pregnant woman is somehow vulnerable and needing protection. We have seen this most commonly expressed when we ask maternity care providers why they do not discuss stillbirth during pregnancy, and an extremely common response is 'I don't want to cause anxiety/worry'. However, there are a number of ways that midwives can address the topic of stillbirth throughout pregnancy without inducing worry (see Figure 17.1 for examples).

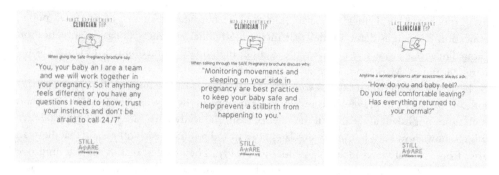

FIGURE 17.1 Suggested ways to talk about stillbirth throughout pregnancy

Source: Adapted from aim high pregnancy care timeline, with kind permission Still Aware

The perception that a pregnant woman will be filled with worry at being told about stillbirth is an assumption and not based on fact. Interestingly, when providing information directly to pregnant women we have found they welcome the information. In this case, knowledge is power.

The challenge of including an ongoing discussion about stillbirth into routine antenatal care

Those who travel on planes frequently would automatically be able to 'assume the brace position applicable to your seat' without being told what to do. A first-time flyer would learn the same very quickly because it is part of routine safety information prior to any flight anywhere in the world. Yet in 2010 Crangle estimated that fear of flying or aviophobia resulted in as many as 500 million people worldwide avoiding flying altogether and an even greater number enduring flying with some degree of fear. There is no doubt that providing all passengers with the safety demonstration may trigger anxiety in a few and yet *all* airlines across the globe routinely provide this demonstration as part of their duty of care to the safety of the flying public, and even though we travel often, we are yet to see a person run screaming from the plane! This example provides an analogy for providing routine information to women about how to keep safe in pregnancy as an important part of midwives duty of care. This involves empowering the woman to trust her intuition (Warland, Heazell et al., 2018) monitor strength, frequency and pattern of her baby's movements (Heazell et al., 2017) and settling to sleep on her side from 28 weeks (Warland, Dorrian, Morrison, & O'Brien, 2018) (see Figure 17.1).

We recognise that giving such information can be challenge because it involves breaking the habit of silence, yet as discussed in Chapters 2, 3, 4 and 6 midwives have a duty of care. In this case the duty of care is to routinely discuss the possibility of stillbirth and ways to reduce risk with all pregnant women regardless of their perceived risk status. The information about keeping baby safe in pregnancy needs to be so familiar that it becomes rote.

The challenge of changing habits

It is often said that it takes three months to change a habit. With respect to maternity care there are many habits that may be amenable to change. One of these is the way women are

6 ACTIONS FOR YOUR SAFER PREGNANCY

Avoid comparing your pregnancy to others, every one is different, get to know your baby's normal, you and your baby are a team.

Monitor the frequency of your baby's movement, if anything feels irregular, don't wait, contact your care provider.

Monitor the strength of your baby's movement, if they start to weaken, or feel unusual for your baby, contact your care provider immediately.

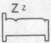

From 28 weeks onwards settle to sleep on your side, if you wake up on your back, don't worry, just settle back to sleep on your side.

Monitor the pattern of your baby's movement, if anything changes, call your care provider straight away.

Trust your instincts and report any concerns or uneasy feelings to your care provider without delay.

stillaware.org

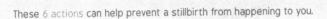
These 6 actions can help prevent a stillbirth from happening to you.

FIGURE 17.2   Six steps for a safer pregnancy

Source: Kind permission Still Aware

asked about fetal movements. Most often this is asked as a closed-ended question, such as 'is the baby moving?' or 'is your baby moving normally?' From the woman's perspective, this only gives her the opportunity to answer either 'yes' or 'no' and in fact the answer can be 'yes' until it is 'no', and when it is 'no' it may be too late to save the baby's life. It may be better, therefore, to ask an open-ended question, such as 'tell me about your baby's movements'. This gives the woman an opportunity to engage with you in a conversation about her baby. It allows her to tell you *who* her baby is and *how* her baby is, as well as empowering her to get to know her baby as an individual, which in turn allows her to report any changes in her unborn baby's behaviour to you.

'I wish someone had told me stillbirth was a possibility' is what we hear people say most often after the stillbirth of their baby. What is also evident is the belief from some care providers that they have spoken about stillbirth in pregnancy to women because they ask women about their baby's movements or encourage them to call. Herein lies the problem. Even with the best of intentions, information *without* also giving the why is just information. It is important to understand what talking about stillbirth actually looks like, rather than what we think it might look like.

The challenge of imparting knowledge

Have you ever had a one-sided conversation? This usually occurs if one person feels as though they have knowledge they might consider the other person doesn't have. This person may

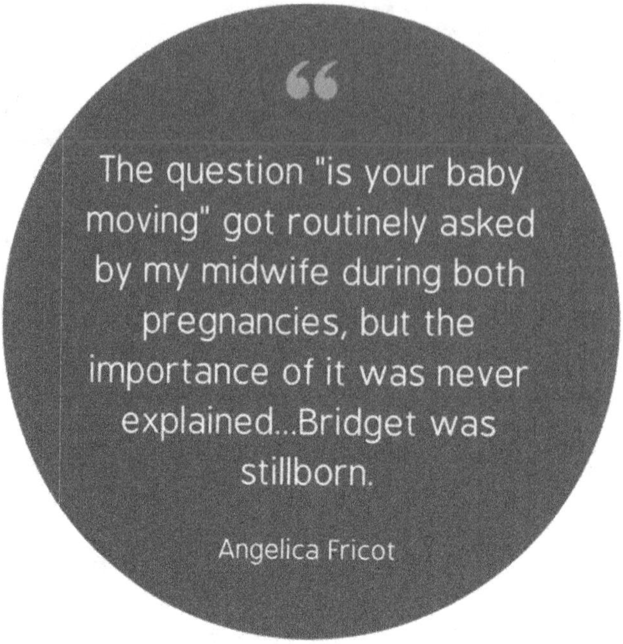

> The question "is your baby moving" got routinely asked by my midwife during both pregnancies, but the importance of it was never explained...Bridget was stillborn.
>
> Angelica Fricot

FIGURE 17.3 Quote shared with permission Still Aware

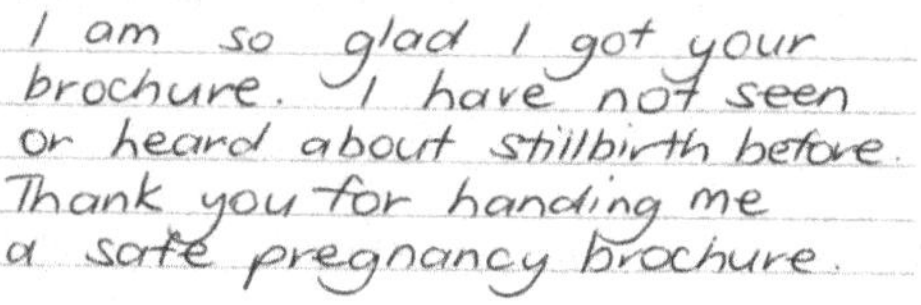

I am so glad I got your brochure. I have not seen or heard about stillbirth before. Thank you for handing me a safe pregnancy brochure.

FIGURE 17.4 Note received from a pregnant woman after reading Still Aware SAFE Pregnancy brochure on stillbirth

be very willing to tell you all about their knowledge and expertise, what they did, what they do, without seeming in the least bit interested in finding out about you or your experiences, knowledge and expertise. What is the most common response to the 'listener' in a one-way conversation? They stop 'listening' such that they are unlikely to recall anything the one-sided conversationalist actually said. Unfortunately, a one-way conversation can also happen during antenatal care. The tendency to hold a one-sided conversation is understandable because midwives often feel that they have a large amount of important information to impart at each visit. But delivering this in a one-sided conversation is not helpful, because the risk is that the woman will stop listening and thus she may miss some important, even lifesaving, information. It is therefore important to involve the woman in helping her discover her own understanding, the information that she needs to keep her and her unborn baby safe. Thus when providing information it is important, at the very least, to check the woman's understanding by asking a question like 'What do you think was the most important thing about what I said to you today?' or 'When would you call me?'

Activity 1

Please read this scenario and choose an answer.

ALTERED FETAL ACTIVITY SCENARIO

Caitlin Ward 30 year old primiparous woman with a singleton pregnancy at 39 weeks. She has recently stopped working. She has had a busy day. She has just gotten ready for bed and realises her baby isn't moving as he normally does at this time of the day. She calls you and after you have determined her age, gravity, parity, gestational week and what has triggered her recent concern) what is your most likely first response?

A] Reassure her, it sounds like she has been busy today and hasn't noticed her baby's movements

B] Ask her how many times her baby has moved today? (your next response will depend on her answer to that question)

C] Suggest she have something sugary to eat or cold to drink to "wake the baby" and ring back if she's still concerned

D] Suggest she concentrate on her baby's movements for the next hour and ring back if she's still concerned

E] Invite her in to be assessed

While it might be tempting to do some of these other options, E is the response which allows the midwife to assess Caitlin's baby and to provide her with reassurance that she has acted as her baby's advocate. She and her baby should be assessed using recognised guidelines and , if all is well, prior to being sent home Caitlin should be informed that if she becomes concerned again or remains concerned that she should not delay in attending care again.

FIGURE 17.5   Scenario 1

The challenge of providing sensitive evidence-based care once stillbirth has occurred

When a baby dies, there are three main times when the midwife may face challenges and need to make decisions about how best to act. These are:

- At the time of diagnosis
- During labour and birth, or at the time of death
- While providing postpartum care.

At each of these times, there are three core principles which, if followed, will likely assist the bereaved parents:

- Good communication
- Provision of privacy
- Care providers partaking in shared decision-making with the bereaved parents.

The challenge of providing good communication

When adults are traumatised, they frequently will regress to the cognitive functional capacity of an eight-year-old, in that they will appear confused and indecisive, with a shortened attention span and trouble concentrating (McKissock & McKissock, 2018). Understanding this makes communication with them much easier, but the challenge is still to provide communication that is easy to understand while not actually treating the parents as if they are children because they are temporarily incapacitated by their grief. Good communication is considered a core competency of the qualified midwife, by most midwifery professional bodies globally (e.g. Butler, Fullerton, & Aman, 2018.) However, good communication can be difficult to maintain when caring for bereaved families while simultaneously managing one's own emotions. It is common for midwives to fear 'saying something wrong' (Warland, 2018), and therefore they may be tempted to say nothing. It is important to understand that there are no magic words to say, but it is crucially important to simply 'be with' the woman and her family because this is generally remembered and often viewed by the parents as more valuable than anything that might be said. If you feel something needs to be said, then simple statements such as 'I'm so sorry' (Pullen, Golden, & Cacciatore, 2012) are usually remembered and appreciated.

It is best to avoid platitudes such as 'this won't happen next time' or 'this is such an unfortunate situation, stillbirth isn't common', as the second author found:

> I remember the midwife looking at me and say 'honestly you are just unlucky, this is so rare'. Instantly I was wracking my mind to figure out what it was that I did wrong. Later my obstetrician came into the room stood at the end of the bed and with an apologetic tone say 'Don't blame yourself. You didn't do anything wrong, things like this happen. I have recently had another woman go through this and she just went on to have another baby. So we'll make sure it won't happen next time'.

Statements like this are unhelpful. Regardless of the perceived rarity, stillbirth does happen, and suggesting that luck had anything to do with it is not helpful. Statements like 'don't blame yourself' are patronising and paternalistic because you are assuming that the mother is actually already blaming herself. If she wasn't thinking that way, she may well afterwards. Additionally, suggesting that 'it won't happen next time' and 'have another baby' glosses over the loss; they are similar to statements like 'move on' and they assume that one life can replace another.

It is also best to avoid asking a newly bereaved parent closed-ended questions such as 'would you like to . . . bathe the baby, dress the baby, undress the baby', as the first author found:

> I was looking after a couple who were in recovery following an emergency caesarean section after a cord prolapse and the baby did not survive. He was a little messy looking and so I said to the dad 'would you like to bathe your baby?' Of course he said 'no'! Realising my mistake I proceeded to get the bath ready and when I was about to put the baby into the bath asked the father if he had a camera. He went and got the camera and then I said 'would you please hold the baby while I take a picture of him in the bath?' He agreed. I took my time fiddling with the camera and before he knew it he was bathing his baby when moments before he had said 'no'. This reminded me to never, ever ask parents a closed-ended question because in this case 'no' didn't actually mean 'no'.

When providing sensitive care, such as following a stillbirth, it is, of course, important to also take into account cultural and spiritual needs and language barriers. This involves not only the use of interpreters but also access to information in the bereaved person's first language.

The challenge of providing privacy

It is important to understand that bereaved parents need privacy but not abandonment (Ellis et al., 2016). When parents initially learn that their baby has died, it may be tempting for the midwife to leave them alone to 'give privacy', but Pullen et al. (2012) indicate that most parents appreciate their midwife staying with them for a while. If it is necessary to leave them alone, then one way to reassure the parents that you are not abandoning them is to provide them with an explanation as to why you are leaving, when you will return, and how they can contact you in the meantime. Parents may also appreciate being asked if they would like some privacy for religious or cultural reasons. For example, some families may wish to pray together or want a cultural elder or religious leader to be present.

The challenge of shared decision-making

It is very common to hear newly bereaved parents say 'They let me' or 'they didn't let me' – for example, 'they let me (or didn't let me) . . . hold the baby . . . bathe the baby . . . take the baby outside . . . take the baby home', but when they use this language it implies that the parents did not consider they had control or agency over what they were able to do with their own baby. These kinds of statements support evidence that suggests that many bereaved parents consider their care providers seemed to have failed to notice their state of mind and/or to respond to their needs and requests (Downe, Schmidt, Kingdon, & Heazell, 2013). Once again, thinking of the parents as having the functional capacity of an eight-year-old helps the midwife, to provide options for shared decision-making that are gently proposed, alongside support and time to consider those options. Best evidence indicates that midwives need to be honest and promptly give parents all information available in order to help them feel that they have participated in decision-making, as well as provide a sense of control over the situation (Ellis et al., 2016; Warland, 2018).

BOX 17.1   SHARED DECISION-MAKING

Examples of shared decision-making are:

Pain relief for labour and birth

If as a midwife you have access to pain relief, it may be tempting to sedate and or over-medicate in order to try to avoid adding the physical pain of birth to the significant emotional pain the mother is already enduring. However, many mothers remember, often with regret, not being entirely 'with it' in the time after birth, such that their memory of that precious time is not as clear as they would want.

Quote from the first author's personal experience:

> They offered me an epidural but I didn't want one. I said that I'd use the shower, as I had done for my other births. No one thought to warn me that this might not be a good idea. I had traumatic flashbacks every time I had a shower for months after the birth.

Location for post-birth care

If within a hospital setting, the issue may arise of deciding where to locate the parents for post-birth care. This is a time to ensure shared decision-making occurs, because some parents may choose to avoid hearing the cries of newborn babies altogether while others may wish to be located in a busy birth suite or postnatal unit specifically so they can be reassured by those same cries. While many may report finding the cries of newborn babies distressing (Nordlund et al., 2012; Kelley 2012), it is best not to assume what the parents want to do. A few hours before the time for transfer say something like

> we need to make a decision as to where to go now. You have the choice of the postnatal ward or the women's health ward. If you choose to go to the postnatal ward you will be able to hear cries of newborn babies; the woman's health ward will be quieter. Have a think and let me know what you would like me to do. If you change your mind at any stage, that is fine.

Organising other children

Another time when parents can feel they have been denied shared decision-making is for care of their other children. It can be tempting to think they are a 'bother' and other family members may think that babysitting is one way they can help the parents. However, this is another time when parents need to be asked what they would like to do, as one bereaved mother whose own mother wanted to provide babysitting said, 'please don't as this will remove me from reality, because they are helping me stay grounded'.

Seeing and holding the baby

The exception to offering parents choice within the context of shared decision-making after stillbirth is regarding facilitating them seeing and holding their baby. Over the past 40 years there has been a paradigm shift in 'best' practice. In the 1970s and 1980s, in many parts of the world, parents were discouraged or even prevented from seeing their baby after death by maternity care providers, who did this believing that they were protecting the parents from psychological stress. However, then a shift of practice standards arose, driven by bereaved parents themselves, which resulted in many countries encouraging the practice. Then one small study (Hughes, Turton, Hopper, & Evans, 2002) was published suggesting negative psychological sequalae in a group of parents who saw and held their stillborn baby and the pendulum swung the other way, with guidance suggesting that parents be asked if they wanted to see and hold their baby (Warland, Davis et al., 2011). However, following further research (Kingdon, Givens, O'Donnell, & Turner, 2015) it is now the case that seeing and holding the stillborn baby is once again facilitated by midwives. Even so in some high-income countries, such as Spain, these practices are still not routine (Cassidy, 2018) and sometimes in LMICs the baby's body is still disposed of without any recognition or ritual, such as naming, funeral rites, or the baby being held by the mother (Frøen et al., 2011).

SEEING AND HOLDING THE BABY SCENARIO

Danielle and Mike arrived at your hospital a couple of hours ago in early labour. Unfortunately When Danielle arrived there was no fetal heart. As she was in early labour with her 3rd baby she was transferred to birth suite and she is slowly progressing, in your care, since then.

Between contractions she says to you:

"What will the baby look like?"

Your response should be something like

"I don't know but it will be ok, we will meet your baby together"

You can't actually know what the baby will look like and it is best to avoid giving parents details that they actually don't want, or need

FIGURE 17.6 Scenario 2

The problem with denying parents the opportunity to see and hold their baby after stillbirth is that it is counterintuitive. There is never any question that parents want to see and hold their baby immediately after a live birth. In fact it would be considered very odd by most parents if they were asked by their midwife if they wanted to see and hold their baby after birth. Midwives across the globe simply birth the live baby directly into the parents' waiting arms without question. It is therefore counterintuitive to suggest that bereaved parents would not benefit from the same assumptive care; in fact evidence from systematic review (Kingdon, Givens, O'Donnell, & Turner, 2015) as well as expert opinion supports this view (Warland, Davis et al., 2011).

There is one notable exception to this strategy and that is when working in contexts constrained by tradition, culture or spiritual belief, in this case the care of the parents may need to 'conform to the regulating power of the context in which they find themselves' (Popoola, Skinner, & Woods, 2018 p. 44). However, unless such contact is precluded by culture tradition or spiritual belief, it is best to avoid asking the parents if they want to see and hold their baby and simply and naturally birth the stillborn baby into the parent's arms.

Conclusion

In this chapter we have outlined the challenges of providing midwifery care in the context of stillbirth. First we outlined some strategies midwives might use to raise and discuss the topic of stillbirth in pregnancy. We highlighted that this information should be given as a matter of routine, regardless of perceived risk and in whatever context the midwife is working. Whilst giving information, it is imperative that midwives and health professionals are cognisant of the language they use, as insensitive or inappropriate words may have a life-long impact on the woman and/or her partner and family.

Then we provided three core principles of care when a baby dies, namely communication, and facilitating privacy, and shared decision-making. Strategies to enhance best practice are to avoid platitudes and closed-ended questions and instead empower and enable the parents to actively parent their baby in the small amount of precious time that is available to them. The strategies we offer throughout this chapter are a work in progress. Research and practice in the area of stillbirth is rapidly changing across the globe and strategies offered were based on the best available evidence at the time of publication.

References

Butler, M.M., Fullerton, J.T. and Aman, C., 2018. Competence for basic midwifery practice: Updating the ICM essential competencies. *Midwifery, 66*, pp. 168–175.

Cassidy, P.R., 2018. Care quality following intrauterine death in Spanish hospitals: Results from an online survey. *BMC Pregnancy and Childbirth, 18*(1), p. 22.

Crangle, M., 2010. *Conquer your fear of flying.* Gill & Macmillan, Dublin.

Downe, S., Schmidt, E., Kingdon, C. and Heazell, A.E., 2013. Bereaved parents' experience of stillbirth in UK hospitals: A qualitative interview study. *BMJ Open, 3*(2), p. e002237.

Ellis, A., Chebsey, C., Storey, C., Bradley, S., Jackson, S., Flenady, V., Heazell, A. and Siassakos, D., 2016. Systematic review to understand and improve care after stillbirth: A review of parents' and healthcare professionals' experiences. *BMC Pregnancy and Childbirth, 16*(1), p. 16.

Filby, A., McConville. F. and Portela, A., 2016. What prevents quality midwifery care? A systematic mapping of barriers in low and middle income countries from the provider perspective. *PLoS One, 11*(5), p. e0153391. https://doi.org/10.1371/journal.pone.0153391

Flenady, V., Wojcieszek, A.M., Middleton, P., Ellwood, D., Erwich, J.J., Coory, M., Khong, T.Y., Silver, R.M., Smith, G.C., Boyle, F.M. and Lawn, J.E., 2016. Stillbirths: Recall to action in high-income countries. *Lancet, 387*(10019), pp. 691–702.

Frøen, J.F., Cacciatore, J., McClure, E.M., Kuti, O., Jokhio, A.H., Islam, M., Shiffman, J. and Lancet's Stillbirths Series Steering Committee., 2011. Stillbirths: Why they matter. *Lancet, 377*(9774), pp. 1353–1366.

Hauck, F.R. and Tanabe, K.O., 2008. International trends in sudden infant death syndrome: Stabilization of rates requires further action. *Pediatrics, 122*(3), pp. 660–666.

Heazell, A.E.P., Warland, J., Stacey, T., Coomarasary, C., Budd, J., Mitchell, E.A. and O'Brien, L.M., 2017. Stillbirth is associated with perceived alterations in fetal activity – Findings from an international case control study. *BMC Pregnancy and Childbirth, 17*, p. 369. doi:10.1186/s12884-017-1555-6

Hughes, P., Turton, P., Hopper, E. and Evans, C.D.H., 2002. Assessment of guidelines for good practice in psychosocial care of mothers after stillbirth: A cohort study. *Lancet, 360*(9327), pp. 114–118.

Kelley, M.C. and Trinidad, S.B., 2012. Silent loss and the clinical encounter: Parents' and physicians' experiences of stillbirth –A qualitative analysis. *BMC Pregnancy and Childbirth, 12*(1), p. 137.

Kingdon, C., Givens, J.L., O'Donnell, E. and Turner, M., 2015. Seeing and holding baby: Systematic review of clinical management and parental outcomes after stillbirth. *Birth, 42*(3), pp. 206–218.

McClure, E.M., Saleem, S., Goudar, S.S., Moore, J.L., Garces, A., Esamai, F., Patel, A., Chomba, E., Althabe, F., Pasha, O., Kodkany, B.S., Bose, C.L., Berreuta, M., Liechty, E.A., Hambidge, K., Krebs, N.F., Derman, R.J., Hibberd, P.L., Buekens, P., Manasyan, A., Carlo, W.A., Wallace, D.D., Koso-Thomas, M., . . . Goldenberg, R.L. 2015. Stillbirth rates in low-middle income countries 2010–2013: A population-based, multi-country study from the Global Network. *Reproductive Health, 12*(Suppl 2), pp. S7–S15.

McKissock, M. and McKissock, D., 2018. *Coping with grief* (5th ed.) ABC Books, Australia.

Nordlund, E., Börjesson, A., Cacciatore, J., Pappas, C., Randers, I. and Rådestad, I., 2012. When a baby dies: Motherhood, psychosocial care and negative affect. *British Journal of Midwifery, 20*(11), pp. 780–784.

Popoola, T., Skinner, J. and Woods, M., 2018. Stillbirth bereavement care in constrained contexts: Implications for a family-focused care. *Journal of Pediatrics and Child Health, 54*(S1), p. 44. doi:10.1111/jpc.13882_109

Pullen, S., Golden, M.A. and Cacciatore, J., 2012. 'I'll never forget those cold words as long as I live': Parent perceptions of death notification for stillbirth. *Journal of Social Work in End-of-Life & Palliative Care, 8*(4), pp. 339–355.

Skadberg, B.T., Morild, I. and Markestad, T., 1998. Abandoning prone sleeping: Effect on the risk of sudden infant death syndrome. *Journal of Pediatrics, 132*(2), pp. 340–343.

Warland, J., 2013. Keeping baby SAFE in pregnancy: Piloting the brochure. *Midwifery, 29*(2), pp. 174–179.

Warland, J. 2018. Bereavement and perinatal loss. In Glover, P., Lewis, L., McNeill, L., Costins, P., Warland, J., Kew, C., Bradfield, Z., Kuliukas, L., Staff, L., Burns, V., Mannix, T., Taylor, A., Lee, N. and Brady, S. (Eds.), *Midwifery* (1st ed.) Wiley, Qld, pp. 368–384.

Warland, J., Davis, D. L., Ilse, S., Cacciatore, J., Cassidy, J., Christofferson, L. and Vannacci, A., 2011. Caring for families experiencing stillbirth: A unified position statement on contact with the baby. An international collaboration. *Illness Crisis & Loss*, 20(3), pp. 295–298.

Warland, J., Dorrian, J., Morrison, J. L. and O'Brien, L. M. 2018. Maternal sleep during pregnancy and poor fetal outcomes: A scoping review of the literature with meta-analysis. *Sleep Medicine Reviews, pii*, S1087-0792(17)30013-8. doi:10.1016/j.smrv.2018.03.004. [Epub ahead of print].

Warland, J. and Glover, P., 2015. Talking to pregnant women about stillbirth: Evaluating the effectiveness of an information workshop for midwives using pre and post intervention surveys. *Nurse Education Today*, 35(10), pp. e21–e25.

Warland, J., Heazell, A.E.P., Stacey, T., Coomarasary, C., Budd, J., Mitchell, E.A. and O'Brien, L. M., 2018. 'They told me all mothers have worries', stillborn mother's experiences of having a 'gut instinct' that something is wrong in pregnancy: Findings from an international case control study. *Midwifery*, 62, pp. 171–176.

PART III

Decision-making within the context of the socially and culturally constructed maternity care environment

18

MIDWIFERY DECISION-MAKING

Feeling safe to support women's choice in the maternity care environment

Lyn Ebert

Chapter overview

Midwives need to feel safe to support women and fully engage in midwifery decision-making. When midwives do not feel their professional body of knowledge is valued and they do not feel safe to advocate for the woman, they may release midwifery responsibility, shifting the responsibility for choices and decision-making. This chapter explores midwifery decision-making within the context of the socially and culturally constructed maternity care environment. Information presented in this chapter is derived primarily from a study examining how midwives work with and support women in an attempt to facilitate choice within maternity services often focused on meeting institutionally required outcomes[1] (Ebert, 2012). Although this study is Australia-based, which is a high-income country, the findings can be applied to middle- and low-income countries and the diversity of midwifery models of care provisions within all three incomes levels.

The two concepts discussed in this chapter are 'feeling valued' and 'feeling safe'. Both concepts are essential in order for midwives, irrespective of geographical location or model of care, to facilitate the midwife–woman partnership and create an environment that supports mutual responsibility in relation to decision-making within maternity care encounters.

Introduction

Woman-centred care is an internationally recognised concept and is also the name of a philosophy of maternity care which gives priority to the wishes and needs of the user, that is, the childbearing woman (International Confederation of Midwives [ICM], 2014a). The word midwife means 'to be with woman', so by its very nature midwifery means to hold the woman at the centre of care. While placing choice of and control for care options with the woman are viewed as fundamental to woman-centred care (Morgan, 2015), a woman's choice is enhanced or restricted by the information presented, services available, and care options offered by the individual healthcare professional. Midwives can also be restricted in their ability to fully engage in midwifery decision-making, resulting in a lack of woman-centred care and professional satisfaction

Control and choice

Between 2009 and 2012 I undertook a study exploring the concept woman-centred care as experienced by socially disadvantaged women (*n* = 17), registered midwives (*n* = 31) and student midwives (*n* = 28) (Ebert, 2012). Data was collected primarily through focus groups over multiple locations in Australia, including metropolitan and rural, and from a range of diverse maternity care provisions such as tertiary and midwifery-led centres. A major finding was that women have a different understanding of what constitutes woman-centred care than midwives have. While women spoke of the actions and interactions within individual maternity care encounters as being either woman-focused or not, midwives and students spoke of models of care that either support or hinder woman-centred care.

All three participant groups in this study (women, midwives and student midwives) appeared to understand that there is a hierarchy of control within the maternity care environment, with midwives having limited power or control within the maternity care environment. Doctors were seen to have more authoritative control over clinical decision-making than midwives, and midwives were seen to have greater control than women. Student and registered midwives also communicated that local health district management has control over and influences midwifery practice including workplace policies, models of care provided and decision-making processes. This view is supported by studies and reviews undertaken in various midwifery contexts globally (Smith, 2016, Daemers et al., 2017, Healy, Humpreys and Kennedy, 2016).

Control and choice is restricted through limiting options made available, the contextual environment and/or the individual healthcare professional. Women are for the most part, 'told' what 'choice the system wants them to make'. Midwives are not able to support women to take control of their maternity care encounters because midwives do not have control within maternity care encounters when doctors seek control of decision-making. In Wanda's story (Box 18.1), Wanda describes how the doctor took control of the maternity care encounter. The midwife attempted to advocate for the woman. However, the woman was not considered, and the midwife's professional knowledge was dismissed. The woman and midwife had no voice in decision-making. Such disempowerment is discussed in Chapter 6.

BOX 18.1 WANDA'S STORY

WANDA: 'I was at this birth and we were supporting her as best we could and the doctor was just about to do an episiotomy and I thought, now hold on a minute, you need to tell her, you need to say look, I have to do this. I got into trouble for that, [doctors] they're used to calling the shots, "it's my way or the highway" '.

Women often view pregnancy and childbirth as a physically and emotionally vulnerable time in their life. Women will often place the power for decision-making with the midwife to ensure a healthy outcome for their baby and expect the midwife to advocate for their needs. Midwives may not know this transfer of power and responsibility for decision-making has occurred. Women, who silently defer control to the midwife, may be viewed by the midwife as negligent in their assumed inability to engage in decision-making processes. Conversely, women seeking to maintain a sense of power and control within their maternity care encounters, choosing not to conform to institutional policies and protocols or cultural expectations by questioning the preferred options offered, may be seen as irresponsible. Furthermore, the midwife's clinical competence and professional accountability is questioned if women make choices outside the expected and respected values of the maternity service. Responsibility for birth outcomes and women's choices, regardless of decision-making processes, is habitually positioned with the midwife (see Chapter 3).

Feeling valued

The midwife, as the link between the woman and the contextual environment within which she/he practices, needs the midwifery role of guide and guardian to be seen as important and respected by colleagues, management and other health professionals. This is often not the case when a midwife is silenced by the perceived power structures of the health service. In Olga's story (Box 18.2), Olga voices her concerns with the risk discourse and coercion of the woman to conform to the desired course of action. Again, the woman was not considered, and the midwife's professional knowledge was not valued. The woman and midwife had no voice in decision-making.

BOX 18.2   OLGA'S STORY – PART 1

OLGA: *'The part I find challenging to my own personal profession because I would never put someone at risk* [is when] *you've got a medical team coming in* [saying] *"Your baby will die and you could as well if we don't hurry up and get this baby out" . . ., so you have to be the person that negotiates between the two and I look at it as a lose-lose situation. No-one's really getting what they want because either they cave in and go with the hospital's protocol or they say no and then the hospital is the one whose protocols aren't being followed'.*

The midwives in my study communicated that managerial and medical control over midwifery models of care demonstrated not only a failure to value the needs of women but also demonstrated a failure to value midwifery as a profession (Ebert, 2012). The midwives wanted to feel their professional knowledge and decision-making processes were valued by midwifery colleagues, management and other healthcare professionals. They communicated that their professional survival, however, was dependent on valuing and meeting the needs of the doctor, not the needs of the woman – 'it's my way or the highway'. Doctors were viewed to have power over women and midwives. Doctors choices are valued higher and therefore they are the principle decision-maker. Midwives understand that their choices are less valued, so they shift responsibility of choice to those who will make the final decision – the medical staff. Midwives who maintain a medicalised framework of interaction within the maternity care encounter are less likely to be marginalised by medical colleagues or senior midwives and management (Pollard, 2010). Considering the need to preserve their sense of midwifery worth, it is understandable that a midwife might steer the midwife-woman interaction and decision-making process.

Within any maternity care environment around the world that values a medical model of care, the provision of woman-centred care requires the midwife to challenge the values sanctioned by their midwifery and medical colleagues as well as management. According to Hollins Martin and Bull (2006), midwives that oppose the dominate workplace values expose themselves to workplace conflict with the risk of professional intimidation and social group exclusion. The risk is often deemed to be so high that conformity ensues. Pollard (2010), however, suggests that midwives may employ a medicalised framework of interaction to be recognised and accepted as a professional. It is every midwife's desire to be accepted and valued as a professional, yet it is this desire that motivates them to adopt the valued ways of acting and reacting within the maternity care encounter.

Two decades ago, Fahy (1998) asserted that the problem-solving management styles of maternity care environments frame midwives' ways of working. Midwives working within a problem-solving maternity care environment were more likely to 'do things to' the woman. 'Doing to' ensures institutional processes and results can be mapped and measured. Fahy also claimed that midwives who practise in ways that enable them to be 'with woman' are seen by management and colleagues to be 'doing nothing' (Fahy, 1998). Little appears to have changed in midwives' understandings and ways of working in hospital-based maternity care environments across the globe in the last two decades.

Fahy (2008) contends that when we are aware our movements and behaviours are being monitored, we moderate our actions to align with the dominant group, the group with power. In order to be professionally safe, midwives may need to align themselves with contextual institutional management specifications and expectations and a task-focused environment. The midwife demonstrating a valuing of workplace requirements gains a sense of being valued by management – a 'good' worker. However, midwives acknowledge here that their professional ideologies (woman-centred care) are placed at risk as a result of providing task-centred care. The woman is not valued, and the midwife understands midwifery professional ideologies and ways of practising are not valued. Therefore, it is not safe to work in such a manner.

Institutionally focused decision-making

Midwives around the world understand that hospital management has control over what services and supports are available to women, and that the needs of individual women are not always taken into consideration. Women are required to follow the hospital's operational processes. The woman is not a valued part of the system, but rather seen as a visitor:

> Most women do as they are told. They are in the system. They don't butt the system . . . partly because they haven't got any other information, they don't know and they only get the information we give them so if we tell them it has to be done, then they do it.
>
> *(Midwife Helen)*

Midwives see they are positioned on the front line in the conflict between service users, the woman, and maternity service management and or their medical colleagues. Midwives cannot feel 'valued' in maternity services that prevent midwives from working in models of maternity care that align with their professional and personal ideologies. Midwives' inability to work autonomously or to their full scope of practice as defined by the ICM hinders their ability to meet the needs of the woman (ICM, 2014b). The midwife is not safe to go against the dominant values of the workplace culture. Institutionally focused and medically orientated models of care demonstrate that management and institutional needs take precedence over women's needs and that women's needs, and midwifery work is not valued.

Professional belonging

Group pressure to voice a collective view can be strong in maintaining professional identity. Stapleton et al. (2002) found that midwives employed and promoted self-censorship to reduce the risk of undermining their midwifery colleagues. Deery (2009) goes on to say that midwives constantly calibrate their performances depending on who they are interacting with. She describes midwifery work as a drama played out within the cultural context of the maternity care environment, with midwives assuming a particular stage persona around colleagues that maintains their observed allegiance with the group's professional identity. Professional groups, including midwifery, have an image to uphold. Although the midwifery discipline's underlying principles and philosophies of woman-centred care and partnership are valued and therefore held to be true for the group, individual workplace contexts also have a socially constructed culture which may, collectively, uphold a different and dominant localised value system. When a group member disrupts the united front, impression management for the group is disturbed. Midwives who voice a different view to their localised professional group can be socially excluded and intimidated. Midwives need to conform, and the culturally dominant professional image needs to be maintained. Midwives advocating for a woman's choice or seeking to provide all possible care options may be shunned by the group. In Rosie's story (Box 18.3), Rosie recalls how she is questioned by her colleagues when the woman has made an informed decision, based on Rosie providing all care options. Rosie is aware responsibility for any poor birth outcomes will be placed with her.

BOX 18.3   ROSIE'S STORY

ROSIE: 'I've been questioned as to whether you gave the woman the right information, "Did you make this decision, are you sure it was an informed decision, you gave her the appropriate information?" I've been disrespected by my colleagues. . . . It can be really hard sometimes'.

Midwives may be unwilling to furnish control to the woman when they see their ability to have control within maternity care encounters is already limited. Midwives may not feel safe to 'allow' the woman to have control over choice, placing control for decision-making with the woman, when decisions are seen to directly affect their professional standing within the maternity environment. Midwives participating in my study spoke of the 'witch-hunt' culture with midwifery colleagues, medical staff and management scrutinising every aspect of the midwife's actions and decisions when decision-making resulted in choices that were outside the expected and accepted care options (Box 18.4).

BOX 18.4 OLGA'S STORY – PART 2

OLGA: 'I don't actually have a problem with it, as long as it's documented that that's what the woman wanted. But, I don't like the witch hunt society that the hospital creates. When a woman chooses not to follow their advice and it's not witch hunting the woman, it's witch hunting the midwife'.

However, midwives do not always support women's choices. When women challenge hospital or cultural rules, midwives will often exercise their position of institutional or professional authority to encourage conformity. Midwives are seen as the enforcers of disempowering rules and regulations. Midwives may support and enforce hospital or cultural rules because they understand the rules are equally about ensuring they, midwives, act in accordance with operational requirements. This understanding is supported by Hollins Martin and Bull (2006), who found that midwives can feel obliged to follow hospital rules and policies, fearing the consequences of challenging the practices and beliefs of more senior staff. The fear of litigation and being ostracised by colleagues maintains conformity of written and unwritten rules. While Hollins Martin and Bull (2006), provide an explanation as to why midwives might encourage conformity of rules by women and their midwifery colleagues, Porter and colleagues (2007) suggest that some midwives can be uncomfortable with shifting the balance of power towards the woman during decision-making processes. Placing the balance of power for decision-making with the woman can result in the midwife being vulnerable. Enforcing rules and regulations maintains a sense of control for the midwife. The midwife, therefore, must be willing to give up their position of power in order for the woman to have greater control and choice.

Maintaining ignorance around choice and care options, therefore, positions a greater degree of control with the midwife, affording a measure of protection from professional and personal persecution within the maternity care environment. Midwives are shielded to some extent against blame when they maintain control around decision-making. Being shielded from shame or blame is dependent upon the level of control and choice afforded to the woman and degree of adherence to the health service's preferred directives of care. Figure 18.1 reveals the shame and blame decision-making framework that promotes the midwife's need to maintain control over decision-making within maternity care encounters.

Feeling safe

Within midwifery literature, the terms 'safe' and 'safety' are primarily used to discuss the physical health of the woman and/or her baby. The context for application of these terms is most often in relation to birthing outcomes or the birthing environment. However, this concept is becoming increasingly visible in the literature pertaining to mental health issues and pregnancy (Eagle Williams, 2011; Marks, McConnell and Baker, 2005), emotions in midwifery (Hunter, 2005, 2006, 2009) and the psychological stress of midwifery work (Copp, 2010; Klein, 2009). Studies tend to focus on a particular midwifery context, such as continuity of midwifery care models of practice (Gu, Zhang and Ding, 2011, Goffinet, 2005), the labour

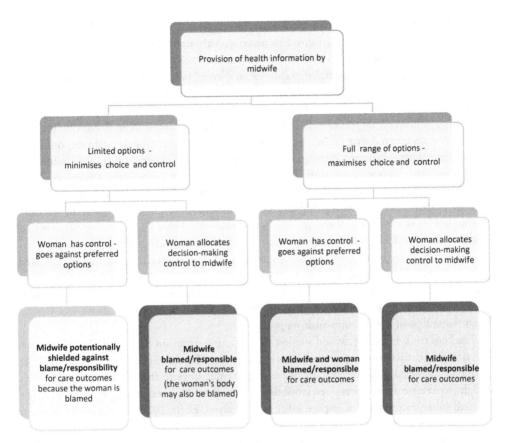

FIGURE 18.1 Shame and blame decision-making framework

and birthing event (Leinweber and Rowe, 2010, John and Parsons, 2006) or workplace practices and environment (Knezevic et al., 2011).

The term 'feeling safe' within this chapter describes a state within a maternity care encounter in which the woman and midwife can interact without fear of perceived or actual psychological (or physical) harm. The woman is guarded and guided by the midwife to experience maternity care encounters in a manner she chooses and makes healthcare decisions, free from controversy. Feeling safe in the context of maternity care is comparable with the concept of cultural safety, which requires healthcare professionals to create conditions that enable the less powerful to comment with safety. The aim of cultural safety is to benefit those who nurses and midwives serve, with the potential to ultimately improve experiences for the service user (Johnstone and Kanitsaki, 2007). Similarly, the midwife needs to be guided and guarded by maternity service management to work autonomously to the midwife's full potential within the model of care in which they practice free from controversy.

Releasing responsibility

Women around the world trust their midwife to provide the information and guidance that facilitates optimal maternity care outcomes. Any desire to question the midwife is minimised when the midwife, viewed as the expert, advises a course of action with an authoritative presence, portraying the course of action as best practice. Although women in my study articulated that midwives failed, at times, to guide them in their choices, the women understood that midwives had a greater body of knowledge and that midwives' knowledge was superior in relation to childbearing than their own (Ebert, 2012). These women persisted, therefore, in transferring or releasing responsibility for maternity care decisions to the midwife, even when the midwife ignored their need for information in order to participate fully in the decision-making process.

Women understand that midwives and other healthcare professionals retain responsibility for maternity care decisions throughout the entire childbirth continuum, while midwives understand that responsibilities shift throughout the childbirth continuum. Midwives in my study voiced that women have greater control over maternity care choices during pregnancy and the postnatal periods, with a shift in control and responsibility for choice to the midwife during labour and birthing. Some midwives communicated that an acceptance of increased responsibility for decisions made during labour and birth by midwives was due to the consequences of choice being more immediate, observable and measurable. Midwives expressed that their midwifery colleagues as well as other health professionals placed the responsibility for variations from normal progress in labour and birthing as well as poor birth outcomes with the midwife, not with the woman. Positioning of blame with the midwife was seen to occur regardless of the decision-making processes.

Findings from my study would suggest that differing decisions by a midwife and woman can transpire early within a maternity care encounter without the other's knowledge. While women transferred responsibility for maternity care decisions to the midwife, the midwives sought to release or re-locate responsibility to women. Neither player in the encounter seemed aware transference of responsibility had occurred (Ebert, 2012). Furthermore, women transferred the responsibility for maternity care decisions to healthcare professionals during the first maternity care encounter, with responsibility for maternity care decision-making not fully reclaimed until discharge from the maternity service, after giving birth. In other words, the woman's only sense of control was to decide to give any health-related decisions away, to the midwife. Consequently, the woman decided to retain control over her non-health-related maternity decisions. Women therefore act in a similar manner to health professionals. They make a referral regarding their maternity care to a person deemed, by them, to be more qualified when decisions are outside their scope of knowledge or practice. Midwives need to understand that a considered and responsible choice has been made by the woman to ensure the best outcome for herself and her baby.

Midwifery discourse and decision-making

Despite the focus of midwifery being 'with-women' and woman-centred, verbal communication styles differ according to location and organisation of care (McCourt, 2006). Midwives working within organisational premises, under the direct supervision of their employer, follow a professional 'client–healthcare worker' model of communication (McCourt, 2006). The midwife initiates, controls and concludes the conversation. The client listens, asks appropriate questions and provides relevant information upon request. Verbal communication reflects a task-orientated approach, using language aligned with the corporate body. Although midwives report their role as facilitating choice and empowering women through partnership and effective communicative relationships (Leap, 2000), incongruence in midwives' internal discourses or expressed values regarding the woman–midwife relationship and their expressed discourses regarding clinical practice can occur in such environments. Student midwives in my study (Ebert, 2012) understood that while midwives espoused the woman–centred care philosophy, they often practised a medically focused model of care.

> Midwives pretend, under the umbrella of being a midwife clinic, but it's actually medicalised, most of it is obstetric based, like they [the women] just come to the hospital clinic. Women don't make choices; the doctors make them for them.

These students recognised that midwives, in this environment, do not work in partnership with women. They work in partnership with the medically focused institution and do not offer care choices outside the models available or those decreed by the medical staff. Midwives' ability to engage in midwifery decision-making processes with women is hindered in medically dominated environments.

The environment within which the woman–midwife interaction occurs is created out of policies and procedures dictated by federal, state and local authorities. Women and midwives enter into a unique relationship and yet are bound by a set of socially constructed rules and perspectives about behaviours expected and accepted throughout their partnership. They initiate and play the game 'Doing My Job'. Both parties require certain patterns of behaviour for the partnership to be deemed successful. In cooperation, the woman and midwife follow the game plan. Midwives undertake the role of 'just doing my job' while the woman reciprocates with the 'I'm silently conforming' role until the game ends when the baby is born and the partnership is completed. Power and discipline is maintained by the organisation.

In following activity, readers are asked to read a quote by a woman, shortly after having birthed (Ebert, 2012). The maternity care encounter portrayed focuses on the interaction between a medical officer, registered midwife and a woman. Thinking about the model of care and the cultural, political and socioeconomic milieu of the geographical location in the world where you currently practise midwifery, answer the proposed questions. You may wish to draw on relevant chapters in this book.

BOX 18.5 SUZIE'S STORY – LINKED ACTIVITY 1

Activity

SUZIE: 'The doctor was performing my perineal repair and I could still feel it, and I'm looking at the midwife, I was crying and she's going "I know" and I'm thinking why you can't say anything. She [the midwife] didn't say anything she was just, I don't know. Cause he'd jumped in and said, "I will do it" and she was supposed to do it'.

1 What power dynamics or sociocultural factors may have influenced the interaction and decision-making processes in this encounter?
2 Reflect on similar interactions that you have witnessed or been involved in and consider the implications for the healthcare professionals involved and the potential impact on the woman.

3 Reflect on the power dynamics and or sociocultural factors that shape the work-place environment in which you practise. How are maternity care encounters and decision-making processes influenced?
4 What personal and professional attributes do you possess that either help or hinder your ability to effectively engage in midwifery decision-making?
5 What insights have you gained from this chapter (and book) that you can use to support midwifery decision-making when exposed to this type of situation?

Conclusion

A hospital, like any organisation, has values that are both shaped by and maintained through management styles and strategies that ensure employee alignment with values (Afsar, Cheema and Saeed, 2017). Potential managers are recruited and remunerated while employees are rewarded for portraying organisationally sanctioned values. This in turn sets a preferred way of being within the organisation. Health service structures that value medically orientated work practices and managerial style operating processes will impact on the midwife's ability to practice woman-centred care. Health and maternity service management need to encourage a shift in the workplace culture to one that positions the woman at the centre of care, both within the individual maternity care encounter and the organisation of maternity services. The midwifery body of knowledge needs to be recognised and valued within the maternity care environment by medical staff and management. Midwives need to be considered the lead maternity care provider within maternity services and refer to their medical colleagues when necessary. Mutual respect between the professions needs to be implemented within the maternity care environment and supported by management.

Midwives need to be safe to be woman-centred in their practice. A valuing of the woman and midwifery ways of being need to become the dominate workplace culture. When the midwife, regardless of the midwifery context, feels valued and safe in the care they provide, they can guide and guard the woman to have a positive maternity care experience. Midwives need to negotiate respectfully with the woman at the commencement of every maternity care encounter concerning the degree of participation in decision-making that the woman wants. Seeking the woman's input into her desired level of engagement in decision-making processes demonstrates a valuing of the woman's need to feel safe in her choices. Freeman and Griew wrote of a shared woman-midwife decision-making process in 2007, stating that it had the potential to give women an active voice in their maternity care and to influence woman-midwife relationships and institutional norms (Freeman and Griew, 2007).

Mutually respectful relationships between the midwifery and medical professions and maternity care management can facilitate decision-making processes that encourage midwives to support the woman in her choice. Shared responsibility for decision-making processes, based on a woman-centred philosophy, can diminish the current shame and blame framework. Decision-making processes in the maternity care environment need to be evidence-based and woman-centred. One decision-making algorithm that meets this criteria is Page's (2002) five steps for putting science and sensitivity into practice (Box 18.6). When the maternity care environment and management value decision-making processes based on evidence as well as the needs of the individual woman, with the woman an active partner in the decision-making process, the midwife can feel guided and guarded in her role to guide and guard the woman.

BOX 18.6 PAGE'S FIVE STEPS FOR EVIDENCE-BASED MIDWIFERY CARE

Page's five steps for evidence-based maternity care that includes the woman as a partner in decision-making processes are:

- Finding out what is important to the woman and her family
- Using information from the clinical examination
- Seeking and assessing evidence to inform decisions
- Talking it through
- Reflecting on outcomes, feelings and consequences (Page, 2002, p. 47).

Note

1 Names presented in this chapter are pseudonyms.

References

Afsar, B., Cheema, S. & Saeed, B. 2017. Do nurses display innovative work behavior when their values match with hospitals' values? *European Journal of Innovation Management*, 21, 157–171.

Copp, E. 2010. Ways to deal with stress and become calm and confident instead. *MIDIRS Midwifery Digest*, 20, 30–32.

Daemers, D., Van Limbeek, E., Winjnen, H., Nieuwenhuijze, M. & De Vries, R. 2017. Factors influencing the clinical decision-making of midwives: A qualitative study. *BMC Pregnancy and Childbirth*, 17.

Deery, R. 2009. Community midwifery 'performances' and the presentation of self. In Hunter, B. & Deery, R. (eds.), *Emotions in midwifery and reproduction*. Hampshire: Palgrave Macmillan.

Eagle Williams, L. 2011. The right assessment and support will help vulnerable young mothers to achieve a positive outcome. *MIDIRS Midwifery Digest*, 21, 84–87.

Ebert, L. 2012. *Woman-centred care and the socially disadvantaged woman: An interpretative phenomenological analysis*. Doctor of Philosophy Thesis, NSW: University of Newcastle.

Fahy, K. 1998. Being a midwife or doing midwifery? *Women and Birth*, 11, 11–16.

Fahy, K. 2008. Power and the social construction of birth territory. In Fahy, K., Foureur, M. & Hastie, C. (eds.), *Birth territory and midwifery guardianship: Theory for practice, education and research*. Edinburgh: Butterworth Heinemann Elsevier.

Freeman, L. & Griew, K. 2007. Enhancing the midwife-woman relationship through shared decision making and clinical guidelines. *Women and Birth*, 20, 11–15.

Goffinet, F. 2005. *Primary predictors of preterm labour* [Online]. Available at: http://0-www3.interscience.wiley.com [accessed May 23, 2019].

Gu, C., Zhang, Z. & Ding, Y. 2011. Chinese midwives' experience of providing continuity of care to labouring women. *Midwifery*, 27, 243–249.

Healy, S., Humpreys, E. & Kennedy, C. 2016. Midwives' and obstetricians' perceptions of risk and its impact on clinical practice and decision-making in labour: An integrative review. *Women and Birth*, 29, 107–116.

Hollins Martin, C. & Bull, P. 2006. What features of the maternity unit promote obedient behaviour from midwives? *Clinical Effectiveness in Nursing*, 9, e221–e231.

Hunter, B. 2005. Emotion work and boundary maintenance in hospital-based midwifery. *Midwifery*, 21, 253–266.

Hunter, B. 2006. The importance of reciprocity in relationships between community-based midwives and mothers. *Midwifery*, 22, 308–322.

Hunter, B. 2009. Mixed messages: Midwives' experiences of managing emotions. In Hunter, B. & Deery, R. (eds.), *Emotions in midwifery and reproduction*. London: Palgrave Macmillan.

International Confederation of Midwives. 2014a. *Philosophy and model of midwifery care* [Online]. The Hague. Available at: www.internationalmidwives.org/our-work/policy-and-practice/icm-defini tions.html [accessed January 3, 2019].

International Confederation of Midwives. 2014b. *Scope of practice of the midwife* [Online]. The Hague. Available at: www.internationalmidwives.org/our-work/policy-and-practice/icm-definitions.html [accessed January 3, 2019].

John, V. & Parsons, E. 2006. Shadow work in midwifery: Unseen and unrecognised emotional labour. *British Journal of Midwifery*, 14, 266–271.

Johnstone, M. & Kanitsaki, O. 2007. An exploration of the notion and nature of the construct of cultural safety and its applicability to the Australian health care context. *Journal of Transcultural Nursing*, 18, 247–256.

Klein, M. 2009. The phoenix midwife. *MIDIRS Midwifery Digest*, 19, 177–181.

Knezevic, B., Milosevic, M., Golubic, R., Belosevic, L., Russo, A. & Mustajbegovic, J. 2011. Work-related stress and work ability among Croatian university hospital midwives. *Midwifery*, 27, 146–153.

Leap, N. 2000. Journey to midwifery through feminism: A personal account. In Stewart, M. (ed.) *Pregnancy birth & maternity care*. Edinburgh: Books for Midwives.

Leinweber, J. & Rowe, H.J. 2010. The costs of 'being with the woman': Secondary traumatic stress in midwifery. *Midwifery*, 26, 76–87.

Marks, L., Mcconnell, J. & Baker, M. 2005. Broader skills for working with perinatal depression. *Community Practitioner*, 78, 280–282.

Mccourt, C. 2006. Supporting choice and control? Communication and interaction between midwives and women at the antenatal booking visit. *Social Science & Medicine*, 62, 1307–1318.

Morgan, L. 2015. Conceptualizing woman-centred care in midwifery. *Canadian Journal of Midwifery Practice*, 14, 9–15.

Page, L. 2002. *The new midwifery: Science and sensitivity in practice*. London: Churchill Livingstone.

Pollard, K. 2010. How midwives' discursive practices contribute to the maintenance of the status quo in English maternity care. *Midwifery*, 27, 612–619.

Porter, S., Crozier, K., Sinclair, M. & Kernohan, W. G. 2007. New midwifery? A qualitative analysis of midwives' decision-making strategies. *Journal of Advanced Nursing*, 60, 525–534.

Smith, J. 2016. Decision-making in midwifery: A tripartite clinical decision. *British Journal of Midwifery*, 24, 574–580.

Stapleton, H., Kirkham, M., Thomas, G. & Curtis, P. 2002. Evaluating informed choice. Midwives in the middle: Balance and vulnerability. *British Journal of Midwifery*, 10, 607–611.

19

WOMAN CENTRED-CARE AND SHARED DECISION-MAKING IN MIDWIFERY CARE

Marianne Nieuwenhuijze

Chapter overview

Involving women in the decision-making process is an important part of respectful, woman-centred care in the perinatal period as promoted in the worldwide White Ribbon Alliance campaign (2012). In this chapter, we explore what shapes women's experience of childbirth in the perinatal period. We specifically look at shared decision-making as a way to promote woman-centred care.

Introduction

> Puck clearly remembers the birth of her first child, nearly two years ago. It was a positive experience and she had a healthy child. However, she still wonders why certain interventions were done and how little she was told about them or consulted before doing them. Now that she is pregnant again, she really feels this should be different in the upcoming birth.

Stories like Puck's are common when you talk with women a year after birth; they have settled in their new life and start looking back, wondering why their midwife or other care providers did certain things. They often indicate they felt little control and were not involved in decisions that were made during care in the perinatal period. Studies have shown that women's feelings are less positive about birth when they look back after a longer period, and that it takes more than a healthy child to have a lasting positive childbirth experience (Greenfield, Jomeen & Glover, 2019; Rijnders et al., 2008).

Irrespective of where in the world a woman is located, the experience of childbirth is exceptional for each woman. It has short- and long-term implications for herself, her family and society (Bishanga et al., 2019; McKenzie-McHarg et al., 2015, Larkin, Begley & Devane, 2009) and leaves clear memories up to 20 years after the event, as the unique study of Simkin (1992) showed. A significant factor positively correlated to satisfaction with childbirth and birth experiences is women's sense of control that over time comes forward in studies from around the world (Greenfield, Jomeen & Glover, 2019; Mirghafourvand et al., 2019; Downe et al., 2018; Meyer, 2013; Hendrix et al., 2009). Being involved in decision-making enhances women's sense of control and positive feelings about herself, the birth experience and care.

Women's experience of childbirth

Women have described childbirth as an intense powerful life experience that affects their life and being (Olza et al., 2018). Studies done in different countries all over the world, show that women include physical elements (the course of the pregnancy and birth), emotional elements (their own feelings, thoughts and behaviour) and social elements (the interaction with their surroundings, e.g. their partner and professionals) when evaluating their birth experiences (Downe et al., 2018; Larkin, Begley & Devane, 2009). This also includes women's involvement in decision-making about their own care and that of their baby. Similar elements influence their experiences of the antenatal and postnatal period, as the whole period is a major transition to motherhood (Downe et al., 2016). The intensity of the experience can effect a sense of vulnerability in a woman, requiring stronger connections with others and a greater need for personal and professional support (Olza et al., 2018; Seefat-van Teeffelen, Nieuwenhuijze & Korstjens, 2011).

There can be profound discrepancies between how midwives look upon the event and how a woman evaluates her experience. What midwives regard as normal may be evaluated as a negative or even a traumatic experience by women and vice versa (Beck, 2011; Freedman et al., 2018). Women may even experience care during this period as a violation of their integrity and human rights, where they themselves have become invisible and an instrument for reproducing their child (Gebremichael et al., 2018; Lokugamage & Pathberiya, 2017). This violation can be physical (e.g. performing vaginal examination without the woman's permission) or verbal (e.g. using patronising language).

The way women experience the perinatal period has short- and long-term implications for their own health and well-being, as well as for that of their babies, families and society. A positive experience contributes to women's sense of accomplishment, self-esteem, feelings of competence and well-being as well as enhancing maternal-child attachment and positive descriptions of the baby (Aune et al., 2015; Hildingsson et al., 2011). A negative experience can severely influence women's emotional well-being, causing post-traumatic stress symptoms or disorders and depressive mood (Greenfield, Jomeen & Glover, 2019; McKenzie-McHarg et al., 2015). This may have adverse effects on the relationship with their partner and the bond with their baby (Elmir et al., 2010). Negative experiences are also associated with avoidance of further postnatal care, searching alternative care options in the next pregnancy, fear of childbirth, avoidance of a subsequent pregnancy, the wish for an elective caesarean section or the choice for a home birth in future births (Greenfield, Jomeen & Glover, 2019; Bishanga et al., 2019; Sigurðardóttir et al., 2019; Rigg et al., 2018; Çapik & Durmaz, 2018; Nilsson et al., 2012).

The experience of childbirth is influenced by a number of factors, including women's health, social environment and cultural background, the course of her pregnancy and birth, and the care offered by professionals (Çalik, Karabulutlu & Yavuz, 2018; Bhattacharyya et al., 2018; Henderson et al., 2018; Overgaard, Fenger-Grøn & Sandall, 2012; Larkin, Begley & Devane, 2012). What matters to women in childbirth was explored in systematic qualitative review of 35 studies from low-, middle- and high-income countries (Downe et al., 2018).

This included giving birth to a healthy baby in a safe environment with practical and emotional support from birth companions and competent, reassuring, kind staff. Most women wanted a physiological labour and birth while acknowledging that birth can be unpredictable and frightening, and that they may need 'to go with the flow'. If interventions were needed or wanted, women wanted to retain a sense of personal achievement and control through active decision-making. Other studies also found that sense of control was a significant factor associated with satisfaction and a positive birth experience (Greenfield, Jomeen & Glover, 2019; Mirghafourvand et al., 2019; Downe et al., 2018; Meyer, 2013; Hendrix, 2009).

Sense of control in childbirth

In a concept analysis, Meyer (2013) explored what defining attributes are of control in childbirth. These included (1) a woman's sense of being an active participant in the decision-making process; (2) her access to information around the events related to her birth; (3) her personal security in the sense of trust, respect and support from her provider; and (4) physical functioning relating to her sense of control over her body, emotions and pain. Women express that they want to participate in decisions regarding their care in pregnancy and childbirth, but the degree of involvement may vary depending on a woman's individual preferences and circumstances (Declercq et al., 2013; Seefat-van Teeffelen et al., 2011). A woman's involvement also seems to arise from the feeling that she is informed and can challenge decisions if the need arises. Even from feeling supported enough by trusted people present 'to let go' of their control (Parratt & Fahy, 2003). Having a sense of control – as in having the possibility to influence or be actively involved in what is happening during this life-changing period – seems key to a positive experience of pregnancy and childbirth.

Women's involvement in decision-making

Given the importance of the experience and the value of sense of control, midwives need to consider how they can play a positive role in inviting each woman to be actively involved in her care and participate in decision-making.

Decision-making is a process in which those making the decision use various types of 'evidence' to make a choice (Noseworthy, Phibbs & Benn, 2013). In healthcare, this process is no longer regarded as a one-way activity. Neither the old patriarchal approach in which the care provider makes all the decisions and decides what is essential information, nor the notion of informed choice where the provider gives all the information leaving the decision entirely with the woman, seems to meet the needs of many women. There is a relational notion between the woman and her midwife involved in coming to a decision (Noseworthy, Phibbs & Benn, 2013). Most women want to participate in decision-making and they want genuine choice (Declercq, Cheng & Sakala, 2018). They want to take responsibility for their own health, but also value the expertise and advice from their midwife (Declercq et al., 2013; Seefat-van Teeffelen, Nieuwenhuijze & Korstjens, 2011; Howarth, Swain & Treharne, 2011). Being involved contributes to their feeling of strength and preparedness to face the challenges of starting a family. A joint process between the woman and her midwife, aimed at mutual understanding to come to a decision, is the way to move forward (Nieuwenhuijze & Kane Low, 2013). This approach is advocated by the model of shared decision-making (Elwyn et al., 2017).

Shared decision-making

Shared decision-making is defined as

> an approach where clinician and patient share the best available evidence when faced with the task of making decisions, and where the patient is supported to consider options, to achieve his/her informed preferences.
>
> *(Elwyn et al., 2010, p. 971)*

In the process towards a decision, there is an interactive exchange of professional information (evidence and expertise regarding options, including benefits, harms and uncertainties) and personal information (circumstances and preferences), including an exploration of values, goals, background of preferences and beneficial solutions for the given situation. The process

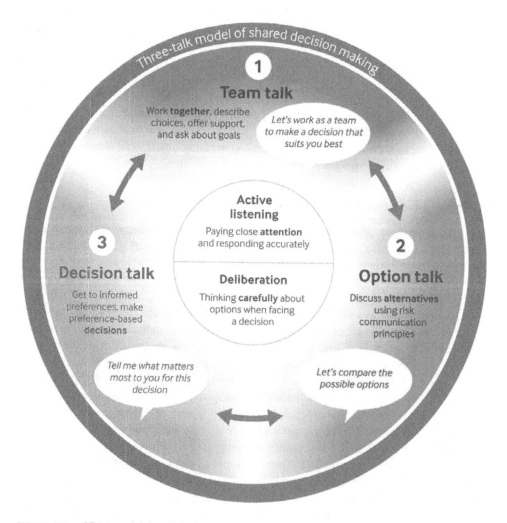

FIGURE 19.1 SDM model for clinical practice (Elwyn et al., 2017)

allows a woman to build towards a well-informed decision that fits her needs and circumstances (Nieuwenhuijze & Kane Low, 2013). Those needs and circumstances can be personal, but are also influenced by her environment, the community and culture she is a part of.

The model of shared decision-making (Elwyn et al., 2017) is described and its strengths and limitations discussed in Chapter 1. I will be drawing on this model and its three talks to demonstrate the importance of shared decision-making for woman-centred care.

Shared decision-making for woman-centred care in midwifery

Irrespective of geographical location or model of care, there are many situations during pregnancy, childbirth and the postnatal period where shared decision-making is feasible, for example in decisions around place of birth, birth after caesarean section, external version for breech presentation, birthing positions and induction/augmentation of labour. In principle, it can be applied to every decision where options, including watchful waiting, are present. To enable a woman's involvement in the decisions, the midwife plays an important role in supporting and informing the woman. She starts the dialogue, presents information on options and invites the woman to express her values, preferences and needs for support and information. To facilitate the woman to disclose what matters to her, a trusting relationship between her and her midwife is of great importance.

Experts identified four professional competences that are required to practice shared decision-making in maternity care (Nieuwenhuijze et al., 2014):

1 Establish a relationship and open dialogue with the woman (and her partner) based on respect and recognition of cultural diversity
2 Evaluate available evidence and experience, and provide the woman with accurate, honest information in the context of her individual situation
3 Activate and enable the woman to participate in the decision-making process, support her to deliberate about the options and to express her preferences and views
4 Reduce tension and guide the process to reach a well-informed decision.

Use of the three talks of shared decision-making in midwifery practice

After establishing that the course of the pregnancy or birth requires a decision, the three talks in Elwyn's model of shared decision-making can be used to support the woman to come to an informed preference and decision. The process is influenced by psychological and social factors, which need attention in order to create space for an effective dialogue between the woman and her midwife. Only when the woman feels that safe and pressing worries are addressed can she give her full attention to what is discussed. For example, it is not useful to discuss options for prenatal screening if the woman is worried whether her pregnancy is still intact because she just had some bleeding. The midwife needs to gain a deeper understanding of the woman and her environment through carefully listening to the woman. The challenge is that not all models of care allow for enough time and continuity of care. The community midwife in a village in Ghana, who knows the whole family, can have a deeper understanding of the woman than the hospital-based midwife can gain in a fragmented care system in a western country. Midwives often assume that certain groups of women (e.g. with a lower level of education) do not want to be involved in decision-making. However, studies show that most of these women do want to participate (Ebert et al., 2014).

Shared decision-making in midwifery practice is not a one-size-fits-all approach: pregnant women differ in their preferences for involvement and needs for support, depending on their individual characteristics, sociocultural contexts and support from their personal networks (Noseworthy, Phibbs & Benn, 2013).

Within the three-talk model of shared decision-making (Elwyn et al., 2017), the first talk is the *team talk*, where the woman and the midwife take a step back from the situation. Together, they check whether the woman has a clear understanding of the issue requiring a decision. It also needs to be clear to the woman that a choice is needed, that options are available and what timeframe is available for the decision. The availability of options may differ depending on resources within high-, middle- and low-income countries. Some women have difficulty with sharing in the decision-making, because they are less literate regarding health or have difficulty understanding numbers or the concept of risk (Ebert et al., 2014). Others may come from a cultural background that lacks a tradition of individuals being involved in decisions, for example India, where a woman's voice is secondary to that of a male. If the woman is hesitant to be involved, the midwife ensures that she feels supported, not left alone with the responsibility for the decision, and tries to address her concerns. Subsequently, the midwife explores what the woman already knows and if there are any misconceptions. The support given to the woman in this phase is attentive to uncertainties and confusions the woman might have.

In the next talk, the *option talk*, dialogue and exchange are central. After listing the options, including 'watchful waiting', the exchange involves evidence-informed and experience-based information on the options (benefits and harms) as well as the exploration of the woman's personal goals, values and preferences. Decision aids are supportive for presenting the information and explaining outcomes for each option. The presentation of this information may different depending on resources and needs of the audience, for example, the colourful paintings of mother and child clinics in India. Whatever the context, these presentations of information cannot replace the dialogue and the trustful relationship between the woman and her midwife that allows exchange of further information. At the end of this talk, all the information is summarised. The support given to the woman in this phase is attentive to the woman's need for information that is tailored to her circumstances, her understanding of the information and the time necessary to process the information.

If possible, a *deliberation* phase gives the woman time to consider the information and understand her options. The midwife can guide her to other reliable sources of information. Often a woman will feel the need to discuss her decision with others. Acknowledging this need is important for a good shared decision-making process.

In the *decision* talk, the midwife and the woman focus on the preferences and move to a decision. Subsequently, a plan for making that decision possible is discussed and the whole process is evaluated. The support given to the woman in this phase is attentive to her feeling confident with her choice and ensuring that, where feasible, she feels the freedom to revisit her choices and change her decisions.

Additional recommendations for improving the quality of the shared decision-making process in maternity include (Ebert et al., 2014; Nieuwenhuijze et al., 2014):

- *Communication*: strive for an open dialogue with respect, empathy and use of understandable language

- *Information*: offer honest, complete, evidence-informed information adjusted to the woman's level of understanding, discuss uncertainty – evidence may be lacking and outcomes are not always predictable at the individual level
- *Midwife*: be prepared to discuss decisions several times, check if there is a clear understanding of what is discussed and agreed, respect a woman's autonomy and explicitly obtain a woman's consent when taking actions, make sure that other care providers are informed about a woman's decisions
- *Birth*: start preparation for decisions in birth during antenatal care, make the woman aware that unforeseen events can occur and that time for decision-making may be limited; explore a woman's expectations and preferences; during birth explain what is happening and that action is required – even if those explanations must be brief in acute situations; always seek a woman's consent; discuss the situation and decisions again after the birth.

Conclusion and recommendations

The process of shared decision-making in midwifery care is valuable in promoting optimal health outcomes for a woman and her baby. It is a significant part of woman-centred care, recognising the woman as a full participant in the care around her pregnancy and birth. In using shared decision-making as a dialogue between a woman and her midwife, the conversation includes a broad range of elements that bear on the final decision women make in care. Shared decision-making as a process offers opportunities to enter into discussions that maintain the integrity of all of the individuals involved. How this process is actually shaped depends on available resources, the cultural context and the woman's needs, but always puts the woman and her child in the centre of care. Additionally, midwives' open approach to shared decision-making in the perinatal period contributes to women's skills for adequate woman-professional communications and is not only an investment for their present pregnancy but can also support them in future encounters with health professionals outside maternity care.

References

Aune, I., Torvik, H. M., Selboe, S. T., Skogas, A. K., Persen, J. and Dahlberg, U. (2015) Promoting a normal birth and a positive birth experience – Norwegian women's perspectives. *Midwifery* 31(7), pp. 721–727.

Beck, C. T. (2011) A meta-ethnography of traumatic childbirth and its aftermath: Amplifying causal looping. *Qualitative Health Research* 21(3), pp. 301–311.

Bhattacharyya, S., Srivastava, A., Saxena, M., Gogoi, M., Dwivedi, P. and Giessler, K. (2018) Do women's perspectives of quality of care during childbirth match with those of providers? A qualitative study in Uttar Pradesh, India. *Global Health Action* 11(1), 1527971, pp. 1–12.

Bishanga, D. R., Massenga, J., Mwanamsangu, A. H., Kim, Y. M., George, J., Kapologwe, N. A., Zoungrana, J., Rwegasira, M., Kols, A., Hill, K., Rijken, M. J. and Stekelenburg, J. (2019) Women's experience of facility-based childbirth care and receipt of an early postnatal check for herself and her newborn in North-western Tanzania. *International Journal of Environmental Research and Public Health* 16(3), pii: e481.

Çapik, A. and Durmaz, H. (2018) Fear of childbirth, postpartum depression, and birth-related variables as predictors of posttraumatic stress disorder after childbirth. *Worldviews of Evidence Based Nursing* 15(6), pp. 455–463.

Çalik, K. Y., Karabulutlu, Ö. and Yavuz, C. (2018) First do no harm – Interventions during labor and maternal satisfaction: A descriptive cross-sectional study. *BMC Pregnancy Childbirth* 18(1), p. 415.

Declercq, E. R., Cheng, E. R. and Sakala, C. (2018) Does maternity care decision-making conform to shared decision-making standards for repeat cesarean and labor induction after suspected macrosomia? *Birth* 45(3), pp. 236–244.

Declercq, E. R., Sakala, C., Corry, M. P., Applebaum, S. and Hemlich, A. (2013) *Listening to mothers III: Pregnancy and birth.* New York: Childbirth Connection.

Downe, S., Finlayson, K., Oladapo, O., Bonet, M. and Gülmezoglu, A. M. (2018) What matters to women during childbirth: A systematic qualitative review. *PLoS One* 13(4), pp. e0194906.

Downe, S., Finlayson, K., Tunçalp, Ö. and Gülmezoglu, A. M. (2016) What matters to women: A systematic scoping review to identify the processes and outcomes of antenatal care provision that are important to healthy pregnant women. *BJOG: An International Journal of Obstetrics & Gynaecology* 123(4), pp. 529–539.

Ebert, L., Bellchambers, H., Ferguson, A. and Browne, J. (2014) Socially disadvantaged women's views of barriers to feeling safe to engage in decision-making in maternity care. *Women and Birth* 27(2), pp. 132–137.

Elmir, R., Schmied, V., Wilkes, L. and Jackson, D. (2010) Women's perceptions and experiences of a traumatic birth: A meta-ethnography. *Journal of Advanced Nursing* 66, pp. 2142–2153.

Elwyn, G., Durand, M. A., Song, J., Aarts, J., Barr, P. J., Berger, Z., Cochran, N., Frosch, D., Galasiński, D., Gulbrandsen, P., Han, P. K. J., Härter, M., Kinnersley, P., Lloyd, A., Mishra, M., Perestelo-Perez, L., Scholl, I., Tomori, K., Trevena, L., Witteman, H. O. and van der Weijden, T. (2017) A three-talk model for shared decision making: Multistage consultation process. *British Medical Journal* 359, pp. 1–7.

Elwyn, G., Laitner, S., Coulter, A., Walker, E., Watson, P. and Thomson, R. (2010) Implementing shared decision making in the NHS. *British Medical Journal* 341, pp. 971–973.

Freedman, L. P., Kujawski, S. A., Mbuyita, S., Kuwawenaruwa, A., Kruk, M. E., Ramsey, K. and Mbaruku, G. (2018) Eye of the beholder? Observation versus self-report in the measurement of disrespect and abuse during facility-based childbirth. *Reproductive Health Matters* 26(53), pp. 107–122.

Gebremichael, M. W., Worku, A., Medhanyie, A. A., Edin, K. and Berhane, Y. (2018) Women suffer more from disrespectful and abusive care than from the labour pain itself: A qualitative study from women's perspective. *BMC Pregnancy Childbirth* 18(1), p. 392.

Greenfield, M., Jomeen, J. and Glover, L. (2019) 'It can't be like last time' – Choices made in early pregnancy by women who have previously experienced a traumatic birth. *Frontiers in Psychology* 10(56), pp. 1–13.

Henderson, J., Carson, C., Jayaweera, H., Alderdice, F. and Redshaw, M. (2018) Recency of migration, region of origin and women's experience of maternity care in England: Evidence from a large cross-sectional survey. *Midwifery* 67, pp. 87–94.

Hendrix, M., Van Horck, M., Moreta, D., Nieman, F., Nieuwenhuijze, M., Severens, J. and Nijhuis, J. (2009) Why women do not accept randomisation for place of birth: Feasibility of a RCT in the Netherlands. *BJOG: An International Journal of Obstetrics & Gynaecology* 116, pp. 537–542.

Hildingsson, I., Nilsson, C., Karlström, A. and Lundgren, I. (2011) A longitudinal survey of childbirth-related fear and associated factors. *Journal of Obstetric, Gynecologic, and Neonatal Nursing* 40, pp. 532–543.

Howarth, A. M., Swain, N. and Treharne, G. J. (2011) Taking personal responsibility for well-being increases birth satisfaction of first time mothers. *Journal of Health Psychology* 16, pp. 1221–1230.

Larkin, P., Begley, C. M. and Devane, D. (2009) Women's experiences of labour and birth: An evolutionary concept analysis. *Midwifery* 25, pp. e49–e59.

Larkin, P., Begley, C. M. and Devane, D. (2012) 'Not enough people to look after you': An exploration of women's experiences of childbirth in the Republic of Ireland. *Midwifery* 28, pp. 98–105.

Lokugamage, A. U. and Pathberiya, S. D. (2017) Human rights in childbirth, narratives and restorative justice: A review. *Reproductive Health* 14(1), p. 17.

McKenzie-McHarg, K., Ayers, S., Ford, E., Horsch, A., Jomeen, J., Sawyer, A., Stramrood, C., Thomson, G. and Slade, P. (2015) Post-traumatic stress disorder following childbirth: An update of current issues and recommendations for future research. *Journal of Reproductive and Infant Psychology* 33(3), pp. 219–237.

Meyer, S. (2013) Control in childbirth: A concept analysis and synthesis. *Journal of Advanced Nursing* 69, pp. 218–228.

Mirghafourvand, M., Mohammad Alizadeh Charandabi, S., Ghanbari-Homayi. S., Jahangiry, L., Nahaee, J. and Hadian, T. (2019) Effect of birth plans on childbirth experience: A systematic review. *International Journal of Nursing Practice* e12722, pp. 1–9.

Nieuwenhuijze, M.J. and Kane Low, L. (2013) Facilitating women's choice in maternity care. *Journal of Clinical Ethics* 24, pp. 276–282.

Nieuwenhuijze, M.J., Korstjens, I., de Jonge, A., de Vries, R. and Lagro-Janssen, T. (2014) On speaking terms: A Delphi study on shared decision-making in maternity care. *BMC Pregnancy and Childbirth* 14, p. 223–244.

Nilsson, C., Lundgren, I., Karlström, A. and Hildingsson, I. (2012) Self-reported fear of childbirth and its association with women's birth experience and mode of delivery: A longitudinal population-based study. *Women and Birth* 25(3) pp. 114–121.

Noseworthy, D., Phibbs, S. and Benn, C. (2013) Towards a relational model of decision-making in midwifery care. *Midwifery* 29, pp. e42–e48.

Olza, I., Leahy-Warren, P., Benyamini, Y., Kazmierczak, M., Karlsdottir, S.I., Spyridou, A., Crespo-Mirasol, E., Takács, L., Hall, P.J., Murphy, M., Jonsdottir, S.S., Downe, S. and Nieuwenhuijze, M.J. (2018) Women's psychological experiences of physiological childbirth: A meta-synthesis. *BMJ Open* 8, e020347. doi:10.1136/bmjopen-2017-020347.

Overgaard, C., Fenger-Grøn, M. and Sandall, J. (2012) The impact of birthplace on women's birth experiences and perceptions of care. *Social Science & Medicine* 74, pp. 973–981.

Parratt, J. and Fahy, K. (2003) Trusting enough, to be out of control: A pilot study of women's sense of self during childbirth. *Australian Journal of Midwifery* 16, pp. 15–22.

Rigg, E.C., Schmied, V., Peters, K. and Dahlen, H.G. (2018) A survey of women in Australia who choose the care of unregulated birthworkers for a birth at home. *Women and Birth* pii: S1871–5192 (18)30660–7.

Rijnders, M., Baston, H., Schönbeck, Y., van der Pal, K., Prins, M., Green, J. and Buitendijk, S. (2008) Perinatal factors related to negative or positive recall of birth experience in women 3 years postpartum in the Netherlands. *Birth* 35, pp. 107–116.

Seefat-van Teeffelen, A., Nieuwenhuijze, M. and Korstjens, I. (2011) Women want proactive psychosocial support from midwives during transition to motherhood: A qualitative study. *Midwifery* 27, pp. e122–e127.

Sigurðardóttir, V.L., Gamble, J., Guðmundsdóttir, B., Sveinsdóttir, H. and Gottfreðsdóttir, H. (2019) Processing birth experiences: A content analysis of women's preferences. *Midwifery* 69, pp. 29–38.

Simkin, P. (1992) Just another day in a woman's life? Part II: Nature and consistency of women's long-term memories of their first birth experiences. *Birth* 19, pp. 64–81.

White Ribbon Alliance. (2012) Respectful maternity care: The universal rights of childbearing women. Accessed on January 2019: www.who.int/woman_child_accountability/ierg/reports/2012_01S_Respectful_Maternity_Care_Charter_The_Universal_Rights_of_Childbearing_Women.pdf

20

COLLABORATIVE DECISION-MAKING FROM A WOMAN'S PERSPECTIVE

Daniela Drandić and Magdalena Kurbanović

Chapter overview

The collaborative decision-making process in maternity care depends on the model of care being practiced. In a midwifery model of care, such as teams/caseload (hereinafter referred to as caseload) or private/independent midwifery care, there is space and time for the midwife and woman get to know each other during pregnancy. They both have the time to decide whether they fit each other's values and priorities regarding autonomy and decision-making, and if they feel it's necessary, they have the opportunity to decide not to work together. Conversely, within a hospital setting, a midwife and woman may have to forge a relationship within the constraints of a 'shift' with little or no room to seek out another care provider if their values are not compatible. Due to the nature of the situation, decision-making in midwifery-led care is more likely to put the woman at the centre of the decision-making process, while hospital-based midwifery is more likely to put the organisation and/or healthcare provider at the centre.

Introduction

From early childhood, girls around the world are traditionally taught to conform to the wishes of authority and discouraged from asking questions about authoritative knowledge. Authority is often embodied by a white, male figure who 'knows best' for everyone. This paternalism is not limited to high-income countries but it is a global issue. When faced with healthcare choices, it is not unusual for many women to simply accept their (male) healthcare provider's opinion without question, using the paradigm where conformity is required to achieve optimal outcomes (Turner, 1987). This is exacerbated during maternity care, where modern discourse is focused on risk and choice, effectively alienating for women who are made to feel that they are not qualified to make important decisions and should rather defer to the 'experts' (Ebert et al., 2014), but which also deems them selfish for wanting to exercise their own choice.

Although women of childbearing age want more information and to actively participate in decision-making than any other group (Goldberg, 2009), they need to have an enabling environment where they feel safe to actively participate in decisions about their care (Ebert et al., 2014). At the same time, midwives who care for women during the childbearing year also need to be empowered and comfortable in their role as a guide in this process. If for some reason the midwife does not feel safe, it may hinder information exchange, effectively preventing a woman from participating in decision-making (Ebert et al., 2014). Collaborative decision-making requires both participants to feel comfortable in their roles (Ebert et al., 2014). Women place great importance on collaborative relationships with their healthcare providers; a Canadian study found that the vast majority of women (90.8%) stated that it was either very important or important to them that they lead decision-making about their maternity care (Vedam et al., 2017). The value of these relationships is especially important for women from vulnerable groups. This type of relationship is especially valued when provided by midwives, as demonstrated by Swedish research (Berg et al., 1996). Yet in countries where gender and health inequalities are more pervasive, such as Africa or India, empowering women to feel safe in a maternity setting or with a midwife to co-share decision-making is more difficult (Ghose et al., 2017; Sultana et al., 2017). The impact of gender responsive healthcare to improve the global health of women is being targeted by groups such as UNAIDS, UNWOMEN (formerly UNIFEM) and UNFPA, PAHO, WHO, and the World Bank, Futures Group, International Centre for Research on Women (ICRW), Population Council and EngenderHealth (Bloom and Arnoff, 2012).

We will explore how a midwife's working environment and her own values shape how she influences a woman's decision-making processes and how a woman's values, culture and beliefs' shape her preferred decision-making process.

Midwives and collaboration with colleagues

How colleagues affect decision-making processes

Even though midwifery is regarded as an autonomous profession, in many parts of the world midwifery is still very much dominated by a medical model. Such a scenario may well apply to many countries around the globe, for example Central and Eastern European countries, where despite their formal compliance with European Union (EU) directives, the reality in clinical practice is very different in that obstetricians are still legally responsible even for physiological childbirth (Mivšek, Baškova and Wilhelmova, 2016).

In medically dominated environments such as hospitals, a strict hierarchy exists where decisions are governed by organisational rules and protocols that must be followed rigidly (Porter et al., 2007). In such an environment, the midwife's decision-making processes will tend to reflect not only the institution's protocols and evidence-informed care but also the adopted philosophy and attitudes towards childbirth. The need to belong is an integral part of human nature, and social acceptance in the context of the work environment is integral for healthcare workers' self-esteem and for their survival and well-being in the environment they are working in (Baumeister, 2011), resulting in a tendency to adopt the decision-making practice that is acceptable at the institution. When faced with differing opinions with the authority figure, midwives can often follow the path of obedience and prioritise it over advocating for woman's personal preferences (Hollins Martin and Bull, 2004, 2005, 2006; Porter et al., 2007). The authority figure can also be a fellow midwife, and in some studies senior midwives were able to influence decision-making process of other midwives, irrespective of whether the midwife had built a relationship with woman she was caring for and understood her birth values and preference (Hollins-Martin and Bull, 2005). They did this by assuming the lead in the woman's care with a disregard for women-centred care (Hollins-Martin and Bull, 2005; O'Connel and Downe, 2009).

Another factors that impacts collaborative or shared decision-making is the heavy workloads midwives experience in some work environments – such as simultaneously providing care for more than one labouring woman and at the same time spending a significant amount of time on documentation, managing technology, often in settings where fragmented care is dominant and the midwife only meets women for a very short time during their childbearing journeys. A hectic environment and fragmented care together make it difficult for midwives to create a trusting relationship with women they are caring for. Consequently, midwives may not have the opportunity to engage with women in a meaningful way that facilitates understanding their values, wants and needs or sharing relevant information, contributing to inadequate opportunities for women to be included in decision-making. This may be further hindered by the number of professionals within a multidisciplinary team that have input in a woman's care plan (and their hierarchical relationship), as each member brings their own characteristics, biases and values to the process. A delicate balance must be struck, as collaboration between midwives and other maternity care professionals is crucial for facilitating the decision-making process and ensuring women's choices are respected (Behruzi et al., 2017).

The length of a midwife's working experience has a significant influence on collaboration with other professionals and in turn on decision-making process. Inexperienced nurses (and by extension, inexperienced midwives) are often guided by rules and are oriented by task completion, while more experienced colleagues have an intuitive grasp of the situation and place the utmost importance on meeting the patient's actual concerns and needs, even when that means planning and negotiating for a change in the plan of care (Alligood, 2014). While inexperience can lead to bureaucratic decision-making, experience can also hinder including women in the decision-making process. Referred to as 'inertial power of tradition', this happens when more experienced midwives can be inflexible regarding some aspects of care that were not present during their training and larger part of their career, which may or may not have included the midwifery philosophy of woman-centred care (Porter et al., 2007).

Apart from midwives' personal characteristics, their perceptions of the women they are caring for can also have a negative impact on collaborative decision-making. Midwives may label some women as not wanting to be involved in decision-making, assuming that these particular women would rather adapt a passive role and hand their autonomy over to someone else – like a perceived healthcare expert. By taking charge over decisions and assuming an authoritarian approach, these midwives believe they are in fact adhering to the woman's choice (Porter et al., 2007). In some more extreme cases, midwives may even deem certain women as not being capable of being involved in decision-making on account of lacking enough credible knowledge about childbirth, consequently labelling them as an inappropriate partner for collaborative decision-making (Porter et al., 2007).

Since collaborative decision-making is a way of enabling an evidence-based, women-centred approach, it is very important for midwives to be aware of factors that influence these processes so they can help women feel involved and make sure informed decisions they make are reflective of their personal values regarding childbirth rather than that of the midwife.

The role of supporters in labour and birth

There are many advantages of continuous labour support in hospital settings that has been well documented, including shorter labours, higher rates of spontaneous vaginal delivery, lower rates of medical interventions and positive birth experience (Bohren et al., 2017; Hodnett et al., 2012). As a result, increasing number of hospitals around of world are facilitating and encouraging women to have access to companions at birth. The World Health Organization (2018) recommends a companion of choice (support person) for all women throughout labour and childbirth (WHO, 2018) Therefore it is important to consider the role that support person has in the decision-making process. The support person can come in the form of a midwife, doula or birth partner from the woman's social network who can be a friend, female relative or in many cases the woman's partner. The support person can create a positive context thought merely being present and providing birthing women with emotional and physical support, but also can play an important role as an advocate that ensures her wishes and decisions are honoured (Kainz, Eliasson and von Post, 2010). Therefore it is important they share the same values, or at least that the support person knows and respects the birthing woman's values. This is not always entirely straightforward, however, as is discussed in Chapter 21.

For some women, hospital births can be stressful since they are often highly medicalised, subjected to institutional routines and high rates of intervention, usually attended by unfamiliar personnel and lacking privacy and intimacy (Baker et al., 2005; Harris and Ayers, 2012; Murray-Davis et al., 2014; Sigurdardottir et al., 2019). Feeling overwhelmed may result in women deferring decision-making to those they perceive as experts. Although this may seem pragmatic in the short term, in the long term it may not be as a woman's perception of control and participation in decision-making during labour and childbirth have a significant impact on how she perceives her birth experience (Goldberg, 2009; Macfarlane, Rocca-Ihenacho and Turner, 2014), and in lower-resource countries, this has an even greater effect on a woman's long-term reproductive health and decisions such as birth interval (Osamor and Grady, 2016). There is also evidence that mode of delivery can have impact on the father's perception and stress level, meaning fathers experience higher levels of stress when a lot of interventions are used, such as operational delivery and caesarean section (Chan, Paterson and Brown, 2002; Keogh et al., 2006).

Even though research suggests that the presence of a support person has a positive influence on labour outcomes (Bohren et al., 2017), McGrath and Kennell (2008) demonstrated that support provided by fathers alone provided did not have the same degree of positive effect as support given by an experienced doula. (The role of the doula is discussed in Chapter 21.) Whilst fathers' presence at the birth had a positive effect on pain medication administration and labour length, the suggestion was that fathers are too emotionally involved and experience their own anxiety and distress as they observe the pain and process of labour (Ip, 2000). Nevertheless, being present at the labour did lead fathers to take a more active and controlling role in decision-making (Ip, 2000).

Decision-making is a very complex process, especially when more than one person is involved. It is important for midwives and other healthcare professionals to acknowledge that and to provide emotional support and guidance not only for women they care for but for their birth partners. One potential strategy is childbirth education programmes that address effective decision-making and take in consideration the needs of the expectant fathers as well as mothers (Lothian, 2007; Simpson, Newman and Chirino, 2010; DeJoy, 2011).

Caseload midwifery

Practicing in midwifery-led models of care provides midwives with a much higher degree of autonomy with regard to the scope and type of care they provide to women; however, even here midwives often feel that many areas of decision-making are under the control of obstetrics (Healy, Humphreys and Kennedy, 2016). An Irish study found that midwives themselves can even undermine their own autonomy in order to avoid being implicated in adverse outcomes (Healy, Humphreys and Kennedy, 2016). Although midwives who practice as private practitioners or using the caseload model are regarded as the most autonomous, the degree to which midwives they are able to make decisions freely is dependent on the way the system they are working in is organised, its hierarchies and the extent to which midwives are regulated by the medical model of care.

Hierarchy and the lack of understanding and significance of midwifery-led care, as well as lack of systematic support has resulted in more midwives relegating their own autonomy to that of more powerful obstetricians (Levy, 1999) – in some cases to the point where midwives feel that obstetricians do not have trust in their decision-making capabilities (Healy, Humphreys and Kennedy, 2016). The dominance of the medical model in maternity care can permeate and undermine the decision-making processes of midwives – the dominant group's views become the acceptable norm, and those of groups who are less powerful become subversive (Levy, 1999). A consequence of this is that the information provided to pregnant and birthing women is then different, substantively affecting the decision-making process (Coxon et al., 2017; Levy, 1999). No matter their values, desires or evidence-based care, or even the model of care they are using, the systems providing maternity care to women make it difficult for them to achieve true autonomous, unbiased decision-making.

Women's values and decision-making

Women who have a clear idea of how they want to give birth before they become pregnant usually do not seek out information to weigh the risks and benefits of this choice, and even actively discount information that is not in accordance with their already made choice (Regan, McElroy and Moore, 2013). Many sources of information are available to women before and during pregnancy. An American study identified four major categories of information that women used to inform their birthing choices: (1) the birth stories of other women or attending a birth themselves (nearly three-quarters of women responding that this was helpful in deciding how they wanted to birth); (2) childbirth classes; (3) healthcare providers; and (4) written materials such as books, journals and resources on the internet (Regan, McElroy and Moore, 2013). In lower-resource settings, women do not usually make decisions about maternity care autonomously, and family members, especially husbands and mothers-in-law, have a large influence whether and where women seek maternity care (Osamor and Grady, 2016).

In both high- and low-resource countries, a woman's social status also has a great effect on the resources available to her and those she is available to seek out, and despite the fact that they want to actively participate in their care, women who are less educated, less wealthy and have disabilities often have fewer choices about maternity care options available to them (Ebert et al., 2014; Malouf, Henderson and Redshaw, 2017; Osamor and Grady, 2016). This can be because healthcare providers withhold information from them in order to make the women's choices congruent with their own, or because the healthcare provider does not want to relinquish the decision to the woman, for fear of then having to take responsibility for a possible adverse outcome (Healy, Humphreys and Kennedy, 2016; Walsh, 2005). Without information and healthcare providers who are willing to facilitate their choice, women may delegate the responsibility for decision-making to those who they see as belonging to the healthcare system (physicians, midwives) because they believe themselves to be outsiders to the healthcare culture and decision-making processes (Ebert et al., 2014).

Healthcare providers are influential in regards to making decisions about childbirth – with one American study showing that nearly one-fifth of women found healthcare providers to be an important source of information (Regan, McElroy and Moore, 2013). However, there is a large discrepancy in the amount, type and relevance of information women receive, depending on their chosen caregiver; those cared for prenatally by midwives were presented with numerous options and reported that discussion on type of birth was a theme over numerous visits; on the other hand, women who received care from physicians reported that they were not forthcoming with information about birth choices, often stating that it was up to the woman to ask informed questions and expect answers, as opposed to having the physician provide information during appointments (Regan, McElroy and Moore, 2013).

Informed consent integral to decision-making

Despite legal and ethical requirements which are discussed in Chapters 3 and 4, informed consent is not always understood in the same way by all healthcare providers, nor is it always administered in a consistent way (Goldberg, 2009). Many healthcare providers consider informed consent to be a simple signature on a consent form when it is in fact a dynamic process of exchanging information as the clinical situation progresses, all the while involving patients in decisions without the use of coercion (Goldberg, 2009; Kukura, 2018).

Women face a number of barriers when trying to achieve informed decision-making. Some of these are institutional – midwives may not have the power to clearly state their opinions, but feel that they must comply with those of the more powerful medical professionals (Levy, 1999). Not having an opportunity to have meaningful and understandable discussions about their care with healthcare providers is another barrier which disproportionately affects women with disabilities (Malouf, Henderson and Redshaw, 2017;) and women from minority groups (Jomeen and Redshaw, 2013). Maternity care facilities and practices that continue to use practices that are not based on evidence and healthcare providers who refuse to implement the informed decisions made by their clients are further barriers that are unfortunately disproportionately encountered by women from vulnerable groups (Stirling, Vanbeisen and McDougall, 2018).

In order to make an informed decision, a patient must have access to a healthcare provider who has expertise grounded in evidence and possesses the ability to communicate in a manner that allows them both to express views and concerns freely. An integral component to informed decision-making that is often overlooked is the right to refuse what is being offered, without the guarantee that a healthcare provider will respect and respond to a woman's decisions without any repercussions for the woman, informed decision-making is moot (Human Rights in Childbirth, 2018).

Decision-making (and consequently, informed consent) where the healthcare user is the ultimate decision-maker can be at odds with a medical-risk based model of maternity care because it puts the responsibility for outcomes on healthcare user, not the healthcare provider (Healy, Humphreys and Kennedy, 2016). Healthcare providers who were taught or practice in the medical model of care are often uncomfortable with this type of 'delegating' of responsibility, believing that decision-making should rest with the healthcare provider as the person who 'knows best' (Healy, Humphreys and Kennedy, 2016; Walsh, 2005). Noteworthy, however, is that many healthcare users are also uncomfortable with the idea of making choices for themselves, by themselves, especially when the stakes are high, as they are in maternity care (Jomeen, 2006).

Frameworks for change

One solution with the potential to implement informed decision-making, especially in settings where the change towards empowering women in healthcare will not likely come from the systems, is Twelve Steps to Safe and Respectful Mother Baby Care, launched in 2018 by a collaboration of international experts and organisations, which includes global umbrella organisations from the fields of obstetrics, midwifery and paediatrics and based on the latest evidence in maternity care (International Childbirth Initiative, 2018). The 12 steps emphasise the importance of informed choice, autonomy and avoiding care that is not based on evidence, including the implementation of a midwifery model of care, which is linked to higher rates of satisfaction and better outcomes, especially when caseload midwifery is practiced (Allen et al., 2015; Ebert et al., 2014; McRae et al., 2018; Renfrew et al., 2014). Implementing this standardised, recognised and validated program has the potential to change maternity care in the same way that the baby-friendly hospital initiative transformed breastfeeding support in maternity facilities. It also has the potential to change rigid hierarchies that exist in many maternity systems, especially those where hospital and obstetric care are dominant. By opening up these systems to increased collaboration and putting the woman at the centre of care, there is a real possibility to transform systems.

Another solution, or tool, to implementing informed decision-making in maternity care is to measure women's autonomy in decision-making and monitor it over time in a given setting. This is possible using tools such as the Mother's Autonomy in Decision Making (MADM) scale (Vedam et al., 2017). Being able to monitor with a standard tool over time, implementing actions to make sure the values reported by women are consistently increasing or remain favourable, has the potential not only to increase women's satisfaction with care but also to increase their own health behaviours and outcomes (Shay and Lafata, 2014). It may also affect at a system level by reducing the overuse of procedures and increase the sustainability of healthcare systems (Vedam et al., 2017).

Finally, it is imperative that midwifery education all over the world begins empowering midwives to be more than medical assistants, encouraging them to create relationships with the women they care for and to practice evidence-based care.

Conclusion

The importance of including women in decision-making must not be underestimated. Shared decision-making is closely tied to positive outcomes including satisfaction with care, management of health behaviours and health outcomes (Vedam et al., 2017; Shay and Lafata, 2014). Involving women in decision-making in maternity care increases a woman's sense of responsibility for her own health and that of her infant, both during and after pregnancy (Harrison et al., 2003; Vedam et al., 2017).

Increasing access to the midwifery-led models of care is a key way of increasing women's decision-making and consequently improving their health. The short- and long-term benefits decision-making provides for women, their infants, families, communities and healthcare systems, which include increased satisfaction, reduction in the overuse of interventions and procedures and as a result, improved sustainability of healthcare systems (Legare et al., 2012), need to be high on the maternity agenda.

At the same time, it is imperative to understand and actively work to remove the barriers women face to receiving balanced, evidence-informed information about care choices in pregnancy and childbirth. This is especially true of women from vulnerable groups, women with lower levels of education and from lower resource settings. There must be an improved balance in responsibility between healthcare providers and women if the goal of appropriate care and involvement in decision-making is to be achieved (Healey et al., 2017). Far from a 'nice to have' element in maternity care, informed decision-making has the potential to transform experiences and systems.

References

Allen, J. et al. (2015). 'Does model of maternity care make a difference to birth outcomes for young women? A retrospective cohort study', *International Journal of Nursing Studies*, Elsevier Ltd, 52(8), pp. 1332–1342. doi:10.1016/j.ijnurstu.2015.04.011

Alligood, M. (2014). *Nursing Theorists and Their Work*. 8th ed. St. Louis: Mosby, Elsevier, pp. 124–125.

Baker, S. R. et al. (2005). '"I felt as though I'd been in jail": Women's experiences of maternity care during labour, delivery and the immediate postpartum', *Feminism & Psychology*, 15(3), pp. 315–342. doi:10.1177/0959-353505054718

Baumeister, R. (2011). 'Need to belong theory', In: P. VanLange, A. Kruglanski and E. Higgins, ed., *Handbook of Theories of Social Psychology*. Thousand Oaks: Sage Publications Ltd, pp. 121–140.

Behruzi, R., Klam, S., Dehertog, M., Jimenez, V. and Hatem, M. (2017). 'Understanding factors affecting collaboration between midwives and other health care professionals in a birth center and its affiliated Quebec hospital: A case study', *BMC Pregnancy Childbirth*, 17(1), p. 200.

Berg, M., Lundgren, I., Hermansson, E. and Wahlberg, V. (1996). Women's experience of the encounter with the midwife during childbirth. *Midwifery*, 12(1), pp. 11–15.

Bloom, S. and Arnoff, E. (2012). Gender and health data and statistics: An annotated resource guide. [online] Chapel Hill: MEASURE Evaluation. Available at: www.measureevaluation.org/resources/publications/ms-12-52 [accessed 19 February 2019].

Bohren, M., Hofmeyr, G., Sakala, C., Fukuzawa, R. and Cuthbert, A. (2017). 'Continuous support for women during childbirth', *Cochrane Database of Systematic Reviews* (7), CD003766. DOI: 10.1002/14651858.CD003766.pub6

Chan, K. and Paterson-Brown, S. (2002). 'How do fathers feel after accompanying their partners in labour and delivery?' *Journal of Obstetrics and Gynaecology*, 22(1), pp. 11–15.

Coxon, K. et al. (2017). 'What influences birth place preferences, choices and decision-making amongst healthy women with straightforward pregnancies in the UK? A qualitative evidence synthesis using a "best fit" framework approach', *BMC Pregnancy and Childbirth*, 17(1), pp. 1–15. doi:10.1186/s12884-017-1279-7

DeJoy, S. B. (2011). The Role of Male Partners in Childbirth Decision Making: A Qualitative Exploration with First-Time Parenting Couples. Graduate Theses and Dissertations. University of South Florida. http://scholarcommons.usf.edu/etd/3720.

Ebert, L., Bellchambers, H., Ferguson, A. and Browne, J. (2014). 'Socially disadvantaged women's views of barriers to feeling safe to engage in decision-making in maternity care', *Women and Birth*, 27(2), pp. 132–137. doi:10.1016/j.wombi.2013.11.003

Ghose, B. et al. (2017). 'Women's decision-making autonomy and utilisation of maternal healthcare services: Results from the Bangladesh Demographic and Health Survey', BMJ Open, 7(9), pp. 1–9. doi:10.1136/bmjopen-2017-017142

Goldberg, H. (2009). 'Informed decision making in maternity care', *Journal of Perinatal Education*, 18(1), pp. 32–40. doi:10.1624/105812409X396219

Harris, R. and Ayers, S. (2012). 'What makes labour and birth traumatic? A survey of intrapartum "hot-spots"', *Psychology & Health*, 27(10), pp. 1166–1177. doi:10.1080/08870446.2011.649755

Harrison, M. J., Kushner, K. E., Benzies, K., Rempel, G. and Kimak, C. (2003). 'Women's satisfaction with their involvement in health care decisions during a high-risk pregnancy', *Birth*, 30(2), pp. 109–115.

Healy, S., Humphreys, E. and Kennedy, C. (2016. 'Midwives' and obstetricians' perceptions of risk and its impact on clinical practice and decision-making in labour: An integrative review', *Women and Birth*, 29(2), pp. 107–116. doi:10.1016/j.wombi.2015.08.010

Hodnett, E., Gates, S., Hofmeyr, G. and Sakala, C. (2012). 'Continuous support for women during childbirth', *Cochrane Database of Systematic Reviews*, (7). CD003766. doi:10.1002/14651858.CD003766.pub4

Hollins Martin, C. J. and Bull, P. (2004). 'Does status have more influence than education on the decisions midwives make?' *Clinical Effectiveness in Nursing*, 8, pp. 133–139.

Hollins Martin, C. J. and Bull, P. (2005). 'Measuring social influence of a senior midwife on decision making in maternity care: An experimental study', *Journal of Community and Applied Social Psychology*, 15, pp. 120–126.

Hollins Martin, C. J. and Bull, P. (2006). 'What features of the maternity unit promote obedient behaviour from midwives?' *Clinical Effectiveness in Nursing*, 952, pp. e221–e231.

Human Rights in Childbirth. Right to informed consent. Human Rights in Childbirth. [Online] (2018). Available at: http://humanrightsinchildbirth.org/index.php/2018/08/08/right-to-informed-consent/ [Accessed 2 February 2019].

International Childbirth Initiative [Online] (2018). Available at: https://www.internationalchildbirth.com/ [Accessed 23 Feburary. 2019].

Ip, W. Y. (2000). 'Relationships between partner's support during labour and maternal outcomes', *Journal of Clinical Nursing*, 9(2), pp. 265–272.

Jomeen, J. (2006). 'Choices for maternity care are they still "an illusion"?: A qualitative exploration of women's experiences in early pregnancy', *Clinical Effectiveness in Nursing*, 9(2), pp. e191–e200.

Jomeen, J. and Redshaw, M. (2013). 'Ethnic minority women's experience of maternity services in England', *Ethnicity & Health*, 18(3), pp. 280–296.

Kainz, G., Eliasson, M. and von Post, I. (2010). 'The child's father, an important person for the mother's wellbeing during the childbirth: A hermeneutic study', *Health Care for Women International*, 31, pp. 621–635.

Keogh, E., Hughes, S., Ellery, D., Daniel, C. D. and Holdcroft, A. (2006). 'Psychosocial influences on women's experience of planned elective cesarean section', *Psychosomatic Medicine*, 68, pp. 167–174.

Kukura, E. (2018). 'Obstetric violence', *Georgetown Law Journal*, 106(3), pp. 721–801.

Legare, F., Turcotte, S., Stacey, D., Ratte, S., Kryworuchko, J. and Graham, I. D. (2012). 'Patients' perceptions of sharing in decisions', *Patient*, 5(1), pp. 1–19.

Levy, V. (1999). 'Midwives, informed choice and power: Part 1', *British Journal of Midwifery*, 7(9), pp. 583–586.

Lothian, J. A. (2007). 'Listening to mothers II: knowledge, decision-making, and attendance at childbirth education classes', *Journal of Perinatal Education*, 16(4), pp. 62–67.

Macfarlane, A. J., Rocca-Ihenacho, L. and Turner, L. R. (2014). 'Survey of women's experiences of care in a new freestanding midwifery unit in an inner city area of London, England: 2. Specific aspects of care', *Midwifery*. Elsevier, 30(9), pp. 1009–1020. doi:10.1016/j.midw.2014.05.008

Malouf, R., Henderson, J. and Redshaw, M. (2017). 'Access and quality of maternity care for disabled women during pregnancy, birth and the postnatal period in England: Data from a national survey', *BMJ Open*, 7(7), pp. 1–12. doi:10.1136/bmjopen-2017-016757

McGrath, S. K. and Kennell, J. H. (2008). 'A randomized controlled trial of continuous labor support for middle-class couples: Effect on cesarean delivery rates', *Birth*, 35(2), pp. 92–97.

McRae, D. N. et al. (2018). 'Reduced prevalence of small-for-gestational-age and preterm birth for women of low socioeconomic position: A population-based cohort study comparing antenatal midwifery and physician models of care', *British Medical Journal – BMJ Open*, 8(e022220), pp. 1–11. doi:10.1136/bmjopen-2018-022220

Mivšek, P., Baškova, M. and Wilhelmova, R. (2016). 'Midwifery education in Central-Eastern Europe', *Midwifery*, 33, pp. 43–45.

Murray-Davis, B. et al. (2014). 'Deciding on home or hospital birth: Results of the Ontario choice of birthplace survey', *Midwifery*. Elsevier, 30(7), pp. 869–876. doi:10.1016/j.midw.2014.01.008

O'Connell, R. and Downe, S. (2009). 'A metasynthesis of midwives' experience of hospital practice in publicly funded settings: Compliance, resistance and authenticity', *Health: An Interdisciplinary Journal for the Social Study of Health, Illness and Medicine*, 13(6), pp. 589–609.

Osamor, P. and Grady, C. (2016). 'Women's autonomy in health care decision-making in developing countries: A synthesis of the literature', *International Journal of Women's Health*, 8, pp. 191–202.

Porter, S., Crozier, K., Sinclair, M. and Kernohan, W. G. (2007). 'New midwifery? A qualitative analysis of midwives' decision-making strategies', *Journal of Advanced Nursing*, 60(5), pp. 525–534.

Regan, M., McElroy, K. G. and Moore, K. (2013). 'Choice? Factors that influence women's decision making for childbirth', *The Journal of Perinatal Education*, 22(3), pp. 171–180. doi: 10.1891/1058-1243.22.3.171

Renfrew, M. J. et al. (2014). 'An executive summary for The Lancet series on midwifery': Midwifery is a vital solution to the challenges of providing high-quality maternal and newborn care for all women and newborn infants, in all countries', *Lancet*. June, pp. 1–8.

Shay, A., and Lafata, J. (2014). Where is the evidence? A systematic review of shared decision making and patient outcomes. *Medical Decision-Making*, 35(1), pp. 114–131.

Sigurdardottir, V. L. et al. (2019). 'Processing birth experiences: A content analysis of women's preferences', *Midwifery*, 69, pp. 29–38. doi:10.1016/j.midw.2018.10.016

Simpson, K. R., Newman, G. and Chirino, O. R. (2010). 'Patients' perspectives on the role of prepared childbirth education in decision making regarding elective labor induction', *Journal of Perinatal Education*, 19(3), pp. 21–32. doi:10.1624/105812410X514396

Sultana, Z. et al. (2017). 'Factors influencing decision-making in pregnancy and institutional delivery', *International Journal of Integrated Care*, 17(5), pp. 1–2.

Turner, B. (1987). *Medical Power and Social Knowledge*. London: Sage Publications.

Vedam, S. et al. (2017). 'The Mother's Autonomy in Decision Making (MADM) Scale: Patient-led development and psychometric testing of a new instrument to evaluate experience of maternity care', *PLoS One*, 12(2), pp. 1–17. doi:10.1371/journal.pone.0171804

Walsh, D. (2005). 'Professional power and maternity care: The many faces of paternalism', *British Journal of Midwifery*, 13(11), p. 708.

Woolhouse, S., Brown, J. and Lent, B. (2004). Women marginalized by poverty and violence: How patient-physician relationships can help. *Canadian Family Physician*, 50(10), pp. 1388–1394.

World Health Organisation. (2018). Recommendations: Intrapartum care for a positive childbirth experience. Geneva, Licence: CC BY-NC-SA 3.0 IGO.

21

THE DOULA-MIDWIFE PARTNERSHIP

Friend or foe – how to work collaboratively

*Elaine Jefford, Renee Adair, Tina Morrison
and Hannah Dahlen*

Chapter overview

The authors wish to acknowledge there is no intended criticism of our fellow midwives or doulas. As midwives, doulas, academics and researchers we do, however, have a responsibility to acknowledge that albeit potentially contentious, friend or foe, the doula-midwife partnership needs to be explored. This chapter explores the unique role a doula and a midwife play within a woman's childbearing journey and how the doula and midwife are educated to meet the needs of women, and the potential impact this can have on decision-making while providing safe and quality care. The similarities, differences, strengths and limitations between the two roles are highlighted and how, at times, this leads to tension.

Introduction

The term doula is a Greek word meaning 'women's servant helper' and is used to describe people (most are women) who are experienced in providing non-medical support (Campbell et al., 2007; Stevens et al., 2011). Doulas have been described in the literature as lay people who may or may not have received some form of training and remain with women to attend to their emotional and physical comfort needs during labour, birth and/or the immediate postnatal period (Bohren et al., 2017; Rosen, 2004). Historical literature informs us that the role of the doula emerged from women acting as handmaidens offering emotional support and companionship to childbearing women. After the 1970s the term doula was recognised internationally (Steel et al., 2015). Since that time, numerous doula organisations have been born across the globe giving rise to the many versions of doulas now seen worldwide. Recently there has been the rise of the 'Death Doula' role, who provides care and support to those who are dying, such as the Lifespan Doula Association (2017) and the Australian Doula College (2017); however this aspect of doula care is outside the scope of this chapter.

Midwifery and the doula

Within the maternity field, doulas may provide support to a woman and her family during one aspect of her childbearing journey, for example antenatal support, birth support or postnatal support, while some doulas provide care across the whole childbearing continuum or a combination of more than one aspect. Nevertheless a unified definition for the role of a doula is lacking, as each organisation, irrespective of whether it is a high-, middle- or low-income country, offers their unique interpretation of the doula role. Global consensus has been achieved for some areas, recognising that doulas offer physical and emotional support across the childbearing continuum. In other words, irrespective of the model of care a woman engages with, where midwives may be unable to provide a continuity of care model, the doula can provide a 'doula' model of continuity. Further, doulas provide women with information about care options, giving the opportunity for the woman to be the decision-maker. Although it is globally agreed, a doula will not undertake any medical or clinical task, the reality may be different, however, as there is increasing evidence that some doulas are now moving further into what can only be described as midwifery practice (Rigg et al., 2017, 2018). Compounding this is are four key elements: (1) the debate about what constitutes a clinical task and what does not; (2) the diverse doula philosophies around the globe; (3) the fact that doulas are not overseen by a professional, regulatory or legal body; and (4) the level and duration of doula training/education programs varies enormously. Ultimately, the decision-making between the doula and the woman will be impacted upon, by these key elements either collectively or singly. This will be discussed later in the chapter.

Philosophy of care and impact upon decision-making

Doula

There is a diversity in the doula philosophy. It appears to be a continuum. At one end is the 'woman driven philosophy'; at the other end is the 'doula driven philosophy'. For example, Doulas NorthWest USA (2018) has a 'no birth philosophy or definition or belief system', believing each doula enters every relationship as a blank slate upon which individual woman write their own theories and priorities to guide the doula-woman interactions. A 'doula driven philosophy' focuses on a doula's personal maturity, knowledge and unique view of pregnancy, birth and motherhood (Doula UK, 2018), thus philosophically placing the doula 'front and centre' of the doula-woman relationship (Childbirth International, 2018). A concern with this latter philosophical attitude is the similarity to a patriarchy (in this case, matriarchal) hierarchical structure that fosters a power imbalance. The doula becomes a gatekeeper, based on her own philosophical position. Within this gatekeeper role, the doula may filter what information is presented to the woman or bias the way in the information is present, as many health professional are accused of doing. Consequently, such a gatekeeping role can influence the woman's ability to be an informed decision-maker within her own childbearing journey. Reassuringly, the majority of philosophies offered by doula organisations around the world, however, sit within the middle of the philosophical continuum. At this midpoint, the main objective appears to be focus on empowering women across the childbearing continuum (Australian Doula College, 2017; New Beginnings Childbirth Services, 2011–2018, DONA International, 2018). Within an empowering relationship the doula and woman can foster a climate of reciprocity where ideas, needs and values are exchanged and appropriate information can be given or other resources accessed, thus ensuring the woman is able to make an informed decision. Further, such a doula philosophy within a doula model of continuity can assist with the transition into parenting positively, confidently and emotionally intact (Everson et al., 2018; Lucas and Wright, 2019).

Midwifery

The International Confederation of Midwives (ICM) midwifery philosophy (International Confederation of Midwives, 2014a) was developed by midwives to be used globally. It is recognised by its 132 midwifery associations across 113 countries representing approximately 500,000 midwives. Emancipation of women and fostering women's self-confidence to trust their body's ability to give birth are the foundational blocks upon which midwifery care is enacted, within a partnership relationship with women. Embedded in this is a woman's right to self-determination as well as respectful, personalised, continuous and non-authoritarian care (International Confederation of Midwives, 2014a, 2017, 2018b). These latter elements of midwifery align with some of the key, globally agreed upon elements within the doula philosophies (DONA International, 2018). For example the concept of a woman being emotionally intact post birth is also inherent in both doula and midwifery philosophy. This is particularly important today, as our awareness and knowledge around issues such as fear of childbirth (tokophobia) is developing. A contributing factor for women suffering tokophobia is if she believes she has experienced some form of physical or psychological trauma during any point of her childbearing journey (Streibich, 2018). Unfortunately such experiences and the resultant incidences of postnatal post-traumatic symptom disorder appears to be rising in the high-income world (Simpson et al., 2018) and multiple factors are cited as potential risk factors including obstetrical and childbirth-related complications (Dekel et al., 2018) as well as poor communication and lack of support in the postnatal period (Simpson et al., 2018). If communication is poor within a midwife-woman or doula-woman relationship, it will influence the woman's ability to be an informed decision-maker. Unfortunately, a midwife may hold a philosophical attitude similar to that of patriarchy, which fosters a power imbalance. If so, coupled with poor commination skills, this will inevitably influence the decision-making process and the woman's ability to make informed decisions.

It is imperative therefore, both the midwife and doula engage in empowering practices that optimise a woman's psychophysiological well-being. Midwives and doulas working collaboratively in such a way can create, for the woman, new and previously unconceived ways of interpreting her birthing experience. The term 'genius birth' has been applied to situations whereby a woman has an embodied sense of self, self-trust in her own ability to give birth. In other words 'genius birth' focuses on the intrinsic power during childbirth and is not dependent on the type of birth experienced (Parratt, 2010).

Regulation

The term 'midwifery profession' within this chapter is defined as a person who has undertaken a professional education program. A midwife practises the art and science of midwifery and is an accountable practitioner within the professional standards as set by their regulatory and professional body as well as within the legal system (International Confederation of Midwives, 2013, 2014b, 2017, 2018b; Nursing and Midwifery Board of Australia, 2018a, 2018b). In conjunction with this form of accountability, the midwife also has to navigate the increasing level of accountability to organisational policy and procedures. Consequently, increasing a midwife's activity and focus towards the organisation, thus reducing the emotional work of being a midwife and being with woman (Hunter, 2005, 2010; Rigg et al., 2017).

The concept of midwifery professional accountability should not be seen as irrelevant despite this contested space between meeting the needs of the woman and those of the organisation. Professional accountability is in place to protect women by ensuring midwives have appropriate knowledge and skills for justifiable, safe and effective practice (Australian Nursing and Midwifery Accreditation Council, 2014; International Confederation of Midwives, 2014b, 2017, 2018b; Nursing and Midwifery Board of Australia, 2018a, 2018b). In other words, a midwife is required to demonstrate accountability to the woman, regulatory and legal bodies, employer, profession and themselves. This accountability is not flexible and multiple measures exist to ensure compliance. Ultimately a midwife's accountability is intrinsically linked with a midwife's professional identity. Such accountability does not apply to doulas who at this time remain unregulated.

There has been an emergence in recent years of unregulated birth workers (UBWs) in countries such as Australia, Canada and the United States, and many of these are doulas or were previously registered midwives (Rigg et al., 2019). In several states within Australia, some UBWs attend home births without the presence of qualified professional such as a midwife or doctor. The reason offered is these UBWs in Australia and other countries are filling a national and international gap that has been created by lack of support for home birth, privately practising midwives and continuity of midwifery care models in some countries (Rigg et al., 2015, 2016, 2017, 2018, 2019). This expansion of the doula role into that of birth worker is concerning for two reasons. First, it indicates midwives are not always able to provide the care women are seeking; and second, it is leading to doulas extending their reach into the domain of midwifery and incorporating the clinical skills a midwife is trained to use into their practice.

The first comprehensive mixed methods study into this issue in Australia has just concluded and was led by Elizabeth Rigg and others (2018). An analysis of submissions made to the South Australian Government on a Proposal to Protect Midwifery Practice was conducted when the legislation was first proposed (Rigg et al., 2015). This legislation was introduced after a high-profile coroner's case involving an unregistered midwife in South Australia who was involved in several home births where babies had died. The legislation, which has now been introduced, proposed that only a midwife, student midwife or medical practitioner could take care of a woman by managing the three stages of labour or any part of a stage of labour or provision of health services. Thirty-two submissions were received when a call for public consultation on the proposed legislation was issued. Twenty-five (75%) supported the legislation, five (16%) opposed it and two (6%) were neither for nor against the legislation. Several themes and subthemes were identified as related to one overarching theme titled 'not addressing the root cause'. This theme suggested that respondents believed the proposed legislation did not address the underlying issues that lead women to choose an UBW to attend their birth at home without a midwife. Themes included 'legislative barriers', 'regulatory barriers', 'health system barriers', 'iatrogenic trauma', 'unintended consequences' and 'unclear boundaries'. All of these themes were identified as factors that led women to freebirth with or without UBWs.

Ongoing work from this study has shown that many UBWs are doulas, lay midwives and ex-registered midwives. Women who engage UBWs see them as providing the best of both worlds – that is, birthing at home with a knowledgeable person unconstrained by rules or regulations and who respects and supports the woman's philosophical view of birth. Women perceive UBWs as not only the best opportunity to achieve a natural birth but also as providing 'a safety net' in case of emergencies. When asked what UBWs actually do, many of the skills they carry out are clinical skills which are akin to those carried out by registered midwives (Rigg et al., 2018). Even though UBWs are adamant they are not undertaking midwifery and often rename the clinical skills they are carrying out, it is also clear that the women they care for see them as providing 'true midwifery' and see them very much as midwives but as not aligned to the system but to the woman (Rigg et al., 2018). It could therefore be reasoned such a definition can be applied to other high, middle and low income countries. Fundamentally, however, missing in the current global doula landscape is regulation. The same sort of issues applies to midwifery. In some parts of the world, nurses or Skilled Birth Assistants (SBA) or Traditional Birth Attendants (TBA) may undertake some form of obstetric training ranging from as little as three months, yet identify as midwives.

A symptom of the unregulated doula industry is the lack of agreed national and international guiding documents. This disparity manifests in the practice variations according to individual doulas and/or organisation and thus a doula's scope of practice. When reviewing the doula's scope of practice literature, the majority of organisations appear to focus on limitation of practice rather than scope of practice. For example, the doula does not diagnose or treat, speak on behalf of the woman or perform clinical or medical tasks or alternative/complementary therapies irrespective of previous qualification (Australian Doula College, 2017; DONA International, 2018; International Doula Institute, 2018). However, as stated earlier, this is happening in many parts of Australia and the United States (Rigg et al., 2017, 2018, 2019). In Russia, with the oppressive medicalised approach, doulas have become the new supporters for an underground movement of supported home birth. Where midwifery is oppressed and birth medicalised and women not given choice of care provider and place of birth or choice to have or decline medical intervention, we see doulas increasingly filling the gap (Dahlen et al., 2011; Stevens et al., 2011). Nevertheless, as unregulated workers, doula organisations as well as individual doulas work without boundaries. Such practice is compounded by the fact that, not all doula organisations have a code of conduct, competency standards and/or a code of ethics (Australian Council of Professions, 2018; DONA International, 2018; New Beginnings Childbirth Services, 2011–2018), therefore rendering accountability redundant. On the other hand, caution is needed against the over-regulation of doulas as one of the unique roles they play is being able to be truly woman centred with no other obligations or accountability. The employing of doulas by hospitals in the United States, for example, could be also seen as a way to moderate their role and have them enact the wishes of the institution and not women. A tension exists in regulation between protecting the public and constraining women's right to choice.

Embedded within professional regulation and accountability is the role of advocacy. Advocacy, however, is contentious and multifaceted, especially when linked with doulas, midwives and the midwifery profession. The ICM Code of Ethics for Midwives (2018b) stipulate 'midwives empower women/families to speak for themselves on issues affecting the health of women and families within their culture/society' (p. 1). In other words, advocacy means, women's voices are heard within the field of midwifery (International Confederation of Midwives, 2017). It must be acknowledged, as previously mentioned, some midwives and some doulas, however, practice in an authoritarian manner, thus disempowering women (Rigg et al., 2017).

Advocacy and decision-making

Advocacy appears to be one of the most contested roles within the doula landscape. There appears to be two fractions: first, 'supports the woman to voice her own intentions', thus ensuring the woman's voice is heard. The second faction sees doulas choosing to interpret advocacy as 'speaking for the woman'. The doulas who speak 'for the woman' interpret the woman's desires and speak directly to the care provider upon the woman's behalf (Meadow, 2014). This latter perspective provides the opportunity for the doula to be 'front and centre', introducing her own biases and removing focus from the intended woman-centred care

(Childbirth International, 2018). It would be naïve to believe some midwives do not practice or interpret advocacy in the same way. In other words, in a woman's individual childbirthing journey the 'locus of control' shifts from the woman to the doula or midwife, which means women may feel they have no control about the decisions that are being made or over events happening to them. Nevertheless, this patriarchal (matriarchal) approach is juxtaposed to the midwifery philosophy where the woman is the final decision-maker. The 'locus of control' within the midwifery philosophy sits firmly with the woman and the role of the midwife is to facilitate this by entering a partnership relationship where power is shared and decisions are negotiated from a stance of women being fully informed of the potential benefits and risks each decision, action or non-action. As midwives, doulas, academics and researchers who support a woman's voice to be heard, the authors question: how can a doula or midwife claim to be providing woman-centred care if the loudest voice is the doula/midwife and the woman's voice is not heard? Rather this method of care renders the woman silent.

To guide a midwife in enacting shared decision-making is their accountability that is set within a regulatory, professional and legal framework (International Confederation of Midwives, 2013, 2014b, 2017, 2018b, Nursing and Midwifery Board of Australia, 2018a, 2018b). A doula, as an unregulated worker, is not accountable within any professional standards or any regulatory or professional body, and as such has no boundaries on the role of being an advocate or the information or subsequent decisions she/he makes on behalf of the woman. Consequently, this may result in unconscious or conscious territorial behaviour between individual doulas, as well as a doula and the midwife, with the woman at the centre of the conflict (McLeish and Redshaw, 2018).

All these concepts are discussed further in the first section of this book, Chapters 2, 3, 4 and 6.

Education and training

Doula

Boundaries become further muddied within the doula arena with the enormous disparity around education or training. The global doula training landscape varies vastly on whether a trainee is required to undertake supervised practice which includes attendance at birth. For example, USA Doula Training International (DONA, 2018) require three supervised births and 16 hours of post-partum support for two families. The training organisation Australian Doulas College (Australian Doula College, 2017) require three supervised births. The National Childbirth Trust (UK) (2018) has no requirements. In other words any person may call themselves a doula and charge a fee for service irrespective of undertaking any specific training. In some organisations this is limited to care within the birth or the postnatal period, whilst some other organisations cover the entire childbearing journey. Whilst some doulas having undertaken some level of unaccredited training, their training organisation does not require any further development activities or recertification (Childbirth International, 2018). It is worth noting although there is no requirement for recertification, the Australian Doula College (2017) is the only global provider offering a nationally accredited doula qualification. This global disparity may be a symptom of an unregulated workforce.

Midwifery

Midwives, as part of a regulated profession, must achieve a specific level of midwifery education and practice. The ICM have set global standards for midwifery education (2013) and the essential competencies of basic midwifery practice (2018a). These documents provide the minimum standards and competencies a person must achieve before being able to call herself a midwife anywhere in the world. Although these provide basic foundations for midwifery educational programs around the world, individual countries are able to and many have, set additional standards and competencies a person must achieve before being entitled to call themselves a midwife. In order to protect the public a midwife's scope of practice is limited by the level of education attained. The ICM definition of a midwife (2017) offers a scope of practice that covers the whole of the childbearing journey and is applicable globally, irrespective of whether the midwife practices in a high-, middle- or low-income country or the model of care provision. Midwifery education and practice is further supported through the professional/regulatory standards and codes of practice and ethics relevant to that country (see Chapter 2). Additionally, regulatory bodies in some countries, require midwives to undertake regular professional development and/or recertification.

Consequently, we suggest, the term 'professional' and doula are separate entities, and should remain so until the issues of regulation, accountability and level of training are rectified in order to ensure and promote safe, quality care (please refer to Chapter 2).

Continuity of care

Recent research has shown a key element that increases women's satisfaction during childbirth is midwife-led continuity of care (Sandall et al., 2015; World Health Organization, 2018). Further, such research, shows that midwifery-led continuity of care also increases spontaneous vaginal births, increases satisfaction, reduces medical intervention and the likelihood of experiencing preterm labour. There is some evidence midwifery-led continuity of care can also be protective when women are in stressful situations or socially disadvantaged (Simock et al., 2018; Vedam et al., 2019, McRae et al., 2018). Simpson et al. (2018) have taken this further, showing PTSD may be modified in continuity of care relationships. Yet there is no research to date directly linking midwifery – led care explicitly with the term tokophobia. Rather, it is implicit in that the benefits of physical, emotional and social support for women by a midwife or a doula, can enhance their belief in their ability to birth, can result in empowering effects on a woman's psychological experience of physiological childbirth (Lucas and Wright, 2019; Sandall et al., 2015; World Health Organization, 2018).

Whilst a doula cannot lead care, there is research linking their continuous presence with reducing intervention and increasing maternal satisfaction (Spiby et al., 2016; Lucas and

TABLE 21.1 The educational differences between a doula and midwife

Registered Midwife	Doula
Full and part-time options available	
Current registration as RN or specific educational attainment	No prerequisite
Educational program accredited by regulatory body	Untrained
Undergraduate/postgraduate	Face to face classes – 2 days to 9 months
1 to 4 years	Online – 2 months to no time limit
Supervised MW practice experiences including COC in varied environments	Certificate IV Doula support services – (1,143 hours of which 743 supervised) including 3 births

Wright, 2019). The key thread in both doula and midwifery care is that of a 'known person/ carer', including a 'known student midwife' (Jefford et al., 2018) whereby a relationship can develop. Midwife-led continuity of care is embedded in all Australian undergraduate midwifery students who experience woman-centred care as part of continuity of care with their accredited programs (Australian Nursing and Midwifery Accreditation Council, 2014). It is acknowledged, not every midwifery student around the globe is trained in this model of care. Nevertheless there is a global shift towards offering midwifery-led continuity models of care (World Health Organization, 2018)

A tension for midwives, however, is their inability to work within such a partnership ethos when a large proportion of care offered to women occurs in a medicalised fragmented model (Steel et al., 2015). A woman may meet a midwife for the first time, just before birth. This places the woman and the midwife in a vulnerable position whilst they struggle to navigate the contested space between partnership and the unfamiliar. For example, in a patriarchal medical fragmented model of care where a woman is classified as high risk, midwifery care may or may not be less woman-centred and more task-orientated. The midwife wants to fulfil the ethos of midwifery and be 'with woman', yet is compelled to meet the demands of organisational policies and procedures to ensure safe care for such categorised woman: thus herein lies the disconnect midwives suffer. We acknowledge this disconnect is not limited to women deemed high risk, rather the medical model views all birth as pathological (Willis, 1989). Organisational policies and procedures compound this by supporting the increasingly risk-averse culture and thus driving medical intervention in childbirth. This practice censors the enactment of the midwifery philosophy and the midwives' role as guardians of normal, thus stifling the development of the midwife-woman relationship and has the potential to result in unmet needs for women as well as the midwife.

It needs to be acknowledged that a doula may provide the answer to bridging this contested space by being a continuous support for the woman during her childbearing journey (Dahlen et al., 2011; International Doula Institute, 2018). In such cases the doula fills the void by providing emotional support and connecting with the woman, her intrinsic power and embodied sense of self (Parratt, 2010). In other words, the doula is fulfilling their globally agreed philosophy of providing emotional support within a continuous care framework. Yet some midwives may see such actions as adding to their frustration. This may be because the doula's focus is purely on the woman, unlike the midwife who is required to focus on both the woman and the art and science behind each clinical task. This may result in a doula's perception that a midwife is fostering unwanted medical intervention on the woman or even not being woman-centred. A doula offers an option to address this gap by being emotionally present and being 'with woman'. Some midwives may find this challenging and consider this as facilitating further disconnect between midwife and woman, but the reality is medicalised systems that do not place women at the heart have taken the midwifery role and curtailed its potential, and doulas are providing an important service in meeting women's needs (Stevens et al., 2011)

The impact of this territorial behaviour detracts from the belief both doulas and midwives hold, that pregnancy and birth is a physical, emotional and spiritual event in a woman's life has the potential to facilitate a transforming experience for a woman's and her partner. To do this, doulas and midwives need to acknowledge and respect each other's roles and work collaboratively to make a women feel empowered within their birthing experience no matter how that baby comes into the world. To do that, they need to place the woman at the centre of the partnership. The positive effects of a doula care via providing continuous, flexible support has been found effective, especially for marginalised, disadvantaged and medically underserved communities are well documented (Everson et al., 2018; Spiby et al., 2016). Medicaid coverage for doulas is being expanded in New York, where there is high mortality, in an attempt to decrease inequities among childbearing women as well as increasing access to healthcare services (Ferré-Sadurní, 2018). Once within the healthcare services, women need to know their doula and midwife will work together in a non-judgemental professional way, which facilitates her autonomy and builds her trust in herself to birth her baby. One way to do this is through decision-making. Each decision made within this tripartite relationship needs to be transparent so the demands of the birthing environment on all present and how this may or may not influence care provision, including emotional care are shared and understood. By doulas and midwives working collaboratively giving women their voice will facilitate shared decision-making. Through this transparent, shared decision-making, women can be made aware of care options that meet their individual needs, whilst remaining within the boundaries of providing safe and quality care.

Despite the politically contested space, the doula and midwife inhabit what is evident when systems do not meet women's needs in that they will look elsewhere to have these needs met. Doulas are a growing industry providing, in most cases, a much-needed service and providing compassionate relationship-based support in a world where midwives are struggling to fulfil their role of being woman-centred. The Cochrane review (Bohren et al., 2017) on continuous support for women during childbirth included 26 randomised controlled trials and provided data from 17 countries involving more than 15,000 women. Doulas were the most common provider of this support. There is little doubt the benefits for women are significant and include requiring less pain relief, having higher rates of spontaneous vaginal birth, fewer caesarean sections and shorter labours and greater satisfaction. Babies were also better off, with higher five-minute Apgar scores.

Conclusion

The doula-midwife-woman partnership can and should co-exist for the sake of women. There are mutual spaces they all inhabit. Each woman has different needs and different decisions to make, as each woman navigates her own birthing journey. This diversity requires different skills that both the midwife and the doula have that can contribute to meeting these needs. The boundaries that remain blurred, and in some cases are increasingly becoming more blurred, should not be a source of division between doulas and midwives. Rather, they should be a focus for unity where they collaborate and form coalitions to fight for woman-centred care, expansion of choice for all women and shared decision-making. On this, both doulas and midwives are philosophically united, and so they need to manifest this in practice and work together for the sake of women, their babies and families and ultimately the whole of society. Standardised education/training and regulation of doulas will help unite doulas around the globe, strengthening and legitimising their role within the maternity arena.

References

Australian Council of Professions. 2018. *Australian Council of Professions* [Online]. Online: Australian Council of Professions ACN 059 999 914. Deakin, Australian Capital Territory. Available: www.professions.com.au/ [Accessed 12 December 2018].

Australian Doula College. 2017. *Australian Doula College* [Online]. Online: Australian Doula College. Sydney. Available: http://australiandoulacollege.com.au/ [Accessed 12 December 2018].

Australian Nursing and Midwifery Accreditation Council. 2014. Midwife: Accreditation standards. Canberra: Australian Nursing and Midwifery Council.

Bohren, A., Hofmeyr, G., Sakala, C., Fukuzawa, R.K. & Cuthbert, A. 2017. Continuous support for women during childbirth (Review). 7. Cochrane Database of Systematic Reviews: Wiley & Sons Ltd.

Campbell, D., Scott, K.D., Klaus, M.H. & Falk, M. 2007. Female relatives or friends trained as labor doulas: Outcomes at 6 to 8 weeks postpartum. *Birth*, 34, 220–227.

Childbirth International. 2018. *Childbirth International: Training without boundaries* [Online]. Online: Childbirth International. Available: https://childbirthinternational.com/ [Accessed 12 December 2018].

Dahlen, H.G., Jackson, M. & Stevens, J. 2011. Homebirth, Freebirth and doulas: Casualty and consequences of a broken maternity system. *Women and Birth*, 24, 47–50.

Dekel, S., Steuebe, C. & Dishy, G. 2018. Childbirth induced posttraumatic stress syndrome: A systematic review of prevalence and risk factors. *Frontiers in Psychology*, 8.

DONA International. 2018. *DONA International* [Online]. Online: Dona International. Available: www.dona.org/ [Accessed 12 December 2018].

Doula UK. 2018. *Doula UK* [Online]. Online: Doula UK. Available: https://doula.org.uk/ [Accessed 12 December 2018].

Doulas Northwest. 2018. *Doulas Northwest* [Online]. Online: Doulas Northwest. Available: https://doulasnorthwest.com/ [Accessed 12 December 2018].

Everson, C., Cheyney, M. & Bovbjerg, V. 2018. Outcomes of care for 1,892 Doula-supported adolescent births in the United States: The DONA International Data project, 2000 to 2013. *The Journal of Perinatal Education*, 27, 135–147.

Ferré-Sadurní, L. 2018. New York to expand use of doulas to reduce childbirth deaths. *The New York Times*. April 22. https://www.nytimes.com/2018/04/22/nyregion/childbirth-death-doula-medicaid.html

Hunter, B. 2005. Emotion work and boundary maintenance in hospital-based midwifery. *Midwifery*, 21, 253–266.

Hunter, B. 2010. Mapping the emotional terrain of midwifery: What can we see and what lies ahead? *International Journal of Work Organisation and Emotion*, 3, 253–269.

International Confederation of Midwives. 2013. ICM Global standards for midwifery education 2010; amended 2013 Companion Guidelines. International Confederation of Midwives.

International Confederation of Midwives. 2014a. Philosophy and model of midwifery care. The Hague: International Confederation of Midwives.

International Confederation of Midwives. 2014b. Professional accountability of the midwife. Geneva: International Confederation of Midwives.

International Confederation of Midwives. 2017. *Definition of the midwife.* [Online]. Brisbane: International Confederation of Midwives. Available: www.internationalmidwives.org [Accessed 4 September 2015].

International Confederation of Midwives. 2018a. *Essential competencies for basic midwifery practice.* [Online]. International Confederation of Midwives. Available: www.internationalmidwives.org [Accessed 17 December 2018].

International Confederation of Midwives. 2018b. International code of ethics for midwives. The Netherlands: International Confederation of Midwives.

International Doula Institute. 2018. *International Doula Institute* [Online]. Online: International Doula Institute. Available: https://internationaldoulainstitute.com/ [Accessed 12 December 2018].

Jefford, E., Nolan, S., Sansone, H. & Provost, S. 2018. 'A match made in midwifery': Women's perceptions of student midwife partnerships. *Women & Birth.* 912, 1–6.

Lifespan Doula Association. 2017. *End of life doula training* [Online]. Online: Lifespan Doula Association. Available: www.lifespandoulas.com/end-of-life-doula-training/ [Accessed 12 December 2018].

Lucas, L. & Wright, E. 2019. Attitudes of physicians, midwives and nurses about doulas: A scoping review. *American Journal of Maternal Child Nursing*, 44, 33–39.

Mcleish, J. & Redshaw, M. 2018. A qualitative study of volunteer doulas working alongside midwives at births in England: Mothers' and doulas' experiences. *Midwifery*, 56, 53–60.

Mcrae, D., Janessen, P.A., Vedam, S., Mayhew, M., Mpofu, D., Teucher, U. & Muhajarine, N. 2018. Reduced prevalence of small-for-gestational-age and preterm birth for women of low socioeconomic position: A population-based cohort study comparing antenatal midwifery and physician models of care. *British Midwifery Journal Open*, e02222220.

Meadow, S. 2014. Defining the doula's role: Fostering relational autonomy. *Health Expectations*, 18, 3057–3068.

National Childbirth Trust. 2018. *National Childbirth Trust, 1st 1000 days, new parent support* [Online]. Online: National Childbirth Trust. Available: www.nct.org.uk/ [Accessed 12 December 2018].

New Beginnings Childbirth Services. 2011–2018. *New beginnings doula training* [Online]. Online: New Beginnings Childbirth Services. Duffy. Available: www.trainingdoulas.com/ [Accessed 12 December 2018].

Nursing and Midwifery Board of Australia. 2018a. Code of conduct for midwives. Canberra: Nursing and Midwifery Board of Australia.

Nursing and Midwifery Board of Australia. 2018b. Midwife standards for practice. Canberra: Nursing and Midwifery Board of Australia.

Parratt, J. 2010. *Feeling like a genius: Enhancing women's changing embodied self during first childbearing.* PhD Midwifery, Newcastle, NSW.

Rigg, C.E., Schmied, V., Peters, K. & Dahlen, H. 2015. Not addressing the root cause: An analysis of submissions to the South Australian Government on a Proposal to Protect Midwifery Practice. *Women and Birth*, 28, 121–128.

Rigg, C.E., Schmied, V., Peters, K. & Dahlen, H. 2016. Why do women choose an unregulated birth worker in Australia. *BMC Pregnancy and Childbirth, Open*, 1–14.

Rigg, C.E., Schmied, V., Peters, K. & Dahlen, H. 2017. The role, practices and training of unregulated birthworkers in Australia: A qualitative study. *Women and Birth*. 30, S1, pp. 1–47.

Rigg, C.E., Schmied, V., Peters, K. & Dahlen, H. 2018. A survey of women in Australia who choose the care of unregulated birthworkers for a birth at home. *Women and Birth* Nov 29, pii: S1871-5192.

Rigg, E., Schmeid, V., Peters, K. & Dahlen, H. 2019. The role, practice and training of unregulated birth workers in Australia: A mixed methods study. *Women & Birth*, 32(1), e77–e87.

Rosen, P. 2004. Supporting women in labor: Analysis of different types of caregivers. *Journal of Midwifery Women's Health*, 49, 24–31.

Sandall, J., Soltani, H., Gates, S., Shennan, A. & Devane, D. 2016. Midwife-led continuity models versus other models of care for childbearing women. Cochrane Database of Systematic Reviews, (4). Art. No.: CD004667. DOI: 10.1002/14651858.CD004667.pub5.

Simock, G., Laplante, D., Elgbeili, G., Kildea, S. & King, S. 2018. A trajectory analysis of childhood motor development following stress in pregnancy: The QF2011 flood study. *Developmental Psychobiology*, 60, 836–849.

Simpson, M., Schmeid, V., Dickson, C. & Dahlen, H. 2018. Postnatal post-traumatic stress: An integrative review. *Women and Birth*, 31, 367–379.

Spiby, H., Mcleish, J., Green, J. & Darwin, Z. 2016. 'The greatest feeling you get, knowing you have made a big difference': Survey findings on the motivation and experiences of trained volunteer doulas in England. *BMC Pregnancy & Childbirth*, 16, 289–295.

Steel, A., Frawley, J., Adams, J. & Diezel, H. 2015. Trained or professional doulas in the support and care of pregnant and birthing women: A critical integrative review. *Health and Social Care in the Community*, 23, 225–241.

Stevens, J., Dahlen, H. & Jackson, D. 2011. Midwives and doulas' perspectives of the role of the doula in Australia: A qualitative study. *Midwifery*, 27, 509–516.

Vedam, S., Stoll, K., Daphne, N., Mcrae, N., Korchinski, M., Valasquez, R., Wang, J., Patridge, S., Mcrae, L., Elwood Martin, R. & Jolicoeur, G. 2019. Patient-led decision making: Measuring autonomy and respect in Canadian maternity care. *Patient Education and Counseling*, 102 (3), 586–594.

Willis, E. 1989. *Medical dominance: The division of labour in Australian health care.* Sydney: Allen and Unwin.

World Health Organization (WHO). 2018. Recommendations: *Intrapartum care for a positive childbirth experience.* Geneva. Licence: CC BY-NC-SA 3.0 IGO.

22

COLLABORATIVE DECISION-MAKING IN MATERNITY CARE

Marianne Nieuwenhuijze and Jeroen van Dillen

Chapter overview

In this chapter, we describe the collaborative aspects of shared decision-making in maternity care. Both the woman and her midwife are often part of larger systems, in which mono- and multidisciplinary teams of professionals are working with the woman, her partner and/or her significant others around decisions in maternity care, to achieve the best treatment option for her situation and needs. We will explore the importance of a collaborative approach in shared decision-making, the current state of the art around this topic and the challenges involved in moving collaborative decision-making forward in different maternity care settings.

Introduction

Shared decision-making is increasingly accepted as the way to make health decisions in maternity care. Most literature presents shared decision-making as a dyadic process between a woman and her clinician (e.g. midwife or obstetrician) that includes a dialogue on trustworthy information, preferences and values to enable the woman to make a well-informed decision (Elwyn et al., 2017). However, both the woman and her care provider are part of larger systems which have significant influence on choices and decisions made during pregnancy, childbirth and the postnatal period.

Around the world, a pregnant woman will often involve her partner, family member or friend who will support her and influence the decisions she makes. Models of shared decision-making such as Elwyn et al. (2017; as noted in Chapter 1) recognise the importance of supporting others for the patient, in this case the woman, when making decisions. Irrespective of geographical location, a midwife and other care providers are also part of a larger healthcare system where they rely on each other to give a woman the best care for her situation. In practice, this can be organised in mono- or multidisciplinary teams offering shared care or in networks offering sequential care with one care provider referring a woman to another care provider for medical or other reasons.

Independent of the way this is organised, close collaboration between all care providers is necessary to provide a woman with continuity and best quality of maternity care. The implementation of decisions often requires a collaboration of different professionals working with the woman to achieve the best treatment option for her situation and needs. It brings together midwives and obstetricians/physicians, as well as other medical specialists such as a paediatrician/neonatologist, anaesthetist and genetic specialists. In the community setting, this collaboration is broadened with general practitioners or public health nurses, depending on the national or local organisation of maternity care. Other professionals, such as nutritionists, physiotherapists and psychologists, also take part in the care for certain women. This makes shared decision-making a process that often requires interprofessional collaboration between people with different professional backgrounds. Légaré et al. (2011a) defines an interprofessional approach to shared decision-making as

> an interprofessional team, including at least two professionals from different disciplines, identifying best options and facilitating the patient's involvement in decision-making using those options.
>
> *(p. 18)*

Importance of collaborative decision-making

For a woman, the time around childbirth is a dynamic period, where expected and unexpected events will influence the progress of pregnancy and childbirth. Outcomes such as a healthy baby and a woman's positive experience are both important for the short- and long-term well-being of the woman, her baby and her whole family (WHO, 2018). Good-quality services, continuity of care and women's involvement in decision-making play a crucial role in the care for women during the perinatal period to achieve these outcomes (Renfrew et al., 2014).

Downe et al. (2018) performed a systematic qualitative review of 35 studies to inform the WHO intrapartum guideline, with studies conducted in countries all over the world. They found that what matters to most women included giving birth to a healthy baby in a safe environment, with practical and emotional support from birth companions and competent, reassuring, kind staff. Most wanted a physiological labour and birth while acknowledging that birth can be unpredictable and frightening, and that they may need 'to go with the flow'. If intervention was needed or wanted, women wanted to retain a sense of personal achievement and control through active decision-making.

The Cochrane review on models of care for childbearing women (Sandall et al., 2016) found that women who received midwife-led continuity of care had more positive outcomes, including their experience of care. They were less likely to have interventions, such as intrapartum analgesia/anaesthesia, episiotomies or instrumental births. Women's chances of a spontaneous vaginal birth were increased and there was no difference in the number of caesarean births. Women were less likely to experience preterm birth, fetal loss or neonatal death. In addition, women were more often cared for in labour by midwives they already knew. The majority of studies reported a higher rate of maternal satisfaction in midwife-led continuity models of care. The review identified no adverse effects compared with other models. This review was based on 17,674 women at low risk of complications as well as women at increased risk, but not currently experiencing problems.

Although the *Lancet* midwifery series also indicates that midwife-led continuity of care models are the backbone for quality maternal and newborn care, medical obstetric and neonatal services are needed for women and infants with complications (Renfrew et al., 2014). Good collaboration between midwives and medical specialists in a well-organised system is therefore pivotal for quality of maternal and newborn services (Perdok et al., 2015).

Although the findings of the Cochrane review are based on midwife-led care systems in high-income countries, the study of Downe et al. with women from a range of ethnic backgrounds makes it evident that all maternity care needs to assure the possibility of a woman's active involvement in decision-making as well as the experience of continuity in her care. This implies also a collaborative approach to shared decision-making that is more than the agreement between different professionals. It implies a decision-making process that listens to the woman, integrates what matters to her in identifying the best option and makes sure that in implementing the decision there is consistency among all care providers involved in the care.

State of the art on collaborative decision-making

Attention for a collaborative approach to shared decision-making became visible in the literature about a decade ago. Légaré et al. (2008) introduced the term 'interprofessional approach of shared decision-making' in a study protocol on the development of a conceptual model for promoting this approach to shared decision-making.

A model for interprofessional shared decision-making

One of the results in the study by Légaré et al. (2011a) was an interprofessional shared decision-making (IP-SDM) model based on key concepts from shared decision-making and interprofessionalism. Although, the model focuses on the interprofessional context, we think that in mono-disciplinary teams similar issues need consideration to realise continuity of care for women in the shared decision-making process. Especially in larger mono-disciplinary teams, continuity of care is challenging with regard to continuity of care provider, as well as information continuity and management continuity (Perdok et al., 2015). Fontein (2010) found that women in practices with a maximum of two midwives had higher levels of a positive birth experience compared to women in practices with more than two midwives. The women cared for by a smaller team of midwives also had fewer intrapartum interventions. A questionnaire survey among 195 women after giving birth in the Netherlands suggested that experienced continuity of care depends on the care context and is significantly higher for women who are in midwife-led compared to obstetrician-led care during labour (Perdok et al., 2018). The authors stated that it will be challenging to maintain the high level of experienced continuity of care in an integrated maternity care system.

Figure 22.1 visualises the IP-SDM model, including the different actors, the decision-making process and the global context of the environment. This model was validated among stakeholders in primary care in Canada (Légaré et al., 2011b). For this validation process, a video vignette of a pregnant woman and her partner illustrated the model, using their decision-making process about prenatal screening for Down syndrome.

The *environment* is the global context in which the interprofessional shared decision-making process takes place. It includes social norms, organisational routines, government policies and national guidelines.

Actors are the different persons involved in the decision-making process. The patient is central in the decision-making, as symbolised in Figure 22.1. The initiator of the shared

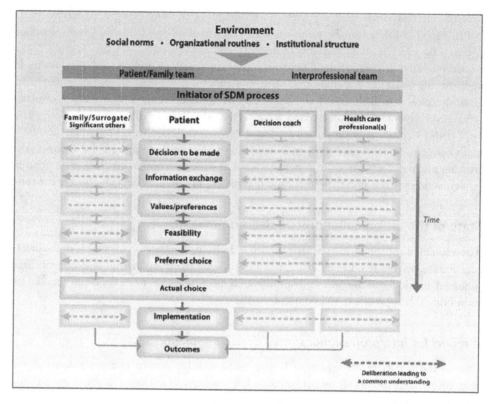

FIGURE 22.1   Interprofessional shared decision–making model (Légaré et al., 2011b)

decision-making process can be any healthcare professional who identifies the health situation and articulates that a decision needs to be made. This can also be the patient coming with a request for specific care. In addition, this model identifies a decision coach who is trained to support the patient's involvement in decision-making. The last column refers to healthcare providers collaborating with the patient either concurrently or sequentially. The family category (the first column) includes relatives, surrogates and/or other people who are important to the patient and can influence the decision-making process.

The *steps in the decision-making* can be found in the second column under the patient and start with the 'Decision to be made', making explicit that a choice needs to be made and inviting the patient to be actively involved and offering support throughout the process.

The aim of the IP-SDM model is to reach agreement among members of an interprofessional team that a decision point exists with one or more potential options, including the option to remain status quo. (A detailed explanation of the model is available at https:// decisionaid.ohri.ca/ip-sdm.html.)

Implementation of interprofessional shared decision-making within a maternity setting

The IP-SDM model offers insight into the process of interprofessional shared decision-making and limits ambiguity around the concepts and roles of actors involved in the process. However, the actual implementation of interprofessional shared decision-making still faces many challenges (Dogba et al., 2016; Dunn et al., 2018). Not every healthcare system can offer designated decision coaches, which means that the explanation of options with pros and cons is left with the healthcare provider. In the context of shortage of staff (midwives and doctors), especially in low resource settings, both time for explanation and for collaborative exchange can be a challenge. Another challenge confers to the coverage of antenatal care. The World Health Organization (WHO) recommends at least four antenatal care visits for all pregnant women. Almost half of pregnant women worldwide do not receive this amount of care (Mbuagbaw et al., 2015). In a study from Indonesia, for example, where a new model for antenatal care including involvement of women and their partners in their care was tested, perceived barriers for this model included financial difficulties, public transport limitations, staff shortage and lack of adequate resources and support from higher (health service) level (Widyawati, 2016).

Additionally, agreement within the interprofessional team on the treatments options offered in the decision-making process can be difficult to achieve. Clinicians built professional opinions about preferred options in care based on research literature, clinical experience, collaboration with other professionals, organisation of care, intuition and ideology, which may result in different views between professional backgrounds (Daemers et al., 2017). In addition, midwives may experience a power imbalance in which they feel less influential than obstetricians. In a study among 102 Dutch obstetricians investigating the curriculum for the doctor of the future, an increase in interprofessional teams was predicted in which the obstetrician was seen as the leader of such a team in maternity care (van der Lee et al., 2011). Furthermore, collaboration between different groups of healthcare professionals is often rooted in historical tensions, which, in addition to perceived power imbalance, can contribute to problems in current collaboration (van der Lee et al., 2014).

How to reach agreement in (inter)professional teams and the time necessary for exchange and debate are challenges to consider. Moral case deliberation can help in dealing with different views on complex issues. It is a collaborative meeting where a group of healthcare professionals jointly reflect on a concrete moral question or dilemma. Essentially, and in contrast to other kinds of (more informal) meetings, a moral case deliberation is structured by a conversation method and moderated by a facilitator, often an ethicist. During the deliberation, professionals have the opportunity to freely articulate and share their stories, experiences, opinions and perspectives. Moral case deliberation brings about changes in practice, mostly for the professional in interprofessional interactions such as feeling related to other professionals, understanding the perspectives of colleagues, and understanding one's own perspective (Haan et al., 2018).

Another issue is when to engage the woman or family in the collaborative shared decision-making process. This is not clearly indicated in the IP-SDM model, and therefore open to debate as articulated in the qualitative study of Dunn et al. (2018). In the context of providing quality maternity care services, meeting basic goals remains challenging in low-income countries. Women encounter many barriers in accessing maternity care (Kyei-Nimakoh et al., 2017). One can image that if basic services are already a challenge, shared decision-making certainly is. The new WHO recommendations for intrapartum care (2018) emphasise women's need for a positive childbirth experience, which should be implemented as a package of care in all settings through kind, competent and motivated healthcare professionals who work in accordance with a human rights-based approach (WHO, 2018).

In the study of Dunn et al. (2018), they explored interprofessional team members' perspectives about the nature of interprofessional shared decision-making in a neonatal intensive care unit (NICU). Participants were nurses, physicians, respiratory therapists and other health professions (pharmacist, occupational and physical therapist, dietician and social worker). All agreed that the process of interprofessional shared decision-making should lead to a well-informed decision and participants feeling valued.

The participants identified four key roles important to interprofessional shared decision-making: (1) a leader who facilitates shared decision-making; (2) a professional who provides information and insight into the case; (3) someone who synthesises and integrates the information together; (4) and the patient (or surrogate) acting as decision-maker. Participants from all groups agreed that interprofessional shared decision-making happens through a collaborative process of working together to identify the options, sharing the process and weighing the facts for a well-informed decision. The participants described consensus as the most common method for reaching a decision. However, consensus meant different things to different people, ranging from finding common ground through understanding to achieving full agreement within the team. In reaching consensus, some professional groups experienced the influence of differences in power position. Strategies to respond to positional power differentials were mentioned, such as (1) being present at meetings as well as being prepared and participating in the discussion with confidence; (2) tailoring the message to the listeners; (3) directing the message to the person who is accountable and in authority; (4) presenting a credible argument supported by evidence; and (5) being persistent.

Participants had mixed thoughts about the moment to involve parents in the decision-making process. Should the team discuss options first in order to present consistent, complete information and clearly articulate the decision to be made to the parents? Or should the parents be present from the beginning to integrate their input and preferences and offer full transparency?

An example of interprofessional shared decision-making within a maternity setting

Based on the IP-SDM model, we developed an example of the interprofessional decision-making process for a woman with a breech presentation at the end of pregnancy. This example is described in the Dutch maternity care context with an autonomous position of both midwives and obstetricians. Healthy women receive care in a midwifery practice and are referred to an obstetrician when complications arise. The reader is invited to internationally contextualise this example to their own clinical environment, acknowledging different forms of collaboration and autonomy in different setting.

BOX 22.1   INTERPROFESSIONAL SHARED DECISION-MAKING: A BREECH PRESENTATION AT THE END OF PREGNANCY

Environment

Shared decision-making is promoted as the norm, but is not yet fully accepted by all professionals. On a regional level, multidisciplinary discussions are ongoing, enhancing a positive attitude towards shared decision-making.

Most Dutch care providers in maternity care accept external version for breech presentation as a treatment option in uncomplicated pregnancy. National guidelines from midwifery and obstetric organisations recommend it as an option. There is general acceptance that a woman makes the actual choice in this situation.

Initiator of SDM process

Laura has had regular check-ups for her first pregnancy with a primary care practice of two midwives. She is now 35 weeks pregnant and everything has gone well. Her baby has been in breech presentation since 30 weeks, but a recent ultrasound did not show any abnormalities. She asks her midwife what consequences this will have for the birth.

Partner	Laura and her baby	Decision coach	Healthcare professionals
Laura is invited to bring her partner	**Decision needs to be made** Laura and her partner receive the information and understand the situation	Her midwife explains the situation and that several options are available	
Partner joins in with questions	**Information to exchange** Laura is asked to summarise the information ('teach back method') and is invited to ask questions	Her midwife describes the options with pros and cons; checks if everything is understood	
Partner is invited to join in	**Values/preferences** Laura tells what is important to her and indicates her preferences	Her midwife asks what is important to Laura	
	Feasibility Laura's questions around the conduct of the procedure are addressed	Midwife and obstetrician have collaborative organised the provision of external versions	
Partner is supportive towards Laura's choice	**Preferred choice** Laura indicates that she prefers a normal birth and would like to have an external version	Her midwife checks if Laura and her partner understand their choice	

Actual choice

After deliberation with her partner, Laura chooses an external version. The obstetrician is informed and agrees with the SDM process.

Implementation

An appointment for an external version is scheduled at the local hospital. In this hospital, an obstetrician and midwife will jointly perform the external version.

Outcomes

At 40 weeks, a healthy baby is born and Laura is very content with the way she and her partner were treated and involved in the decision-making process.

Challenges in interprofessional shared decision-making within a maternity setting

Additional challenges in interprofessional SDM arise when a woman has wishes concerning birthing outside the system (Hollander et al., 2016), for example a home birth in a high-risk pregnancy. In recent years, medical practice has been influenced by increasing amounts of evidence and protocols. Where the medical professional trusts the protocol, some women may choose differently. The motivations of women to choose high-risk birth options are resisting the biomedical model of birth by trusting intuition; challenging the dominant discourse on risk; perceiving birth as an intimate or religious experience; and taking responsibility as a reflection of true control over decision-making (Holten & de Miranda, 2016).

Most professional organisations and the WHO have created guidelines on how to handle situations of perceived maternal-fetal conflict (Hollander et al., 2016). In spite of guidelines, many professionals are still unsure how best to negotiate with women who declined their initial advice. Studying a designated outpatient clinic that aims to increase expertise and improve care for women who opt to birth outside the system revealed positive results. Using a respectful and systematic multidisciplinary approach, in which women feel heard and are invited to explain their motivations for their birth plans, resulted in a plan either within the guidelines or much closer to recommendations than the woman's initial intentions in the greater majority of cases (Van der Garde et al., 2019). In this study, if an agreement was reached on care outside the guidelines and this was deemed to present a challenge for the maternity care team, a moral case deliberation was organised (Haan et al., 2018).

Conclusion

Collaborative decision-making is a desirable approach to involve a woman in her care and enhance her sense of continuity of care when being cared for by different care providers. Good collaboration and communication are essential to achieve collaborative decision-making. However, the implementation involves many challenges. Promoting interprofessional collaboration and education, as well as building a mutual understanding and acceptance of shared decision-making, are the first steps to move this forward. An open dialogue – with curiosity and respect for each other's expertise, values and contribution – will enhance a shared understanding of the best choice for each pregnant woman individually. Essential is an environment that stimulates this as a norm and facilitates practical support, such as time and leadership.

References

Daemers, D.O.A., van Limbeek, E.B.M., Wijnen, H.A.A., Nieuwenhuijze, M.J. and de Vries, R.G. (2017). Factors influencing the clinical decision-making of midwives: A qualitative study. *BMC Pregnancy Childbirth* 17(1), p. 345.

Dogba, M.J., Menear, M., Stacey, D., Briere, N. and Légaré, F. (2016). The evolution of an interprofessional shared decision-making research program: Reflective case study of an emerging paradigm. *International Journal of Integrated Care* 16(3), pp. 1–11.

Downe, S., Finlayson, K., Oladapo, O., Bonet, M. and Gülmezoglu, A.M. (2018). What matters to women during childbirth: A systematic qualitative review. *PLoS One* 13(4), p. e0194906.

Dunn, S.I., Cragg, B., Graham, I.D., Medves, J. and Gaboury, I. (2018). Roles, processes, and outcomes of interprofessional shared decision-making in a neonatal intensive care unit: A qualitative study. *Journal of Interprofessional Care* 32(3), pp. 284–294.

Elwyn, G., Durand, M.A., Song, J., Aarts, J., Barr, P.J., Berger, Z., Cochran, N., Frosch, D., Galasiński, D., Gulbrandsen, P., Han, P.K.J., Härter, M., Kinnersley, P., Lloyd, A., Mishra, M., Perestelo-Perez, L., Scholl, I., Tomori, K., Trevena, L., Witteman, H.O. and van der Weijden, T. (2017). A three-talk model for shared decision making: Multistage consultation process. *BMJ* 359, pp. 1–7.

Fontein, Y. (2010). The comparison of birth outcomes and birth experiences of low-risk women in different sized midwifery practices in the Netherlands. *Women Birth* 23(3), pp. 103–110.

Haan, M.M., van Gurp, J.L.P., Naber, S.M. and Groenewoud, A.S. (2018). Impact of moral case deliberation in healthcare settings: A literature review. *BMC Medical Ethics* 19(1), p. 85.

Hollander, M., van Dillen, J., Lagro-Janssen, A., van Leeuwen, E., Duijst, W. and Vandenbussche, F. (2016). Women refusing standard obstetric care: Maternal-fetal conflict or doctor-patient conflict? Legal and ethical considerations. *Journal of Pregnancy and Child Health* 3(2), pp. 1–4.

Holten, L. and de Miranda, E. (2016). Women's motivations for having unassisted childbirth or high risk homebirth: An exploration of the literature on 'birthing outside the system'. *Midwifery* 38, pp. 55–62.

Kyei-Nimakoh, M., Carolan-Olah, M. and McCann, T.V. (2017). Access barriers to obstetric care at health facilities in sub-Saharan Africa-a systematic review. *Systematic Reviews* 6(1), p. 110. doi:10.1186/s13643-017-0503-x.

Légaré, F., Stacey, D., Gagnon, S., Dunn, S., Pluye, P., Frosch, D., Kryworuchko, J., Elwyn, G., Gagnon, M.P. and Graham, I.D. (2011b). Validating a conceptual model for an inter-professional approach to shared decision making: A mixed methods study. *Journal of Evaluation in Clinical Practice* 17(4), pp. 554–564.

Légaré, F., Stacey, D., Graham, I.D., Elwyn, G., Pluye, P., Gagnon M.P., Frosch, D., Harrison M.B., Kryworuchko, J., Pouliot, S. and Desroches, S. (2008). Advancing theories, models and measurement for an interprofessional approach to shared decision making in primary care: A study protocol. *BMC Health Services Research* 8(1), p. 2.

Légaré, F., Stacey, D., Pouliot, S., Gauvin, F.P., Desroches, S., Kryworuchko, J., Dunn, S., Elwyn, G., Frosch, D., Gagnon, M.P., Harrison, M.B., Pluye, P. and Graham, I.D. (2011a). Interprofessionalism and shared decision-making in primary care: A stepwise approach towards a new model. *Journal of Interprofessional Care* 25(1), pp. 18–25.

Mbuagbaw, L., Medley, N., Darzi, A.J., Richardson, M., Habiba Garga, K. and Ongolo-Zogo, P. (2015). Health system and community level interventions for improving antenatal care coverage and health outcomes. *Cochrane Database Systematic Reviews* Issue 12. Art. No.: CD010994.

Perdok, H., Jans, S., Verhoeven, C., van Dillen, J., Mol, B.W. and de Jonge, A. (2015). Intrapartum referral from primary to secondary care in the Netherlands: A retrospective cohort study on management of labor and outcomes. *Birth* 42(2), pp. 156–164.

Perdok, H., Verhoeven, C.J., van Dillen, J., Schuitmaker, T.J., Hoogendoorn, K., Colli, J., Schellevis, F.G. and de Jonge, A. (2018). Continuity of care is an important and distinct aspect of childbirth experience: Findings of a survey evaluating experienced continuity of care, experienced quality of care and women's perception of labor. *BMC Pregnancy Childbirth* 18(13), pp. 1–9.

Renfrew, M.J., McFadden, A., Bastos, M.H., Campbell, J., Channon, A.A., Cheung, N.F., Silva, D.R., Downe, S., Kennedy, H.P., Malata, A., McCormick, F., Wick, L. and Declercq, E. (2014). Midwifery and quality care: Findings from a new evidence-informed framework for maternal and newborn care. *Lancet* 384(9948), pp. 1129–1145.

Sandall, J., Soltani, H., Gates, S., Shennan, A. and Devane, D. (2016). Midwife-led continuity models versus other models of care for childbearing women. *Cochrane Database of Systematic Reviews* Issue 4. Art. No.: CD004667.

Van der Garde, M., Hollander, M., Olthuis, G., Vandenbussche, F. and van Dillen, J. (2019). Women desiring less care than recommended during childbirth: Three years dedicated clinic. *Birth*, doi:10.1111/birt.12419

Van der Lee, N., Driessen, E. W., Houwaart, E. S., Caccia, N. C. and Scheele, F. (2014). An examination of the historical context of interprofessional collaboration in Dutch obstetrical care. *Journal of Interprofessional Care* 28(2), pp. 123–127.

Van der Lee, N., Westerman, M., Fokkema, J. P., van der Vleuten, C. P., Scherpbier, A. J. and Scheele, F. (2011). The curriculum for the doctor of the future: Messages from the clinician's perspective. *Medical Teacher* 33(7), pp. 555–561.

Widyawati. (2016). The four pillar approach: A new model for iron deficiency anaemia management during pregnancy. Doctoral thesis. Nijmegen NL, Radboud University Nijmegen. https://repository.ubn.ru.nl/bitstream/handle/2066/155828/155828.pdf?sequence=1

World Health Organization (WHO). (2018). *Recommendations: Intrapartum care for a positive childbirth experience.* Geneva. Licence: CC BY-NC-SA 3.0 IGO.

23

DO PERSONALITY TRAITS IMPACT UPON MIDWIVES' DECISION-MAKING AND PRACTICE?

Steve Provost, Anna Smyth, Thejal Rupnarain,
Shahna Mailey, Harvey Ward and Elaine Jefford

Chapter overview

In this chapter, we will draw on empirical research exploring whether certain personality characteristics moderates the quality of clinical decision-making made by midwives and if that influences their midwifery practice. Our research suggests that irrespective of where in the world a midwife is located or in which model of care she works, further examination of the role played by temperamental characteristics of midwives may help them to identify and reflect on the factors influencing their decisions and practice. When identified and reflected upon, a midwife will be better placed to assist women in the collaborative process of childbirth.

Introduction

Little is known about the role of temperament and personality in clinical decision-making. There is some evidence that personality has an influence on medical students decisions with respect to their residency choices (Taber, Hartung, & Borges, 2011) or area of specialisation (Borges & Gibson, 2005; Markert et al., 2008). However, there is little evidence that personality traits described by these measures impact on every-day decisions made in clinical practice. Recent research suggestions that characteristics such as sensitivity to risk and social responsiveness might affect the advice given to patients in oncology and other practices (Batteux, Ferguson, & Tunney, 2017). As a result of these findings, it encourages the view that these factors could play a role in decision-making in midwifery practice.

A number of 'discounting' tasks (delay, probability and social discounting) have been developed as measures of these factors (Madden & Bickel, 2010; McKerchar & Renda, 2012; Osiński, Karbowski, & Ostaszewski, 2015). Measures of temperament that are based on sound biological principles, such as Gray's description of the Behavioural Activation and Behavioural Inhibition Systems (BIS/BAS) (Gray, 1981, 1982) also have the potential to play a role in decision-making. This is because they relate directly to the impact of outcomes (reward and punishment) on behaviour. Yet, there is limited application of these measures within the discipline of midwifery and more specifically related to midwives clinical decision-making.

We sought to examine whether discounting and sensitivity to punishment and reward (the BIS/BAS) moderated the quality of midwives clinical reasoning and subsequent practice. We used a number of brief vignettes derived from a study involving clinical midwives undertaken by Jefford (2012) to ask what clinical reasoning and midwifery practice was exhibited by their peers within each vignette. The midwives who took part in our study were an extremely diverse group. Qualifications ranged from hospital certificates through to PhDs, and all midwives were currently practising across all models of midwifery care, with the majority having worked in more than one model. Duration of time since qualifying as a midwife was between six months and 45 years. The sample were geographically located within metropolitan, regional and rural areas around Australia.

Personality and clinical decision-making

> Personality is defined in the Penguin Dictionary of Psychology (Reber, Allen & Reber, 2009) as the 'Behavioural, emotional, and mental characteristics of an individual that produce consistent patterns of thought, feeling and behaviour (personality, 2009).

It seems reasonable to suppose that these characteristics will influence clinical decision-making in health professionals, including midwives. In 2005, Harris (2005) explored if UK midwife characteristics influenced the care they provided during third stage of labour. She found participating midwives employed complex decision-making processes in order to tailor third stage of labour care to the needs of individual women. Further, each midwife's differing values and beliefs did impact on midwives' care provision. A more recent study (Hadjigeorgiou & Coxon, 2014) explored behaviour of Cypriot midwives. The findings indicate the participating midwives assumed a passive role in order to avoid situations where conflict was anticipated or observed. What these two studies show is that midwives decision-making is affected by individual perceptions, values, and beliefs. Proactive behaviour and midwifery abdication as noted in Chapters 24 and 6 may or may not further influence midwives decision-making. Nevertheless, any application of conventional trait personality inventories, discounting or BIS/BAS is lacking. To date, this link has not been explored in a midwifery setting, and our research is an attempt to fill this gap.

Discounting

The study of discounting began by examining the effect of introducing a delay in the presentation of reward (Madden & Bickel, 2010). It was found that animals (including humans) are very sensitive to delay, and that a small immediate reward is much more potent than a far larger reward delivered after a delay. This phenomenon has been studied extensively in humans utilising what has become known as the 'delay discounting' task (Madden & Bickel, 2010; McKerchar & Renda, 2012). In this task the participant is asked a series of questions taking the form 'would you prefer $x now or $y in z months?' When asked whether they would prefer $10 now or $1,000 in six months, most people would prefer to wait for the larger amount in six months' time. The same might be true if offered $100 now. However as the amount of money offered increases, for example to $500, some people may switch their preference to taking the money now. The point at which a participant will switch their preference to the immediate reward. This is known as the 'point of indifference'. This is the point at which the amount of money on offer now is equal to the value of the larger reward after a delay. In other words, it is the perceived *value* of the delayed reward. If one is asked a series of such questions for different delays in time the point of indifference can be found for each of these times, and if these are graphed you will obtain something like that shown in Figure 23.1, which is a delay discounting function. It illustrates the fact that the value of a sum of money declines sharply (is discounted) as a function of time.

The fact that behaviour appears to be controlled to a greater degree by small immediate rewards rather than longer-term benefits should probably come as no surprise. What is more surprising, perhaps, is the rate at which a person discounts a reward against time, the steepness of the slope, appears to be quite strongly related to the likelihood that the person exhibits behavioural problems related to impulsivity, such as problem gambling and substance abuse (Madden & Bickel, 2010). In terms of midwifery, this offers a way of understanding the role played by delay discounting in a midwife's decision-making processes and how she enacts/reacts to an individual woman. Through this understanding, it may therefore ultimately help a midwife to be better equipped to support the decision-making processes of women in their care as well as their own decision-making. For example, Yoon et al. (2007) found that the level of delay discounting exhibited by pregnant women who disclosed to be smokers at their first antenatal visit predicted the likelihood that they would remain abstinent at 24 months postpartum. Assessing a woman's level of impulsiveness with this simple delay discounting task thus has the potential to identify those women who would be most at risk of relapse, and who may therefore benefit from increased levels of support. This would be particularly critical in communities where levels of smoking are higher and social support for abstinence may be weaker.

A second form of discounting, known as 'probability discounting', has been explored as a possible measure of sensitivity to risk (McKerchar & Renda, 2012). The probability discounting task is effectively very similar to delay discounting, but instead of the choices being framed in terms of the delay to a reward, they are framed in terms of the probability of success. Thus, participants may be asked whether they would prefer to receive $100 for certain, or have a 90% probability of receiving $1,000, and so on. A discounting function can thus be obtained showing how the risk of loss influences the value attached to a sum of money. Although this function is similar to that of delay discounting, its interpretation in terms of optimal behaviour is somewhat different. A shallow discounting curve is characteristic of somebody who is not averse to risk, while a steep curve indicates that the individual is conservative and avoids risk.

Risk sensitivity has been shown to be relevant to 'patient' decision-making within disciplines such as neurology and pharmacology. For example, when multiple sclerosis patients were asked whether or not they would take a new disease-modifying therapy depending upon the likely probability of benefit and risk of side effects, those who were most risk-averse also exhibited poorer treatment adherence (Bruce et al., 2016). In another study, Tompkins et al. (2018) found chronic pain sufferers who were most at risk of opioid abuse discounted the addiction risk of a hypothetical new pain relief drug less steeply than those at lower risk. In Chapter 5, risk within midwifery has been discussed, yet whether risk sensitivity of practitioners might impact on their decision-making and practice is yet to be determined in any discipline, including midwifery.

'Social discounting' refers to the degree that one's behaviour towards another person is influenced by their social distance from you (Osiński, Karbowski, & Ostaszewski, 2015). In order to measure this, participants are first asked to assign a numerical value to people indicating their social distance, using a scale of 1–100, with 1 being somebody that is very close to you (partners or parents, for example) to 100 for somebody that you do not know at all. They are then asked, typically, how much of a sum of money they would share with a person who was at different degrees of separation from them: for example, 'how much of $1,000 would you be willing to share with somebody who was 5 units distance from you?' Interestingly, from a midwifery perspective, social discounting has been shown to be affected by oxytocin (Strang et al., 2017). Strang et al. found that administration of oxytocin to male participants in their study altered the relation between their levels of empathy, increasing the likelihood of them being generous to individuals they were close to. Understanding the process of social discounting and the potential effect it might have on advice given by a midwife in a collaborative decision-making situation will inform questions around professional boundaries, such as whether a midwife should be the primary accoucheur for a member of her family and how this may influence the clinical decisions a midwife makes in such a scenario compared to those when the familiarity boundaries are more distant.

The impact of discounting on clinical decision-making and practice

All three aspects of discounting (delay, probability and social) might be expected to influence clinical decision-making more generally, and more specifically in midwifery. For example, if you think about the internationally accepted midwifery philosophy (ICM, 2014) that birth is a natural physiological event and as midwives we are the guardians of normal (Fahy & Hastie, 2008), thus are reluctant to intervene until necessary. It might therefore be expected that, relative to other health professionals, and on average, the midwife would be low on impulsivity and perhaps less risk-averse. Healey et al. (2017) obtained qualitative data from a purposive sample of midwives working in obstetric-led care, alongside midwifery-led care and community settings suggesting that this is indeed the case, in that obstetricians and midwives differ in terms of their perspective on risk. Sensitivity to risk will also vary among midwives, and as Healey et al. (2016) point out, it may be driven by systemic changes that could negatively impact on the quality of care provided by midwives. This becomes important especially to the decisions a midwife may or may not make when considering the geographical location and contextual environment where autonomy, a midwife's agency and ability to work to their full scope of practice are varied as well as resources including supplies, pay and collaborative practice differ. For example, in an obstetric-led setting in a high-income country where there is no real limit to resources compared to a midwife who practices in a rural setting in a low-income country where there are existing cultural, social and physical inequities.

Risk sensitivity and social distance have been shown to interact in an economic decision-making task (Batteux, Ferguson, & Tunney, 2017). Batteux et al. (2017) first conducted a probability discounting task in which participants had to make decisions for themselves, for a friend (who was present with them) or for another person who was not there. The decisions made for self were more risk-averse than for friends, and those made for others were least risk-averse. This meant that, in terms of the financial decisions made, the decisions made for others were in fact closer to being economically sound than those made for oneself or a friend. In a clinical decision-making context, this implies that the most beneficial outcome might occur when there is greater social distance between the health practitioner and the person to whom they are giving advice. This would be particularly important in the collaborative decision-making context in which midwives work.

Sensitivity to reward and punishment

The role of affect and emotion on decision-making has received considerable attention over recent decades (e.g., George & Dane, 2016). Temperamental differences in affective responsiveness thus have the potential to influence decisions made in a clinical setting. One of the most enduring ideas in psychology is that affective responding is coordinated through the operation of two neural systems concerned with approach and avoidance behaviour (Gray, 1981, 1982). Gray defined these two systems as the behavioural inhibition and behavioural activation systems (BIS/BAS). The BAS is responsive to reward, and its activity results in approach behaviour. The BIS is responsive to punishment, and its activity results in withdrawal. Carver and White (1994) developed an instrument to measure the sensitivity to punishment and reward which an individual might display owing to temperamental differences in the operation of the BIS and BAS. They identified a single factor which corresponded to the operation of the BIS, but found that items relating to sensitivity to reward (the BAS) were best characterised by three factors: reward responsiveness, drive and fun-seeking. Of these, reward responsiveness is the core construct underlying the BAS, and has been shown to be associated with positive psychological functioning more generally (Taubitz, Pedersen, & Larson, 2015). Demianczyk et al. (2014) found that some items of Carver and White's (1994) scale were not reliable when applied to diverse ethnic and racial populations, and they argued that a scale without these items was therefore more appropriate for assessing levels of BIS/BAS activation in populations different to that of the original investigation. In order to maximise the degree to which our results might be of relevance across differing cultures and geographic regions, we adopted this revised instrument for our study.

The role of discounting and temperament in decision-making

Our study was designed to determine whether delay, probability or social discounting and/or sensitivity to reward or punishment were related to the way that midwives judged the quality of decision-making and midwifery practice. A scenario-based procedure was employed in which midwife participants first read three scenarios (presented in a random order) that were collected from practising midwives in a previous study undertaken by Jefford (2012). Participating midwives were asked to make a judgement of the quality of the clinical decision-making and midwifery practice (within the scenarios) on a 7-point Likert scale from 'Very poor' (1) to 'Excellent' (7). They then completed delay, probability and social discounting tasks and a modified version of the BIS/BAS scale (Demianczyk et al., 2014). The questionnaire was distributed by inviting participants who were members of the Australian College of Midwives to the survey located on Qualtrics. Demographic information regarding a number of factors such as age and years of experience was also collected. A total of 59 female midwives provided completed questionnaires. They came from all states and territories of Australia, representing metropolitan, regional and rural communities, and engaged in practice across all possible models (obstetrician-led hospital, stand-alone birth unit, group midwifery practice, etc.). The survey was approved by the Southern Cross University Human Research Ethics Committee.

The points of indifference for the delay, probability and social discounting functions were obtained using an 'investment' scenario, rather than the conventional monetary choice task.

The conventional delay discounting task, described McKerchar and Renda (2012), involves midwifery participants making a number of choices between sums of money which they would prefer to receive immediately or after one of a series of delays (one month, six months, etc.). A modified, five-question discounting task associated with a scenario involving investment was used, as the original discounting task was considered too time consuming. For the discounting task the participants were told to imagine that they had $1,000, and asked to consider how much interest they would have to receive in order to be willing to invest the money for different periods of time (one month, six months, one year, two years and five years). The response to these questions can be used to calculate the points of indifference for the value of $1,000 at these point in time. The probability discounting function was assessed in the same way, by asking how much interest one would have to receive in order to invest $1,000 where there was a specified risk of losing all of your investment (2%, 5%, 10%, 25% or 50%). Finally, in the social discounting task participants were asked how much interest they would need to receive from another person if they were to lend them $1,000 when that person varied in the degree of social proximity to them (1, 5, 20, 50 or 100, on the scale described in the learning activity).

The three clinical midwifery scenarios chosen for the questionnaire were selected to provide a range of judgements regarding the quality of clinical decision-making and midwifery practice, based upon the ratings provided by the international expert panel who 'judged' them for Jefford et al. (2016). The international panel (UK and Australia) consisted of academics, clinical midwives from every model of care offered within the two countries, consumers, and supervisor of midwives (UK only).

The quality of clinical decision-making and midwifery practice

The ratings of the quality of clinical decision-making and midwifery practice made by our participating midwives broadly reflected the differences expected as noted earlier. The average ratings and the standard deviation of the ratings are shown in Figure 23.1. The midwives

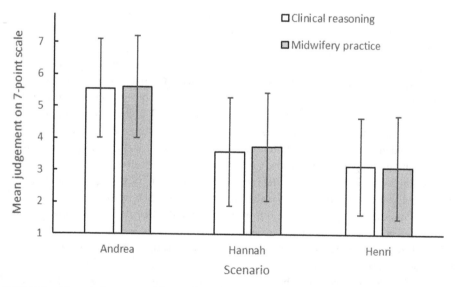

FIGURE 23.1 Mean judgement of the quality of clinical reasoning and midwifery practice

---

BOX 23.1 SCENARIO 1 – ANDREA

Scenario 1 – Andrea

The clinical scenario involving Andrea, a hospital-based midwife, was rated as demonstrating both high-quality decision-making and midwifery practice. It involved Andrea applying the Rebozo technique (Cohen & Thomas, 2015), but instead of using a traditional Mexican scarf she used a towel wrapped around the abdomen. The Rebozo technique can be used for women who are experiencing difficulty being able to push during the final stages of labour (Cohen & Thomas, 2015). In Andrea's scenario the Rebozo technique resulted in a positive clinical outcome.

BOX 23.2 SCENARIO 1 – HANNAH

Scenario 2 – Hannah

This clinical scenario involving Hannah, an independent/private midwife, was rated as demonstrating both low-quality decision-making and midwifery practice. It involved a home birth in which the midwife (Hannah) acceded to the request of the parents to be a 'reassuring' presence at the birth but not to actively participate as they wanted to free-birth this child as they had their others. The 'non-participation' or engagement in Hannah's professional capacity as a midwife, included the failure to check the fetal heartbeat. The outcome of the birth was positive for both mother and baby.

BOX 23.3 SCENARIO 1 – HENRI

Scenario 3 – Henri

The final clinical scenario involving Henri, a midwife who worked in a midwifery-led team model was rated as demonstrating both low-quality decision-making and midwifery practice. It involved a childbirth where the woman was transferred from a midwifery-led model to an obstetric-led hospital as her labour was not progressing as anticipated. Whilst in the hospital the midwife (Henri) excluded other medical staff and the hospital midwives from involvement until a point at which the safety of mother and child were compromised, leading to a negative outcome.

---

participants in our study clearly rated the clinical decision–making and midwifery practice of Andrea to be more aligned with their perception of 'good' midwifery practice to that of Hannah and Henri. However participating midwives did not differentiate the performance of Hannah and Henri, the same way in which the international expert panel within the Jefford et al. (2016) study had done.

The standard deviations of these judgements was quite large as can be seen from this figure, indicating that there were large differences in the ratings given by different individual midwives. This variability in judgement is consistent with the evidence provided by Styles et al. (2011). Furthermore, these differences do not appear to reflect consistent differences in judgements which might be due to some individual midwives being 'tougher' on their midwifery peers than others.

The judgements of clinical decision-making for Andrea and Hannah were correlated, but not very highly, and the judgements for Henri did not correlate with either of the other two scenarios. In other words, the midwives in our study thus appear to be making quite idiosyncratic judgements, and the criteria for these appears to differ on the context provided within each of the three scenario. Given the similarities of the clinical decision-making and midwifery practice judgements, it is tempting to suggest that they are controlled by a single factor, which could possibly be related to whether the participating midwives would have done something similar themselves to the behaviour described in the scenario. Again, this does not seem to have been the case for the international expert panel in Jefford et al.'s (2016) study. A possible explanation, maybe that the international expert panel members, may have been more influenced by professional, legal and regulatory documents (as noted in Chapters 2 and 3) than their own 'gut' responses. If so, then emphasising the importance of adhering to professional, legal and regulatory documents and practice guidelines, perhaps through a checklist similar to the items of the Enhancing Decision-making and Assessment in Midwifery (EDAM) tool (Jefford et al. 2016) (as noted in Chapter 1), might provide for greater consistency in the judgements made across different individuals.

Regardless of the mechanism(s) involved in making these judgements, we found no evidence that they were related to any of the discounting tasks. Discounting functions were obtained for each of the three tasks, which were broadly similar to those described by authors utilising the conventional forced-choice procedure (Madden & Bickel, 2010). The area under the curve of the obtained discounting functions was not significantly correlated with judgements of clinical decision-making or midwifery practice for any of the scenarios (largest $r(47) = -.252$, $p = .085$). While this might not have been particularly surprising for the delay and social discounting functions, we had expected that the participating midwives sensitivity to risk, as measured by the probability discounting task, to have influenced their judgements of the quality of clinical decision-making, at least in those tasks where this was determined to be poor (Hannah and Henri). The rates of discounting for the three tasks also did not correlate with scores on the BIS/BAS, which was also unexpected. It had been anticipated that sensitivity to reinforcement as reflected in the strength of the behavioural activation system would correlate with impulsivity, as measured by the delay discounting task. This was not the case. In fact, the only variable correlated with any discounting function was the length of professional experience of the midwife, which negatively correlated with social discounting ($r(32) = .349$, $p = .05$): more experienced midwives tended to report lower levels of social discounting, indicating that they are less influenced by social distance and more likely to be generous to people that they are not close to socially.

It is possible that this relation interacts with the type of practice in which the midwife is engaged. For example, a midwife in midwifery-led practice may have a different relationship with the woman to those working in a fragmented system such as a large consultant-led hospital. Almost all of the participants in our study, had worked in a variety of care provisions, but there was some evidence that those who had worked in midwifery-led practice had shallower social discounting functions (mean area under the curve = .56) than those who had not (mean area under the curve = .42). This was not, however, statistically significant given the sample size ($t(31) = 1.82$, $p = .079$). If there is a difference between midwives working in different models of care and/or environments, it is of course possible that this may not indicate that the working environment leads to changes in the midwife's level of social discounting: it is possible, instead, that individuals with lower levels of social discounting are attracted to this form of practice. Regardless, further exploration of social discounting and how it may influence the behaviour and career choices of health practitioners, including midwives, seems warranted.

BIS/BAS factors and judgements of clinical reasoning and midwifery practice

This section presents findings related to the midwives clinical decision-making and factors contained within the BIS/BAS tool.

Table 23.1 shows the correlations between the four BIS/BAS factors and judgements of clinical reasoning and midwifery practice. It can be seen from this table that there were relations between the sensitivity to reward and punishment and judgements of clinical reasoning and midwifery practice, but these relations differed for the three scenarios. For the scenario involving Andrea, which was the most highly rated of the three scenarios and which had a positive outcome, there was a substantial correlation between the judgements made for both clinical reasoning and midwifery practice and their level of BAS Reward responsiveness. This relation was not observed for the other two scenarios, but scores on BAS Fun-seeking were correlated with clinical reasoning for Hannah and with midwifery practice for both Hannah and Henri. Thus, those midwives participating in our study who stated that they would be more likely to engage in behaviour purely for the sake of its enjoyment were also more likely to give more positive judgements of the strategy adopted in these two scenarios.

Finally, there was a significant negative correlation between the BIS and judgements of both clinical decision-making and midwifery practice for the Henri scenario. This indicates that the more sensitive a midwife is to punishment the lower their rating of the quality of clinical decision-making was for this scenario. The BIS score was not related to any aspect of the other two scenarios. Henri's scenario involved a situation in which the midwife perceived

TABLE 23.1 Correlations between factors of the BIS/BAS scale and judgements of clinical reasoning and midwifery practice for the three scenarios

	BAS Reward Responsiveness	BAS Drive	BAS Fun-seeking	BIS
Andrea: Clinical reasoning	.472★	.141	.127	.160
Andrea: Midwifery practice	.450★	.083	.217	.209
Hannah: Clinical reasoning	−.024	.176	.277★	−.077
Hannah: Midwifery practice	.029	.199	.371★	.005
Henri: Clinical reasoning	.193	.102	.077	.259★
Henri: Midwifery practice	.221	.201	.334★	.280★

herself to be protecting the mother from intrusions made by other health practitioners, including other midwives, with whom she disagreed. This scenario could be construed to relate more to the social interaction between the midwife and others (doctors, and midwifery staff within the hospital setting), than the relationship she had with the mother. As other health practitioners may be a source of negative feedback regarding a midwife's practice, it is possible that this aspect of the scenario may have caused the participating midwives' sensitivity to punishment to have a greater influence on their judgements than would be the case for the other two scenarios. Alternatively, this scenario is also the only one in which there was a negative clinical outcome, which could also have contributed to this relation.

BOX 23.4   ADELAIDE'S STORY – LINKED TO ACTIVITY 1

Learning activity

We asked our participants to read a scenario drawn from clinical practice such as the one following, and to evaluate what they thought to be the quality of the clinical reasoning and midwifery practice.

   Try this yourself. When looking at this scenario please draw upon the ICM definition of a midwife and the ICM Code of Ethics for Midwives as well as geographical contextual relevant documents.

ADELAIDE

Background to Adelaide's story

Adelaide has worked for 33 years as a midwife. She is currently working in a birth centre attached to a public hospital located in a major city. When the birth unit is quiet, Adelaide is required to work on the hospital's delivery unit where this story occurred.

   Adelaide arrived at 7 a.m. and began caring for Rosalie, a primigravida. Rosalie had laboured all through the night and had been diagnosed, two hours previously, as being in second stage labour. Rosalie had an epidural and a CTG and had been actively pushing following verbal cues from the midwives since full dilation. The whole family were aware that the doctors were planning to conduct an assisted birth shortly.

Adelaide's story

When I entered Rosalie's birthing room, I spent a few minutes getting to know Rosalie, Mike and Joan. I tried to engage them in conversation and basically get a feel of how Rosalie was feeling about the way her labour and birth was progressing. Whilst this was happening, I used all my senses and assessed everything. I looked at Rosalie's position on the bed, her colour, whether she was perspiring, whether she was exhausted or whether she was happy or sad. In essence, I assessed her general well-being and her mental state. I looked at the support people and asked myself, are they in a chair, snoring? Are they exhausted from supporting Rosalie all night? I also assessed the room for clutter or whether it was disorganised. I saw, when Rosalie was pushing, there was a *tiniest little bit* (emphasis) of fetal head on view, but Rosalie was so exhausted after labouring all night that her pushing was not effective at progressing delivery of her baby. I knew the doctors, [once the shift changed in approximately 30 minutes], would come and do an assisted birth.

As Rosalie was pushing with each contraction, I sensed Rosalie did not want to throw the towel in and have an assisted birth. I thought, in this instance, I had to do something; *we* (emphasis) somehow had to push this baby out unassisted. I knew that if I got the lithotomy poles adjusted to suit Rosalie's anatomy and she could just let her knees flop whilst supporting behind the back of her legs she would be able to get much more 'push' into her bottom and get this baby round the bend of the pelvis. My decision was based on looking at the whole picture of Rosalie and my knowledge of the body. I've observed placing the woman in the lithotomy position worked quite a few times in my experience and from observing other midwives. Once I'd made my decision, I actually said to Rosalie, 'would you mind very much if I put your legs into a lithotomy?' I explained to her what I wanted to do.

Outcome

Within 20 minutes of Rosalie agreeing to use the lithotomy poles she birthed her child unassisted.

Your judgements:

For each of these statements indicate the degree to which you agree with a number from 1 (strongly disagree) to 7 (strongly agree).

- I think that Adelaide showed good clinical reasoning.
- I think that Adelaide showed good midwifery practice.

Reflections

Commenting on somebody else's practice can be quite difficult, and our participants found this challenging. This is evidenced by the large differences in the judgements we observed.

So where do these differences come from? People's knowledge of regulations and principles of practice obviously is one source of information that should be used when making these judgements. But if that was the only important factor, then there should be much less variability in the responses than that which we observed.

We hypothesise that at least some of this variability is due to differences in personality. In particular, how individuals respond to the likelihood that they will experience reward or punishment seems to play an important role. This does not only relate to the clinical outcomes obtained, but also relates to how the midwife feels their behaviour will be viewed by other midwives and clinical staff.

Consider your response to the questions relating to clinical reasoning and midwifery practice.

- Were you focused more on what might go right or on what could have gone wrong?
- Is praise from your colleagues very important to you, or do you seek to avoid censure?

We all do both of these things, but some of us are more sensitive to reward or punishment than others. If the level of these factors influence how we judge the actions of others (as our data suggests), then it seems plausible to expect that it will influence how we make decisions ourselves in similar situations.

Can you think of a situation you have faced yourself where your decision might have been influenced by your desire to please colleagues, or avoid their displeasure? In retrospect, do you think you made the best decision at that time?

Conclusion

Although this study was limited to a high-income country (Australia), the findings are important irrespective of geographical location around the world or model of care. This is because this study provides evidence that at least in certain situations, which are not limited to Australia, a temperamental difference in behavioural tendencies influences the judgements which midwives make regarding the quality of clinical decision-making and midwifery practice. Although the exact mechanism by which sensitivity to punishment is having an effect in the Henri scenario is unknown, the presence of this effect encourages the view that 'personality' factors have a role to play in the clinical decision-making process. Whether this implies that temperamental attributes influence clinical decision-making in the real world will require much further research. Our research did not explore how it is that individual differences among midwives may interact with these childbearing women. The expectations and desires of these women concerning childbirth should strongly influence the clinical reasoning and practice of the midwife, and these may well be influenced by temperamental factors measured by the BIS/BAS. Measurement of temperamental differences among expectant mothers and their expectancies regarding childbirth would help to inform this matter. Further development of scenarios which allow the manipulation of these expectancies in order to evaluate their influence on likely clinical decision-making by midwives has the potential to further enhance our understanding of this complex situation.

References

Batteux, E., Ferguson, E., & Tunney, R. J. (2017). Risk preferences in surrogate decision making. *Experimental Psychology, 64*(4), 290–297. Retrieved from https://www.ncbi.nlm.nih.gov/pubmed/28922998. doi:10.1027/1618-3169/a000371

Borges, N.J., & Gibson, D.D. (2005). Personality patterns of physicians in person-oriented and technique-oriented specialties. *Journal of Vocational Behavior, 67*(1), 4–20. doi:10.1016/j.jvb.2003.12.015

Bruce, J. M., Bruce, A. S., Catley, D., Lynch, S., Goggin, K., Reed, D., . . . Jarmolowicz, D. P. (2016). Being kind to your future self: Probability discounting of health decision-making. *Annals of*

Behavioral Medicine, *50*(2), 297–309. Retrieved from https://www.ncbi.nlm.nih.gov/pubmed/266
69602. doi:10.1007/s12160-015-9754-8

Carver, C., & White, T. (1994). Behavioral inhibition, behavioral activation, and affective responses to impending reward and punishment: The BIS/BAS scales. *Journal of Personality and Social Psychology*, *67*, 319–333.

Cohen, S., & Thomas, C. (2015). Rebozo technique for fetal malposition in labor. *Journal of Midwifery & Women's Health*, *60*(4), 445–451.

Demianczyk, A. C., Jenkins, A. L., Henson, J. M., & Conner, B. T. (2014). Psychometric evaluation and revision of Carver and White's BIS/BAS scales in a diverse sample of young adults. *Journal of Personality Assessment*, *96*(5), 485–494. doi:10.1080/00223891.2013.870570

Fahy, K., & Hastie, C. (2008). Midwifery guardianship: Reclaiming the sacred in birth. In K. Fahy, M. Foureur, & C. Hastie (Eds.), *Birth territory and midwifery guardianship* (Chapter 3, pp. 21–38). Glasgow: Elsevier.

George, J. M., & Dane, E. (2016). Affect, emotion, and decision making. *Organizational Behavior and Human Decision Processes*, *136*, 47–55. doi:10.1016/j.obhdp.2016.06.004

Gray, J. A. (1981). A critique of Eysenck's theory of personality. In H. J. Eysenck (Ed.), *A model for personality* (pp. 246–276). Berlin: Springer-Verlag.

Gray, J. A. (1982). *The neuropsychology of anxiety: An enquiry into the functions of the septo-hippocampal system.* New York: Oxford University Press.

Hadjigeorgiou, E., & Coxon, K. (2014). Cyprus 'midwifery is dying . . .'. A qualitative exploration of midwives perceptions of their role as advocates for normal birth. *Midwifery*, *30*, pp. 983–990.

Harris, T. (2005). Midwifery practice in the third stage of labour. (PhD), de Montford University, Leicester. Retrieved from www.dora.dmu.ac.uk/handle/2086/3350

Healy, S., Humphreys, E., & Kennedy, C. (2016). Midwives' and obstetricians' perceptions of risk and its impact on clinical practice and decision-making in labour: An integrative review. *Women and Birth*, *29*(2), 107–116. Retrieved from https://www.ncbi.nlm.nih.gov/pubmed/26363668. doi:10.1016/j.wombi.2015.08.010

ICM. (2014). Core document. Philosophy and model of midwifery care. Retrieved from www.internationalmidwives.org/assets/files/definitions-files/2018/06/eng-philosophy-and-model-of-midwifery-care.pdf

Jefford, E. (2012). Optimal midwifery decision-making during 2nd stage labour: The integration of clinical reasoning into practice. (PhD), Southern Cross University, NSW.

Jefford, E., Jomeen, J., & Martin, C. (2016). Determining the psychometric properties of the Enhancing Decision-making Assessment in Midwifery (EDAM) measure in a cross cultural context. *BMC Pregnancy and Childbirth*, *16*, 95–106.

Madden, G. J., & Bickel, W. K. (2010). *Impulsivity: The behavioral and neurological science of discounting.* Washington, DC: American Psychological Association. 453 pp., ISBN: 978-1-4338-0477-9

Markert, R., Rodenhauser, P., El-Baghdadi, M., Juskaite, K., Hillel, A., & Maron, B. (2008). Personality as a prognostic factor for specialty choice: A prospective study of 4 medical school classes. *Medscape Journal of Medicine*, *10*, 49.

McKerchar, T., & Renda, C. (2012). Delay and probability discounting in humans: An overview. *The Psychological Record*, *62*, 817–834.

Osiński, J., Karbowski, A., & Ostaszewski, P. (2015). Social discounting: Choice between rewards for other people. *Behavioural Processes*, *115*, 61–63. doi:10.1016/j.beproc.2015.02.010

Reber, A. S., Allen, R., & Reber, E. S. (2009). Personality in *The Penguin dictionary of psychology* (4th ed.). [Online]. London: Penguin. Retrieved 23 January 2019, from https://ezproxy.scu.edu.au/login?url=https://search.credoreference.com/content/entry/penguinpsyc/personality/0?institutionId=180

Strang, S., Gerhardt, H., Marsh, N., Oroz Artigas, S., Hu, Y., Hurlemann, R., & Park, S. Q. (2017). A matter of distance-The effect of oxytocin on social discounting is empathy-dependent. *Psychoneuroendocrinology*, *78*, 229–232. doi:10.1016/j.psyneuen.2017.01.031

Styles, M., Cheyne, H., O'Carroll, R., Greig, F., Dagge-Bell, F., & Niven, C. (2011). The Scottish Trial of Refer or Keep (the STORK study): Midwives' intrapartum decision making. *Midwifery*, *27*(1), 104–111. doi:10.1016/j.midw.2009.12.003

Taber, B. J., Hartung, P. J., & Borges, N. J. (2011). Personality and values as predictors of medical specialty choice. *Journal of Vocational Behavior*, *78*(2), 202–209. doi:10.1016/j.jvb.2010.09.006

Taubitz, L. E., Pedersen, W. S., & Larson, C. L. (2015). BAS reward responsiveness: A unique predictor of positive psychological functioning. *Personality and Individual Differences*, *80*, 107–112. doi:10.1016/j.paid.2015.02.029

Tompkins, D. A., Huhn, A. S., Johnson, P. S., Smith, M. T., Strain, E. C., Edwards, R. R., & Johnson, M. W. (2018). To take or not to take: the association between perceived addiction risk, expected analgesic response and likelihood of trying novel pain relievers in self-identified chronic pain patients. Addiction, 113(1), 67–79. Retrieved from https://www.ncbi.nlm.nih.gov/pubmed/28645137. doi:10.1111/add.13922

Yoon, J. H., Higgins, S. T., Heil, S. H., Sugarbaker, R. J., Thomas, C. S., & Badger, G. J. (2007). Delay discounting predicts postpartum relapse to cigarette smoking among pregnant women. *Experimental and Clinical Psychopharmacology*, *15*(2), 176–186. doi:10.1037/1064-1297.15.2.186

24

PROACTIVE BEHAVIOUR IN MIDWIFERY EDUCATION AND PRACTICE

A pre-request for shared decision-making

Eveline Mestdagh

Chapter overview

This chapter will discuss how proactive behaviour can be applied in midwifery education and practice and how it should be a prerequisite of shared decision-making between the woman and the midwife. Individual and contextual antecedents associated with proactive behaviour in midwifery will be discussed. Facilitators and barriers are presented as well as a new midwifery educational program in order to simulate proactive behaviour.

Introduction

The international definition of the midwife clearly indicates the conditions necessary to obtain the professional title 'midwife' and the legally defined scope and settings of midwifery practice (ICM, 2017). (The importance of midwifery regulation is discussed further in Chapter 2.) The international philosophy of midwifery is that of being woman-centred (ICM, 2017). As a skilled and competent health professional, a midwife makes a difference in maternal and neonatal outcomes (Renfrew et al., 2014). One way in which this is achieved is by delineating the current evidence base and integrating it into one's midwifery practice (Carolan, 2011; Fullerton et al., 2011). Halldorsdottir & Karlsdottir (2011) take this further, believing as a prerequisite for true professionalism a midwife must continuously develop herself by following up and integrating newest insights and up-to-date, evidence-informed practices. To keep up to date, midwives need to continuously be involved in and discuss research and the sphere of midwifery practice and be committed to integrate evidence in their provision of woman-centred care (Carolan, 2013). However, Carlson & Plonczynski (2008) found that the majority of healthcare professionals do not consistently put evidence-informed guidelines nor other important research directly into practice, despite the contextual setting for maternal and neonatal care requires it.

In recent years, the context of midwifery practice has grown in complexity, due to rapid evolutions, such as an overload of operational pressure, the need for cost-effective and continuous accessible healthcare, restructuring, savings, centralisation of care, medicalisation of childbirth as well as an overflow of new insights, innovations and availability of evidence related to interventions (Bauer, 2010; Healy et al., 2016; Timmermans et al., 2012). The landscape of the childbearing woman has also become more complex, for example, there are more elderly prima- and multigravida women (Sauer, 2015), increased rates of obesity (Devlieger et al., 2016), and more women are living in very difficult social situations (Briscoe et al., 2016). Accumulatively, the growing complexity along with advancing developments and innovations in midwifery care directly and indirectly influence the working conditions for midwives (Watkins et al., 2017). These changing circumstances expose midwives to work-related stress, which in turn affects midwives emotional and work-related well-being (RCM, 2016). Sidebotham et al. (2015) has implied that stress and burnout in midwives, impacts on workforce retention. In 2018, Geraghty et al. noted that the increasing number of stressors negatively affects the commitment, quality of care and work engagement of midwives. This ever-changing midwifery working field also seems to impact midwives' ability to fully exercise autonomy, and to advocate for women and normal birth. Jefford, Jomeen & Wallin (2018) linked this changing context to where midwifery abdication is inevitable or at least very difficult to prevent. This is discussed further in Chapter 6. What is critical is that emotional well-being of the midwife has been highlighted as an important strategy in maintaining a healthy and motivated midwifery workforce that will continue effectively serving women and their families (Dixon, 2017; Hildingsson et al., 2013).

The labour market, however, is increasingly demanding healthcare practitioners who can work in an innovative context and adapt as necessary (Carman et al., 2010; Lemieux-Charles & McGuire, 2006; European Council, 2011). This potentially increases the challenge to the emotional well-being of midwives and requires midwives, supported by reflective practice, to be proactive (Westerlaken, 2013). Therefore, midwives competences, practice environment and educational programmes need to respond and make appropriate adaptations. In the quest for an answer to the developments and innovations in midwifery and midwifery education, healthcare organisations, universities and governmental institutions mainly focus on operational matters, for example, restructuring of protocols, work areas and financing. Yet, less emphasis is given to underlying aspects of work (processes). The focus of attention should be moved to a possible behavioural change, where the midwife can positively cope and respond to developments and innovative demands of midwifery practice. This chapter links a previously explored concept, albeit in other working areas, proactive behaviour – the midwives' possibility to manage developments and innovations in the context of maternal and neonatal care. Further, facilitating or hindering factors to proactive behaviour in midwifery practice and education will be explored.

Proactive behaviour in midwifery

The roots of the concept of proactive behaviour dates back to the 1960s when research explored motivation theories and where selection of a behaviour is determined by the desirability of the outcome (Vroom, 1964). The focus at this time was mainly on desires, motives and intentions and less on the person who was still placed in a relatively passive position subjected to organisational phenomena. More recently, Grant & Ashford (2008) placed the person in a much more active role in deploying influencing tactics, such as actively seeking feedback, to improve social interactions, working structures and to expand knowledge and skills. These tactics were later called forms of proactive behaviour. Nowadays, organisations request people to be flexible, innovative and act proactively, because they are more likely to redefine and translate their new roles into practice and encapsulate new tasks and goals as the result of continuous alterations in healthcare (Bateman & Crant, 1993; Fay & Frese, 2001; Parker & Sprigg, 1999; Unsworth & Parker, 2003).

Proactive behaviour is described as being committed to self-initiated and change-oriented efforts in work behaviour to enhance personal or organisational effectiveness. In other words, it is about making things happen, anticipating and preventing problems and seizing opportunities rather than passively adapting present conditions (Unsworth & Parker, 2003). Proactive behaviour is used on different levels and varies along several dimensions focusing on form, the intended target, frequency and timing. One can act proactively on an individual level, team level or organisational level (Belshak, 2010; Grant & Ashford, 2008; Parker & Collins, 2010). Proactive behaviour is a universal phenomenon generalisable to multiple professions. All types of actions, ranging from caring for women to work organisation, can be carried out by being more or less proactive. Depending on a variety and combination of a specific individual and contextual factors, everyone can display more or less of proactive behaviours. Parker & Collins (2010), believe the necessary conditions to encourage proactive behaviour is related to the right person, at the right time and in the right context.

In order to understand and apply proactive behaviour into the midwifery field, a concept analysis was performed using Walker & Avant's (2010) eight steps method (Mestdagh et al., 2016). This method helped to understand the evolution of the concept of proactive behaviour in midwifery and made a clear distinction between relevant and irrelevant features.

A midwife who behaves proactively will not look at changes as a barrier or full stop, rather the midwife will seek change as an opportunity to persistently seek ways to improve things, learns from error, and looks for viable alternatives to carry out work as efficiently and effectively as possible. Various individual (e.g. reflecting tendencies, need for achievement) and/or contextual antecedents (e.g. an appreciative team leader, job autonomy) could trigger proactive behaviour in midwives. Additionally, this behaviour has multiple future benefits (e.g. commitment, productivity, organisational success) for the constant evolving nature of reproductive and maternity healthcare.

Proactive behaviour in midwifery students

Study 1

All the antecedents, stemming from the concept analysis, supported the compilation of a questionnaire to determine the influence of individual and/or contextual antecedents; for example job autonomy and control appraisal, towards proactive behaviour in student midwives (Mestdagh et al., 2018). The questionnaire is subdivided into four categories. First, a set of six personal and demographic questions. Second, seven individual antecedents: (1) generalised compliance; (2) affective organisational commitment; (3) proactive personality; (4) change orientation; (5) control appraisal; (6) role breadth self-efficacy; and (7) flexible role orientation. Third, three contextual antecedents: (1) job autonomy; (2) confidence in the possibilities of fellow students; and (3) supportive supervision. And finally, proactive behaviour is assessed using the concept of 'proactive idea implementation' constructed from five components: (1) creating costs and/or (2) time savings; (3) improving quality; (4) achieving improved results; and (5) cooperating more efficiently.

First, second and third year midwifery students' proactive behaviour in Belgium and the Netherlands ($n = 156$ and $n = 421$, respectively), were tested using this questionnaire (Mestdagh et al., 2018; Mestdagh, Van Endert, Van Rompaey et al., 2019). The findings highlighted that the participating midwifery students who have a high role breadth self-efficacy, a higher number of years into the study program, a high trust in their peers and low control appraisal are more likely to show proactive behaviour.

Study 2

In 2017, Belgian and Dutch midwifery students ($n = 55$) who have already completed at least 270 hours of traineeship and thus have observed many midwives in different clinical and ambulatory settings, were interviewed for their experiences (Mestdagh et al., 2018a). These future maternity care providers perceived the existence of proactive behaviour as the result of four key components: (1) the nature-nurture part, referring to the combination of a certain mind-set and self-esteem a midwife must own as well as the learnability of this kind of behaviour; (2) the level of willingness, regulated by the norms and values of the midwife as well as the organisational culture of the team the midwife is working in; (3) the reflective tendencies of the midwife (the importance of reflection is discussed further in Chapter 8); and (4) the time-gaining as well as the limitations of time to always be conscientious and at ease to behave proactively.

In summary, these two studies, involving student midwives in two high-income countries, indicate that proactive behaviour could be a prerequisite for shared decision-making. Although these studies occurred in high-income countries, the implications of this needs to be considered by academics as well as midwives around the world who mentor/preceptor midwifery students within the clinical environment.

Proactive behaviour in midwives

Study 1

The previously mentioned questionnaire was adapted to study proactive behaviour in a group of midwives ($n = 139$) (Mestdagh, Van Rompaey, Colin et al., 2019). Results in this study indicated midwives that have a high role breadth self-efficacy and high job autonomy are more likely to show proactive behaviour. Additionally, independent midwives are more likely behave proactively. Midwives, more than midwifery students, need a high level of control appraisal to have the tendency to show proactive behaviour. Midwives tend to lose some of their level of proactive behaviour after working one year. At the present time, there is no research to help explain why this happens. It could, however, tentatively be hypothesised that erosion of proactive behaviour, after one year, may or may not be due to organisational culture and/or a medicalised model of maternity care. Nevertheless, this erosion has implications for global midwifery decision-making, as if any midwife, irrespective of geographical location or model of care, loses their autonomy thus unable to practise to their full scope, then their decision-making abilities will be limited.

Study 2

To expand and deepen knowledge and understanding about proactive behaviour in midwifery, a large sample of qualified midwives ($n = 102$) in Flanders and the Netherlands were interviewed (Mestdagh Timmermans, Fontein-Kuipers et al., 2019c). From this study, six influencing factors emerged as causal, contextual and conditional factors faced by the midwives in order to enact proactive behaviour in midwifery practice: (1) the need for team consultations; (2) a safe organisational culture; (3) an appreciative midwifery leader; (4) an attitude of lifelong learning; (5) midwives are looking for a way to deal with both challenges in healthcare and (6) the competitive societal system.

To be able to implement the model of shared decision-making into the midwifery practice, proactive behaviour has to be stimulated. The preceding studies provide contextual and conditional factors that influence proactive behaviour. These factors need to be taken into consideration within the global midwifery arena by management, peers and colleagues. By stimulating proactive behaviour, midwifery decision-making can be positively influenced.

Repercussions and challenges of proactive behaviour in midwifery

This chapter does not seek to say that the current midwife or midwifery student is not competent or sufficient. It also does not suggest that change management is a new responsibility of the midwife, and of course, midwives do not need to accept every political statement or change. However, midwives are challenged to find a positive way of dealing with an ever-changing and increasingly pressurised working environment and an increasing culture of accreditation and quality improvement (Stevens & McCourt 2002). What is critical is that midwives are developed as resilient practitioners who feel supported to cope with an ever-changing societal context, this then inevitably impacts on the experiences of both mothers and fathers to be.

Similar and different trends were described in the stimulators of proactive behaviour within the group of midwifery students and the midwives in daily practice. There is an overall need to focus on the individual antecedents of the midwifery student to support proactive behaviour (e.g. stimulating role breadth self-efficacy) and therefore, create a tailored and customised learning environment. Within the practicing midwives, the predominant focus is on the contextual antecedents (e.g. a higher job autonomy and less hierarchical levels in the working area). Overall various individual and/or contextual antecedents possibly trigger proactive behaviour in midwifery. This behaviour is not considered to be a steady state or ready-made behaviour, but could cause multiple effects. Assuming from a contingency approach, the circumstances in which proactive behaviour is shown, can sometimes be more and sometimes be less influenced (Van Linge, 2017).

Within the international midwifery context, the challenges lay in the transfer of recommendations in policymaking, education, clinical midwifery practice and how one can provide mentorship to students and midwives around proactively dealing with these continuing developments.

Political challenges

Care for women and their family is spread over various care professionals. Legally, all (normal) care belongs to the midwifery profession. However, 'normal' midwifery care is overshadowed by medical influences. For all midwives across the globe who work within a medicalised environment, this creates a major political as well as professional challenge especially as midwifery autonomy is important to proactive behaviour. Some of these challenges are discussed in other chapters within this book. It is important, however, to acknowledge that some midwives work in different models of care across the globe, where the midwife is the primary care provider. In such cases, if a woman is low risk and stays low risk, then an obstetrician will not ever be involved in her care. Regardless of model of care, or location around the world, it is suggested midwives, feel the need for an eligible job autonomy and link this as a stimulator to behave proactively. Practicing autonomously provides midwives with more job satisfaction and positively contributes to a good work-life balance (Perdok et al., 2017) and enhances their ability to make decisions as well as shared decision-making with women.

Educational challenges

Midwifery educators around the world nowadays are challenged to facilitate new midwives to be resilient, autonomous, skilled, accountable within multidisciplinary teams and able to continue to learn in ever changing and challenging healthcare systems (CNOs of England Northern Ireland, Scotland and Wales, 2010). Midwifery educators have a key role in helping midwifery students develop resilience, providing them with the skills to handle both workplace and personal stressors. Maintaining the enthusiasm and passion of new midwives entering midwifery practice is challenging when faced with complex and demanding, often underfunded, healthcare settings, staff shortages and an overload of operational pressure. The new midwifery workforce should be educated and supported in transforming healthcare systems (Frenk et al., 2010; Renfrew et al., 2014). The emphasis on continuing professional development is an important future focus for midwifery students (Embo & Valcke, 2017). Additional advanced professional development skills, such as proactive behaviour, have not been sufficiently delineated (Begley et al., 2007). One way to help support student midwives and midwives is that the necessary antecedents, related to proactive behaviour, could be incorporated in the curricula of midwifery educational programs and workplace environment. If proactive behaviour was implemented it could equip midwifery students and midwives with higher role-breadth self-efficacy and autonomy. New learning approaches could challenge the traditional understanding of midwifery education (Hundley et al., 2018). To guide the educational programs in this, an ongoing study called 'PROMIsE' was developed in order to stimulate proactive behaviour (Mestdagh et al., 2018b). At this time no results are available, however it is hypothesised equipping midwifery students with higher role-breadth self-efficacy, autonomy, trust in peers and a lower need for control appraisal, with the aim that the intervention will improve their level of proactive behaviour. We assume that proactive behaviour also is a prerequisite of working towards a more shared-decision midwifery model.

Challenges in midwifery practice

Changes in healthcare (in)directly impact on the future of midwifery education and practice. Midwifery, as a caring profession, carries the potential for burnout if carers are not supported (Sidebotham et al., 2015). The question is whether some of this support can be built through education in order to empower future midwives and help them develop professional resilience. The importance of building resilience, seen as a learned process which is facilitated by a range of coping strategies, including accessing support and developing self-awareness and protection of self, is partnered with a strong sense of professional identity (Hunter & Warren, 2014). Unfortunately, although student midwives enthusiastically embrace these taught competencies, a sobering lack of opportunities to gain clinical practice occurs within health systems that have not yet evolved or are less accessible to midwives. Therefore, practising mid-wives need to be committed to developing this new generation of midwives, supporting them in gaining their confidence and sharing their knowledge (Hundley et al., 2018).

Arising from the studies described in this chapter, midwives do tend to lose part of their proactive behaviour already after one year of working experience. Simultaneously, working experience is required in facilitating proactive behaviour. Experience and knowledge are linked to good clinical reasoning as a necessary condition for optimal and safe midwifery decision-making (Jefford & Jomeen, 2012). The challenge lies in looking for a way to keep midwives proactive after that first year, because proactive behaviour may also well be a pre-requisite for optimal and safe decision-making.

The way a team is composed has some influence on the prevalence of team-learning activities such as trust in peers (Parratt, 2014), which could in turn stimulate proactive behav-iour. The hospital organisational context, irrespective of its geographical location, within which team work however has a significant effect on the prevalence of team learning activities (Timmermans et al., 2012), which in turn is a prerequisite of proactive behaviour. Interest-ingly, midwives who work independently or are community-based are more likely to show proactive behaviour in relation to midwives working in the hospital.

An additional challenge is the empowerment of midwives as leaders. The importance of an appreciative leader was also confirmed by Bailey et al. (2016), stating that supportive supervision of a midwifery leader increases job satisfaction and health worker motivation, which results in a tendency of them displaying proactive behaviour. Empowering leadership broadens the scope of the employees and therefore work more efficiently and tend to behave proactive (Yin et al., 2017).

Finally, a major challenge in care is the diminishing of hierarchical burdens. There is a clear need to shift towards a more open-discussion culture with all partners in the team the mid-wife is working in (Giebels et al., 2016). Therefore, postgraduate programmes of study that focus on interprofessional collaboration, which creates greater insight and respect for each other's job autonomy and focuses on developing a model of shared-governance in midwifery (Derbyshire & Machin, 2011). A safe and supportive organisational culture and midwifery working environment could increase the level of willingness to behave proactively (Belshak, 2010; Edmondson & Walker, 2014).

Conclusion

This chapter has tried to demonstrate the importance of proactive behaviour and its link to create shared-governance and decision-making in midwifery. This concept was studied from different perspectives and tested in a variety of midwifery contexts. Facilitating and hinder-ing factors were explored. Also possible consequences were elaborated and the possibility of using an educational intervention such as of the 'PROMIsE' program to support our future midwives was presented.

References

Bailey, C., Blake, C., Schriver, M., Cubaka, V. K., Thomas, T., & Martin Hilber, A. (2016). A sys-tematic review of supportive supervision as a strategy to improve primary healthcare services in sub-Saharan Africa. *International Journal of Gynecology & Obstetrics, 132*(1), 117–125. doi:10.1016/j. ijgo.2015.10.004

Bateman, T. S., & Crant, J. M. (1993). The proactive component of organizational behavior: A measure and correlates. *Journal of Organizational Behavior, 14*(2), 103–118. doi:10.1002/job.4030140202

Bauer, J. C. (2010). Nurse practitioners as an underutilized resource for health reform: Evidence-based demonstrations of cost-effectiveness. *Journal of the American Association of Nurse Practitioners, 22*(4), 228–231. doi:10.1111/j.1745–7599.2010.00498.x

Begley, C. M., Oboyle, C., Carroll, M., & Devane, D. (2007). Educating advanced midwife practitioners: A collaborative venture. *Journal of Nursing Management, 15*(6), 574–584. doi:10.1111/ j.1365–2834.2007.00807.x

Belshak, F., & Den Hartog, D. (2010). Pro-self, prosocial and pro-organizational foci of proactive behaviour: Differential antecedents and consequences. *Journal of Occupational and Organizational Psychology, 83*, 475–498.

Briscoe, L., Lavender, T., & McGowan, L. (2016). A concept analysis of women's vulnerability during pregnancy, birth and the postnatal period. *Journal of Advanced Nursing, 72*(10), 2330–2345. doi:10. 1111/jan.13017

Carlson, C. L., & Plonczynski, D. J. (2008). Has the BARRIERS Scale changed nursing practice? An integrative review. *Journal of Advanced Nursing, 63*(4), 322–333. doi:10.1111/j.1365–2648.2008.04705.x

Carman, J. M., Shortell, S. M., Foster, R. W., Hughes, E. F., Boerstler, H., Brien, J. L., & O'Connor, E. J. (2010). Keys for successful implementation of total quality management in hospitals. *Health Care Management Review, 35*(4), 283–293. doi:10.1097/HMR.0b013e3181f5fc4a

Carolan, M. (2011). The good midwife: Commencing students' views. *Midwifery, 27*(4), 503–508.

Carolan, M. (2013). 'A good midwife stands out': 3rd year midwifery students' views. *Midwifery, 29*(2), 115–121.

CNOs of England, Northern Ireland, Scotland and Wales. (2010). *Midwifery 2020: Delivering Expectations.* London.

Derbyshire, J. A., & Machin, A. I. (2011). Learning to work collaboratively: Nurses' views of their pre-registration interprofessional education and its impact on practice. *Nurse Education in Practice, 11*(4), 239–244. doi:10.1016/j.nepr.2010.11.010

Devlieger, R., Benhalima, K., Damm, P., Van Assche, A., Mathieu, C., Mahmood, T., . . . Bogaerts, A. (2016). Maternal obesity in Europe: Where do we stand and how to move forward?: A scientific paper commissioned by the European Board and College of Obstetrics and Gynaecology (EBCOG). *European Journal of Obstetrics & Gynecology and Reproductive Biology, 201*, 203–208. doi:10.1016/j. ejogrb.2016.04.005

Dixon, L., Guilliland, K., Pallant, J., Sidebotham, M., Fenwick, J., Mcara-Couper, J., & Gilkison, A. (2017). The emotional wellbeing of New Zealand midwives: Comparing responses for midwives in caseloading and shift work settings. *New Zealand College of Midwives Journal* (53), 5–14. doi:10.12784/ nzcomjnl53.2017.1.5-14

Edmondson, M. C., & Walker, S. B. (2014). Working in caseload midwifery care: The experience of midwives working in a birth centre in North Queensland. *Women and Birth: Journal of the Australian College of Midwives, 27*(1), 31–36. doi:10.1016/j.wombi.2013.09.003

Embo, M., & Valcke, M. (2017). Continuing midwifery education beyond graduation: Student midwives' awareness of continuous professional development. *Nurse Education in Practice, 24*, 118–122. doi:10.1016/j.nepr.2015.08.013

European council. (2011). *Conclusies van de Raad over de modernisering van het hoger onderwijs.* Publicatie-blad van de Europese Unie.

Fay, D., & Frese, M. (2001). The concept of personal initiative: An overview of validity studies. *Human Performance, 14*(1), 97–124. doi:10.1207/S15327043hup1401_06

Frenk, J., Chen, L., Bhutta, Z. A., Cohen, J., Crisp, N., Evans, T., . . . Zurayk, H. (2010). Health professionals for a new century: Transforming education to strengthen health systems in an interdependent world. *Lancet, 376*(9756), 1923–1958. doi:10.1016/s0140-6736(10)61854-5

Fullerton, J. T., Thompson, J. B., Severino, R., & International Confederation of Midwives. (2011). The International Confederation of Midwives essential competencies for basic midwifery practice. An update study: 2009–2010. *Midwifery, 27*(4), 399–408. doi:10.1016/j.midw.2011.03.005

Geraghty, S., Speelman, C., & Bayes, S. (2018). Fighting a losing battle: Midwives experiences of workplace stress. *Women and Birth*. doi: 10.1016/j.wombi.2018.07.012. [Epub ahead of print]Giebels, E., de Reuver, R. S., Rispens, S., & Ufkes, E. G. (2016). The critical roles of task conflict and job autonomy in the relationship between proactive personalities and innovative employee behavior. *Journal of Applied Behavioral Science, 52*(3), 320–341. doi:10.1177/0021886316648774

Grant, A. M., & Ashford, S. J. (2008). The dynamics of proactivity at work. *Research in Organizational Behavior, 28*, 3–34. doi: 10.1016/j.riob.2008.04.002

Halldorsdottir, S., & Karlsdottir, S. I. (2011). The primacy of the good midwife in midwifery services: An evolving theory of professionalism in midwifery. *Scandinavian Journal of Caring Sciences, 25*(4), 806–817.

Healy, S., Humphreys, E., & Kennedy, C. (2016). Midwives' and obstetricians' perceptions of risk and its impact on clinical practice and decision-making in labour: An integrative review. *Women Birth, 29*(2), 107–116. doi:10.1016/j.wombi.2015.08.010

Hildingsson, I., Westlund, K., & Wiklund, I. (2013). Burnout in Swedish midwives. *Sexual & Reproductive Healthcare, 4*(3), 87–91. doi:10.1016/j.srhc.2013.07.001

Hundley, V., Cadée, F., & Jokinen, M. (2018). Editorial midwifery special issue on education: A call to all the world's midwife educators! *Midwifery, 64*, 122–123. doi:10.1016/j.midw.2018.06.013

Hunter, B., & Warren, L. (2014). Midwives' experiences of workplace resilience. *Midwifery, 30*(8), 926–934. doi:10.1016/j.midw.2014.03.010

International Confederation of Midwives. (2017). *International definition of the midwife* (CD2005_001 V2017 ENG).

Jefford, E., & Jomeen, J. (2012). Optimal midwifery decision-making: An empirically grounded model. Paper presented to Nottingham International Conference for Education and Research in Midwifery, Nottingham, UK, 7–8 September, University of Nottingham, Nottingham, UK.

Jefford, E., Jomeen, J., & Wallin, M. (2018). Midwifery abdication –Is it acknowledged or discussed within the midwifery literature: An integrative review. *European Journal of Midwifery, 2*(6), 1–9.

Lemieux-Charles, L., & McGuire, W. L. (2006). What do we know about health care team effectiveness? A review of the literature. *Medical Care Research and Review, 63*(3), 263–300. doi:10.1177/10775 58706287003

Mestdagh, E., Timmermans, O., Colin, P. J., & Van Rompaey, B. (2018). A cross-sectional pilot study of student's proactive behavior in midwifery education: Validation of a developed questionnaire. *Nurse Education Today, 62*, 22–29. doi:10.1016/j.nedt.2017.12.006

Mestdagh, E., Timmermans, O., Fontein-Kuipers, Y., & Van Rompaey, B. (2019). Proactive behaviour in midwifery practice: A qualitative overview based on midwives' perspectives. *Sexual and Reproductive Healthcare*. doi: 10.1016/j.srhc.2019.04.002

Mestdagh, E., Van Rompaey, B., Beeckman, K., Bogaerts, A., & Timmermans, O. (2016). A concept analysis of proactive behaviour in midwifery. *Journal of Advanced Nursing, 72*(6), 1236–1250. doi:10.1111/jan.12952

Mestdagh, E., Van Rompaey, B., Colin, P. J., & Timmermans, O. (2019). A cross-sectional pilot study of midwives' proactive behavior in the midwifery field. *Annals of Nursing Research & Practice*, under review.

Mestdagh, E., Van Rompaey, B., Peremans, L., Meier, K., & Timmermans, O. (2018). Proactive behavior in midwifery: A qualitative overview from midwifery student's perspective. *Nurse Education in Practice, 31*, 1–6. doi:10.1016/j.nepr.2018.04.006

Mestdagh, E., Van Rompaey, B., & Timmermans, O. (2018). Study protocol for 'PROMIsE': Implementation of a curriculum to stimulate PROactive behavior in MIdwifery Education. *European Journal of Midwifery, 2*(10). doi:10.18332/ejm/94653

Mestdagh, E., Van Endert, N., Van Rompaey, B., & Timmermans, O. (2019). What stimulates proactive behaviour of midwifery students during their education? *Archives of Health Science, 1*(1), 104.

Parker, S. K., & Collins, C. G. (2010). Taking stock: Integrating and differentiating multiple proactive behaviors. *Journal of Management, 36*(3), 633–662. doi:10.1177/0149206308321554

Parker, S. K., & Sprigg, C. A. (1999). Minimizing strain and maximizing learning: The role of job demands, job control, and proactive personality. *Journal of Applied Psychology, 84*(6), 925–939.

Parratt, J., Fahy, K. M., & Hastie, C. R. (2014). Midwifery students' evaluation of team-based academic assignments involving peer-marking. *Women and Birth, 27*(1), 58–63.

Perdok, H., Cronie, D., van der Speld, C., van Dillen, J., de Jonge, A., Rijnders, M., . . . Verhoeven, C. J. (2017). Experienced job autonomy among maternity care professionals in The Netherlands. *Midwifery, 54*, 67–72. doi:10.1016/j.midw.2017.07.015

Renfrew, M. J., McFadden, A., Bastos, M. H., Campbell, J., Channon, A. A., Cheung, N. F., . . . Declercq, E. (2014). Midwifery and quality care: Findings from a new evidence-informed framework for maternal and newborn care. *Lancet, 384*(9948), 1129–1145. doi:10.1016/S0140-6736(14)60789-3

Royal College of Midwives. (2016). *RCM campaign for healthy workplaces delivering high quality care.* Caring for You Campaign: Working in Partnership.

Sauer, M. V. (2015). Reproduction at an advanced maternal age and maternal health. *Fertility and Sterility, 103*(5), 1136–1143. doi:10.1016/j.fertnstert.2015.03.004

Sidebotham, M., Gamble, J., Creedy, D., Kinnear, A., & Fenwick, J. (2015). Prevalence of burnout, depression, anxiety and stress among Australian midwives. *Women and Birth, 28*, S27. doi:10.1016/j.wombi.2015.07.093

Stevens, T., & McCourt, C. (2002). One-to-one midwifery practice part 2: The transition period. *British Journal of Midwifery, 10*(1), 45–50.

Timmermans, O., Van Linge, R., Van Petegem, P., Van Rompaey, B., & Denekens, J. (2012). Team learning and innovation in nursing, a review of the literature. *Nurse Education Today, 32*(1), 65–70. doi:10.1016/j.nedt.2011.07.006

Unsworth, K. L., & Parker, S. K. (2003). Proactivity and innovation: Promoting a new workforce for the new workplace. In D. Holman, T. D. Wall, C. W. Clegg, P. Sparrow, & A. Howard (Eds.), *The New Workplace: A Guide to the Human Impact of Modern Working Practices.* (pp. 175–196). Chichester: Wiley.

Van Linge, R. (2017). *Innoveren in de gezondheidszorg [Innovation in health care].* Bohn, Stafleu van Loghum.

Vroom, V. H. (1964). *Work an motivation.* New York: Wiley.

Walker, L. O., & Avant, K. C. (2010). *Strategies for theory construction in nursing* (Fifth ed.). Upper Saddle River: Prentice Hall.

Watkins, V., Nagle, C., Kent, B., & Hutchinson, A. M. (2017). Labouring together: Collaborative alliances in maternity care in Victoria, Australia-protocol of a mixed-methods study. *BMJ Open, 7*(3), e014262. doi:10.1136/bmjopen-2016-014262

Westerlaken, A., Brouns, M., Drost, H., Leerink, B., Meyboom-de Jong, B., Schouten, M., Vos, P., Boomkamp, W., Smid, H., & Zimmerman, A. (2013). *Voortrekkers in verandering in zorg en opleidingen – partners in innovatie. Advies van de verkenningscommissie hbo gezondheidszorg [Pioneers in change in care and education – Partners in innovation].*

Yin, K., Xing, L., Li, C., & Guo, Y. (2017). Are empowered employees more proactive? The contingency of how they evaluate their leader. *Frontiers in Psychology, 8*, 1802. doi:10.3389/fpsyg.2017.01802

25

DEVELOPING THE DECISION-MAKING SKILLS OF STUDENT MIDWIVES IN AN UNDERGRADUATE MIDWIFERY PROGRAMME IN NEW ZEALAND

Lorna Davies and Kendra Short

Overview

The primary focus of this chapter is to explore how student midwives learn to understand and use practice-based reasoning by being introduced to a broad spectrum of approaches and strategies within their undergraduate education. This learning enables them to develop their ability to make practice-focused decisions that will aid them to provide evidence-informed and quality woman-centred care for future clients, their babies and their families, once they are registered as midwives. Although this chapter draws upon the content and framework of a single bachelor of midwifery programme sited within a fairly unique practice context, the more context-specific approaches discussed could be modified for use in any number of educational and practice contexts around the world.

Introduction – setting the scene

We are both registered midwives who work in New Zealand. One of us is a lecturer in midwifery and the other a self-employed community-based midwife who works in both urban and rural settings. Within our roles, we work in partnership to support the development of the decision-making skills of student midwives to prepare them to work as autonomous practitioners.

The context of our working landscape should be explained as it has a considerable bearing on how students develop and utilise decision-making skills. New Zealand has a unique framework for midwifery practice providing a holistic, continuity of carer model that is accessible for most women. The concept of autonomy is deeply embedded in practice (Guilliland and Pairman 1995). At the point of registration, a new graduate is viewed as an autonomous practitioner who may choose to work as a self-employed 'lead maternity carer' (LMC) midwife.[1] The LMC is expected to work autonomously within a scope of practice that includes prescribing and referral rights. In a non-eventful normal pregnancy that precedes a physiological birth and a straightforward postnatal period, the midwife may provide exclusive care. Even if a referral to secondary or tertiary care occurs at any point in the childbirth continuum, the midwife remains the primary carer for the woman. 'Core midwives' operate in similar ways to midwives in any other high-, middle- or low-income country's healthcare system, working in hospitals and other birthing environments and are employed by district health boards. A new graduate midwife can choose either of these options at the point of registration. As a result of this autonomy, practice-based decision-making is a key consideration in any midwifery undergraduate educational curriculum development. Importantly, decisions are primarily made in partnership with women. Therefore, education around decision-making is focused on ensuring both that students have a robust midwifery knowledge base to enable valid information sharing and a strong sense of the impact of their values and beliefs on the information shared and outcomes.

Country-specific factors that impact on decision-making

All countries have contexts that impact on practice-based decision-making in any sphere of healthcare, and specifically on care offered during the childbirth continuum (Lapaige 2009). Some of these result from global phenomena, such as the medicalisation of childbirth, health economics or the choice/risk agenda of neoliberalism (Davies 2017). Others are more local in flavour, and in New Zealand there are some specific historical, sociocultural, economic and political elements that serve to influence the process of decision-making in midwifery. Some of these factors are included in Figure 25.1, although we acknowledge that it would be impossible to provide a definitive list and that there will inevitably be further elements that we do not have the space or time to consider. We do feel, however, that this analysis of key factors that influence the way that midwives practice in relation to decision-making is necessary to understand how we assist student midwives to become skilled practice-based decision-makers.

As Figure 25.1 illustrates, the central focus of midwifery practice in New Zealand is the woman/midwife relationship that is developed within a framework of a partnership between the woman, her family and the midwife (Guilliland and Pairman 1998). Continuity of carer is the modus operandi for delivery of care and this facilitates the relationship-based model of partnership. The model requires that both parties are viewed as equals within the context of decision-making. The midwife brings their specialist knowledge and the woman brings her own specific knowledge, values and beliefs (Guilliland and Pairman 1995).

The bicultural heritage which exists in New Zealand is grounded in the relationship between the indigenous Maori and Pakeha (European). This bicultural context creates a unique quality to decision-making in maternity care as in other spheres of life. The significance of two distinct cultures is strongly present in midwifery frameworks. These in conjunction with standards for practice and competencies, guide midwifery practice and articulate the profession's expectations of its members.

Feminism has played a powerful role in influencing the way that women approach decision-making in New Zealand (Marra, Schnurr and Holmes 2006). The women of New Zealand have been traditionally viewed as having strength and tenacity. Certainly, pre-colonial Maori culture was purportedly based on principles of equality with both women and men viewed as 'essential parts in the collective whole' (Mikaere 1994). Additionally, more socially inclusive and liberal attitudes existed in the early settler community and this created a drive for improvements in the lives of women. The women's suffrage movement won widespread support, and New Zealand became the first country in the world to legislate votes for women

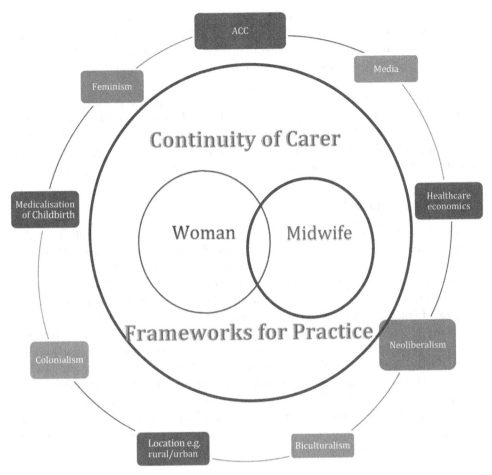

FIGURE 25.1 Central focus of midwifery practice in New Zealand

in 1893. New Zealand has been served by three female prime ministers including Helen Clark, who was the Health Minister during the renaissance of midwifery in the late 1980s and early 1990s. Her support enabled the passing of legislation that decreed that midwifery was an autonomous profession at a time when it had all but been subsumed by nursing.

New Zealand is fortunate to have a no-blame accident compensation scheme under the governance of the Accident Compensation Corporation (ACC). This is a New Zealand Crown entity that provides financial compensation and support to those who have suffered personal injuries. This includes maternity-related injuries and means that midwives like other health practitioners do not have to live in fear of litigation in the way that midwives in countries with similar healthcare provision do (Bismark and Patterson 2006). Notwithstanding, media provides a long-running critique of midwifery and this is generally less than positive, which may result in defensive practice (Davies 2017). Both of these factors again influence decision-making.

Finally, the physical location of the midwife can have a significant impact on assessment and evaluation in practice. Rural practitioners face an array of challenges including, for example, geographical distance, which can be compounded by weather, mobile phone reception and road conditions (Crowther et al. 2016; Gilkison et al. 2018). The location of the available birthing facilities is yet another factor in decision-making here, with some areas having more midwife-led units (MLUs) and others having higher home birth rates (Grigg and Tracy 2012).

We believe that both the midwives who provide formal learning opportunities in an educational facility and those who precept/mentor[2] student midwives in a practice setting need to be cognisant of the impact that these factors and other potential influences have on the way in which they practice and teach. This broad cultural perception also enables students to situate their knowledge so as to understand and meet the needs of the population they are serving.

A quadripartite model

Although the remainder of the chapter will focus on how decision-making skills and strategies are introduced and developed within a bachelor of midwifery programme in New Zealand, the reader is encouraged to see how this knowledge and skills can be translated in their specific contextual setting. We will discuss aspects of the programme and provide empirical examples from our own experiences. The principles introduced can be adapted and applied in a range of other contexts and practice settings.

The acquisition of decision-making skills within the programme involves a quadripartite process where the student is introduced to and fine tunes the requisite skills whilst working with midwifery lecturer, preceptor/mentor midwife and woman/baby/family. All have an equal share in the process and no one form of knowledge takes precedence over the others.

The programme, which is 50% theory and 50% practice-based, is designed to facilitate the development of decision-making by using a scaffolding technique that provides a logical stepped approach across Years 1 to 3 in both their practical and theoretical learning.

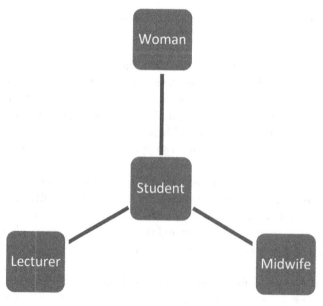

FIGURE 25.2 A quadripartite model of learning

By scaffolding, we mean that basic ideas are revisited throughout the programme and are built upon until the student has a comprehensive understanding. By revisiting progressively throughout their educational experience, the students are provided with different ways of learning whilst the repetition of content leads to increased retention of knowledge and application of skill (Chambers, Thiekötter and Chambers 2013).

Year 1

Walking in the woman's shoes

As established, the partnership model entails that any practice-based decisions are made in full consultation with the woman and her family. This premise is the cornerstone upon which midwifery practice is built in New Zealand. Therefore consideration of the impact of social, emotional, cultural, spiritual, psychological and physical factors when providing care is imperative in the mother-midwife relationship.

Consequently, this is where decision-making in practice is grounded within the programme. During the first year, the student participates in the childbirth journey of women in what are known as 'follow through' experiences. The student follows four women during the year and wherever the women go in relation to the maternity context, the student goes. In this way they can view first-hand the decisions that women make and gain insight into why women make them. In addition to midwifery care environments, the student will be exposed to situations that are relevant to the woman's experience but may not be provided by the midwife directly, for example, antenatal education, ultrasound scans and specialist appointments. The student is sharing as much of the woman's experience, from her point of view, as they are invited to by the woman – they follow the woman, not the midwife. They attend antenatal visits, the birth, if invited by the woman, and the postnatal visits where possible. To make meaning from each experience, the students are required to keep 'logs' as an introduction to clinical record writing and to reflect on these opportunities. They also spend time weekly in small tutorial groups (ākonga),[3] where they are given the time to debrief their experiences to make meaning out of them. The theory components of the course include common challenges to physical well-being in pregnancy and transition to parenthood. The students are also introduced to theories of human growth and development, which encourages them to reflect on their own life and allows them to apply the same principles to the lives of the women that they follow through. The course explores the broader social contexts that influence care for women and finally the complexities of the midwife/woman relationship that underpins the partnership model of midwifery practice in New Zealand.

The following is taken from a log that a first-year student recorded during her practical 'follow through' experience:

> During our birth talk visit at 36 weeks, the midwife asked whether Moira wanted to keep her placenta. Moira and Piripi had spoken to Piripi's mother and grandmother about this and in line with *tikanga māori* (protocol/custom), they wanted the placenta returned to their home *marae* to be buried. Piripi's mother would attend the birth and then take the placenta home with her when she returned home.

During a subsequent ākonga session, the influencing factors for this woman were explored by the student and her peers. Family and cultural tradition was important to this couple and factored into their decision. The discussion progressed to investigate culture, custom, and societal 'norm'; the influence of colonisation and the migration of Maori impacting on the ease of return of the placenta to ancestral land. Further reflection by the student for her portfolio explored personal reasons and her own experience of not keeping her child's placenta and why – including the influence of the medicalisation of childbirth, the treatment of the placenta as 'medical waste', following the societal norm without knowing there was another option.

The concepts of cultural competence and cultural safety[4] are used throughout the programme to explore personal values and beliefs and recognition and discussion of personal bias is interwoven. The effects of both implicit and unconscious bias are increasingly recognised in health generally (Fitzgerald and Hurst 2017). However, in New Zealand, the continuing inequalities and disparities in outcomes for Maori in healthcare show that bias is ongoing and is yet to be fully addressed (Bécares and Atatoa-Carr 2016). For these reasons and to raise awareness, students study the Treaty of Waitangi[5] and the historical and current effects of colonisation on Maori.

Personal reflection is introduced in a formal context in Year 1. The theme of 'stepping into another's shoes' continues during a course that explores epistemology as midwifery ways of knowing. Here students are asked to define and apply the sociological imagination to a personal belief and reflect on and explore the reasons for that belief. The application of this to ongoing midwifery practice is demonstrated in the New Zealand College of Midwives (NZCOM) Code of Ethics and Midwifery Competencies, which expect that a midwife practice without coercion, nor impose her own beliefs on women or their support people (2015, p. 12). Acknowledging personal context promotes understanding between the midwife and woman of the influences on each of their situations, encouraging mutual respect and partnership.

When observing the woman's interactions with people throughout her experience, the student is asked to consider who is seen to make the decisions – the woman, or the health professional?

The following is again a log of a conversation held at a routine antenatal appointment:

> Ellie and her midwife talked about induction today. Ellie said her friend was induced with her first baby because she was overdue, and asked how long she would be allowed to go past her due date. The midwife said the policy at the local unit was to recommend induction at 10 days after the due date.

The student was encouraged by her Kaiako[6] to explore this further – the language used, the power dynamic, the impact of previous experience. Where was the information sharing? Where was the woman's choice in this conversation? Could it even be called a conversation? Who appeared to make the decision?

Throughout the degree, particularly in the first two years, the Kaiako facilitate reflection and debriefing in small groups of students. Students explore the impact of personal context on decision-making, both for the woman and the midwife. Encouraging thought and discussion on the reasons a woman might have made the decision she did assists students to understand different perspectives and ways of knowing. Knowledge of the various impacts on the woman's decision-making can be observed in midwifery practice, then dissected and discussed in a safe environment at weekly ākonga groups. Across millennia, midwives around the world have protected, taught and maintained their skills, knowledge and wisdom in the guise of storytelling (Towler and Bramall 1986). In a contemporary context, we additionally recognise that a narrative approach is an effective method of engaging students with a critical approach that develops and enhances creative decision-making (Gilkinson 2013).

This dynamic approach to learning within the ākonga is based on 'an integration of knowledge that is derived from the art and sciences, tempered by experience and research' (New Zealand College of Midwives [NZCOM] 2015, p. 3). Midwives need to be able to embrace, value and utilise multiple ways of knowing within the decision-making context including scientific, embodied, intuitive, experiential and experimental tenets among others. To achieve this, students need to be able to seek out and employ a range of evidence to support the decision-making process in partnership with women and to engage the skills of critical analysis to discern the value of supporting evidence. Core learning includes an ability to critically appraise a range of different sources of evidence and to articulate knowledge. It also requires an understanding of research principles and methods to determine the quality of information and strength that will enable the students to become evidence-informed practitioners as midwives.

As the students are introduced to midwifery evidence and are becoming more skilled in critiquing material, they are asked to consider the application of their knowledge and understanding, within the context of practice, when sharing information with women and their families. By observing first-hand how ongoing discussions move from initial information sharing to informed decisions, students can apply meaning to the process. The experience of following different women's childbirth journeys helps foster an appreciation for the myriad decisions a woman and her family make as they progress through the childbirth continuum, and also, the wealth of information a midwife must utilise to provide individualised, woman-centred care for those women.

Year 2

Walking alongside the midwife

As the students proceed into their second year, the emphasis moves on to seeing midwifery through the lens of a midwife. The students now move from observer to facilitator of discussions with women and can see first-hand the impact of how midwives can use language and listening to empower women to make informed decisions, or sometimes to coerce them. It is here that the potential for power imbalance in the partnership can be witnessed and then explored in weekly tutor group sessions.

> Sadie, who wanted to use water during VBAC, was informed that it wasn't in the policy by the obstetrician during her consult visit. So disempowering. No decision making on the part of the woman. Fortunately, the LMC midwife had provided some good evidence that supported Sadie's choice and she was able to talk about that.

Students are developing the skill of facilitating discussion with women in an individualised manner and not as a 'patter' of learned information. In so doing they recognise the person in the situation, not the situation itself. They continue to acknowledge the different influences on individual women so that the information shared is discussed in a way that promotes understanding whilst not losing its accuracy and robustness.

A midwife's role in different contexts is also explored, as the second year progresses into complex care situations. Moving from primary care experiences in the first half of the year to clinical placements in secondary and tertiary level hospitals in the second semester exposes the student to very different situations and midwifery roles. Stepping into these different roles means the student can gain insight into what impact this new context has on decision-making, both for the midwife and the woman.

The following is an example of a reflection by a second-year student:

> The LMC midwife handed over care of the woman to the core midwife as she was not epidural-certified. The LMC midwife stayed on throughout the labour in a support role but the core midwife had clinical responsibility. Whilst the core midwife did discuss decisions with the LMC midwife; she was now the lead carer. The decision-making partnership had moved from woman-LMC midwife to woman-core midwife. I could see how difficult it was sometimes for the LMC to not document, prepare equipment, or perform cares. There seemed to be a settling in and adjustment period for her as well as the woman following the handover of care. This could also be due to the increased medicalisation of the labour and more equipment due to the epidural. I really felt for the LMC midwife as I had experienced a handover earlier in the year from a primary care point of view, but now I had to concentrate on my role as core midwife.

The dynamic, ever-changing nature of midwifery around the world is reflected in the breadth of situations the students find themselves in. Exposure to increasingly complex care situations, where the luxury of time is often impossible and the decisions made can have vastly different consequences, changes the focus for the student. The impact of outcome becomes more apparent and the weight of that impact can often smother the importance of the overall experience for the woman. Facilitating conversations in the vastly different environment of the tertiary unit compared to the relative normality of the home as experienced in earlier practical placements can challenge the student. Combined with the reality of meeting women for the first time in fraught situations rather than having time to build a relationship over months, the practical experiences faced in the second half of the year bring many new considerations to the student's thinking.

The differences between informed choice and informed consent are explored in greater depth in the second year. The legal and ethical right to informed choice, or alternatively, informed refusal, is an important part of midwifery care in New Zealand. New Zealand has probably the strongest health consumer legislation in the world and this has a major impact on decision-making. Student midwives need to have a very clear understanding of the information that they are sharing including risks and benefits. The acceptance of care, as well as that declined, needs to be measured, which means that the information shared has to be unequivocal. It is therefore imperative that midwives can share information so that women are fully aware of the possible implications of their decisions. A second-year course encourages the students to explore further epistemological perspectives including, research, historical, legal and ethical dimensions of practice. A legal perspective is introduced in legislation that impacts on practice such as the Health Practitioners Competency Assurance Act (2003). Similarly, the Code of Ethics (NZCOM 2015) is used to provide an ethical framework that informs any decision-making process in midwifery care in New Zealand.

An example of the application of learning in the area of informed consent/refusal is an assignment where the student is asked to write a conversation – in normal language – between themselves and a woman. They are asked to illustrate how they would discuss the issue of group B streptococcus and share information with the woman to enable her to make an informed decision on testing.

Exploring the value of approaching the complexity of collaborative care with an interdisciplinary focus, is achieved using a simulation-based approach. This can be small group role play and scenarios of emergency skills through to elaborate simulation suite type activity in an educational facility. This learning, whilst uncomfortable for many students, enables the practice of skills in a safe, supportive and custom-paced environment that helps the student hone their practical skills. Kitson-Reynolds (2009) states that such interactive decision-making encourages the student to develop procedural knowledge and can expedite the time required to acquire skills of effective decision-making. Importance is placed on dialogue with the woman as well as mastering the practical skills. This includes keeping the woman informed of what is happening; recognising the constant juggle of facilitating informed consent; doing no harm while enabling the woman to feel some control and knowledge of her situation.

Year 3

Learning to be the midwife

The third year of the programme is an apprenticeship year with the student working alongside midwives both in the community and hospital setting for 90% of the academic year. By increasingly taking the lead during midwifery placements in diverse settings the student is enabled to consolidate their learning, applying their knowledge and skills in situations with the safety net of the midwife walking beside them in partnership. The lived experience of being 'out there doing it' forms the foundation for the following year of autonomous practice.

Assignments encompassing the exploration of the lived experience of the placement contribute to the assessment of the students' learning in their final year. A creative piece reflecting an important experience of midwifery for the student acknowledges the art of midwifery and creates an interface between the acquisition of knowledge and its application seen through a personal lens – reinforcing the different perceptions of experience and its impact on personal practice and thus decision-making.

The use of online discussion forums by third-year students facilitates information and experience sharing by students. A particular practice issue is raised by a student, then the rest of the group can provide their own stories, resources, evidence and knowledge. Robust discussion promotes critical thinking of not just research, but contextual and societal influences. This assessment occurs within a three-month placement with one midwife or small practice, so provides plentiful opportunities to take the knowledge gained from collegial discussion and use it in a practical situation. The student then presents one topic as an in-depth case study and subsequent topical discussion with tutors at the end of the paper. They are expected to have explored diverse aspects of the situation demonstrating their information sharing and ways of knowing, and reflection on how this was done so that the woman was empowered to make her own informed decision.

As previously mentioned in this chapter, location can have a substantial impact on decision-making for the woman and the student/midwife. The diverse geographical isolation and topography of many areas of New Zealand can mean that a decision to transfer to a higher-level care institution, for example, may need to be made in vastly different timeframes depending on location and mode of transport. The organisation and travel time component of a helicopter or ambulance transfer from an alpine location is a very real factor in decision-making for remote rural midwives. The students in their final year are exposed to the dynamics of rural midwifery during a six- to eight-week rural placement. During this placement, students encounter the unique influences of the rural environment and must reflect on and use all their (often newfound) appreciation of the rural context to demonstrate knowledge of the lived experience of rural women and midwives in their placement assignment.

Sustainability is a concept that is gaining increasing attention in curricula generally and this includes healthcare education (Goodman 2013). Societal awareness of issues such as climate change, biodiversity and population increase are influencing healthcare decisions and those relating to areas such as parenting. Sustainability is, therefore, becoming a serious consideration in decision-making for the woman/midwife partnership. The students are exposed to sustainability literacy throughout the programme with an introduction to the broad philosophical and socio/cultural/economic and environmental principles of sustainability and are encouraged to consider the contribution that midwifery can make to sustainable healthcare within the frameworks of midwifery practice. In the third year, the students are asked to design and perform a group presentation around the principles of sustainable practice by designing a sustainable practice or workplace using the broad tenets of sustainability.

The epistemological theme is strengthened in the third year where the integral place that research and evidence have in decision-making is consolidated. Research methods, critique and investigation, culminate in a research poster authored by pairs of students with guidance from lecturers. The students' transition to practice is explored in an assignment where different forms of knowledge are defined and the student addresses their progression and application of knowledge in midwifery practice. Midwifery, with its holistic nature, is just one model of care, and knowledge and comparison to technocratic and medicalised models of care and their impact on the woman's maternity experience in other countries and contexts is explored. Reflection, storytelling and demonstrating knowledge of where we have come from both as an individual midwife, and as a profession, reinforces our autonomy and continued growth as a practitioner. The student acknowledges their understanding of self, and the diverse sources of knowledge, from science to intuition, which in turn assists them as midwives to respect and consider women's knowledge.

Conclusion

For this chapter, we have drawn upon the content and framework of a single bachelor of midwifery programme sited within a fairly unique practice context to illustrate how understanding and application of practice-based decision-making can be developed in undergraduate midwifery education. That may at first glance appear to present a narrow perspective. However, we would argue that a comprehensive knowledge and understanding of epistemology relating to midwifery is a universal requirement in terms of informing practice. Similarly, a theoretical and applied knowledge of underpinning scientific principles is without any question a prerequisite to decision-making. The more context-specific approaches discussed could be modified for use in any number of educational and practice contexts. For example, many countries are currently seriously lobbying for continuity of carer models (Perriman, Davis and Fergusson 2018), and others have rural issues that are not dissimilar to those in New Zealand

(Gilkison et al. 2018). The issues relating to sustainability are only likely to increase in the decades to come and impact on practice universally (Davies 2017).

There is a good body of literature relating to clinical decision-making in midwifery but this becomes much less apparent when it comes to how students develop these skills. Furthermore, the research that has been executed tends to be either exploring the role of the midwife in supporting students to become competent decision-makers (Cioffi 2005; Young 2012), or focused on emergency situations (Kitson-Reynolds 2009; Scholes et al. 2012). We concede that the evidence included in the chapter is empirical, and writing it has led us to recognise that there is a dearth of New Zealand specific research on the outcomes relating to decision-making once the students have graduated. Notwithstanding, the analysis has demonstrated how introducing student midwives to decision-making in practice by making the woman the central focus has an understated importance. As Jefford, Fahy and Sundin (2010) state, 'the role of the woman as decision-maker in her own care and how this is negotiated between the woman and the midwife also needs careful research attention'. Undergraduate midwifery education is well placed to drive this standpoint and in so doing ensure that future midwives are approaching decision-making from a woman-centred perspective.

Notes

1 The LMC midwife role is a primary care role that is publicly funded generally community-based. The role aligns with other members of the maternity healthcare professionals and is therefore part of a collaborative workforce (NZCOM Fact Sheet3).
2 We acknowledge that these two terms are used interchangeably in different country settings.
3 Ākonga is a Maori word that has multiple meanings. In this context it means small tutorial style learning group.
4 Cultural competence is integrated into the Midwifery Council of New Zealand competencies for entry to the register of midwives. Cultural competence for midwives requires the application of the principles of cultural safety to the midwifery partnership. Cultural safety is the effective midwifery care of women by midwives who have undertaken a process of self-reflection on their own cultural identity and recognise the impact of their own culture on their practice (Midwifery Council of New Zealand, 2012).
5 The Treaty of Waitangi.
6 Kaiako is a Māori word for facilitator of learning. In this context, the Kaiako is a midwifery lecturer.

References

Bécares, L. and Atatoa-Carr, P. (2016). The association between maternal and partner experienced racial discrimination and prenatal perceived stress, prenatal and postnatal depression: Findings from the growing up in New Zealand cohort study. *International Journal for Equity in Health*, 15, 1: 155.

Bismark, M. and Paterson, R. (2006). No-fault compensation in New Zealand: Harmonizing injury compensation, provider accountability, and patient safety. *Health Affairs*, 25: 278–283.

Chambers, D., Thiekötter, A. and Chambers, L. (2013). Preparing student nurses for contemporary practice: The case for discovery learning. *Journal of Nursing Education and Practice*, 3, 9.

Cioffi, J. (2005). Education for clinical decision making in midwifery practice. *Midwifery*, 14, 1: 18–22.

Crowther, S., Deery, R., Daellenbach, R., Davies, L., Gilkison, A., Kensington, M. and Rankin, J. (2018). Joys and challenges of relationships in Scotland and New Zealand rural midwifery: A multicentre study. *Women Birth*, pii: S1871-5192(17)30321-9. doi:10.1016/j.wombi.2018.04.004

Davies, L. (2017). Midwifery: A model of sustainable healthcare practice? Unpublished Thesis https://ir.canterbury.ac.nz/bitstream/.../Davies,%20Lorna%20final%20PhD%20thesis.pdf

FitzGerald, C. and Hurst, S. (2017). Implicit bias in healthcare professionals: A systematic review. *BMC Medical Ethics*, 18, 1: 19. doi:10.1186/s12910-017-0179-8

Gilkinson, A. (2013). Narrative pedagogy in midwifery education. *Practising Midwife*, 16, 8: 2–4.

Gilkison, A., Rankin, J., Kensington, M., Daellenbach, R., Davies, L., Deery, R. and Crowther, S. (2018). A woman's hand and a lion's heart: Skills and attributes for rural midwifery practice in New Zealand and Scotland. *Midwifery*, 58: 109–116. ISSN 0266-6138

Goodman, B. (2013). Education for sustainability – Principles for nursing curricula. Education Briefing. Plymouth: Plymouth University. www.academia.edu/3109351/Education_for_Sustainability_-_Principles_for_nursing_curricula

Grigg, C. P. and Tracy S. K. (2013). New Zealand's unique maternity system. *Women and Birth*, 26(1): e59–e64.

Grigg, C., Tracy, S. K., Daellenbach, R., Kensington, M. and Schmied, V. (2014). An exploration of influences on women's birthplace decision-making in New Zealand. *BMC Pregnancy and Childbirth*, 14: 1. doi:10.1186/1471-2393-14-210.

Guilliland, K. and Pairman, S. (1995). *The midwifery partnership: A model for practice*. Wellington, NZ: Department of Nursing and Midwifery, Victoria University of Wellington.

Jefford, E., Fahy, K. and Sundin, D. (2010). A review of the literature: Midwifery decision-making and birth. *Women Birth*, 23(4): 127–134. doi:10.1016/j.wombi.2010.02.001

Kitson-Reynolds, E. (2009). Developing decision making for students using interactive practice. *British Journal of Midwifery*, 17, 4: 238–243.

Lapaige, V. (2009). Evidence-based decision-making within the context of globalization: A 'Why-What-How' for leaders and managers of health care organizations. *Risk Management and Healthcare Policy*, 2: 35–46.

Marra, M., Schnurr, S. and Holmes, J. (2006). Effective leadership in New Zealand workplaces: Balancing gender role. In J. Baxter (eds.), *Speaking out: The female voice in public contexts*. Basingstoke, England; New York: Palgrave Macmillan.

Mikaere, A. (1994). *Māori women caught in the contradictions of a colonised reality*. In Waikato Law Review, 2: 125–149.

New Zealand College of Midwives [NZCOM]. (2015). *Midwives handbook for practice* (5th ed.). Christchurch, New Zealand: New Zealand College of Midwives.

Perriman, N., Davis, D. and Fergusson, S. (2018). What women value in the midwifery continuity of care model: A systematic review with meta-synthesis. *Midwifery*, 62: 220–229.

Scholes, J., Endacott, R., Biro, M., et al. (2012). Clinical decision-making: Midwifery students' recognition of, and response to, post partum haemorrhage in the simulation environment *BMC Pregnancy and Childbirth*, 12: 19. https://doi.org/10.1186/1471-2393-12-19

Towler, J. and Bramall, J. (1986). *Midwives in history and society*. London: Croom Helm.

Young, N. (2012). An exploration of clinical decision-making among students and newly qualified midwives. *Midwifery*, 28, 6: 824–830.

INDEX

Note: **Boldface** page references indicate tables. *Italic* references indicate figures and boxed text.

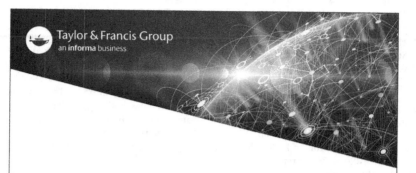

Printed in the United States
by Baker & Taylor Publisher Services